Medical Genetics at a Glance

This title is also available as an e-book.
For more details, please see
www.wiley.com/buy/9780470656549
or scan this QR code:

Medical Genetics at a Glance

Dorian J. Pritchard

BSc, Dip Gen, PhD, CBiol, MSB
Emeritus Lecturer in Human Genetics
University of Newcastle-upon-Tyne
UK
Former Visiting Lecturer in Medical Genetics
International Medical University
Kuala Lumpur
Malaysia

Bruce R. Korf

MD, PhD
Wayne H. and Sara Crews Finley Chair in Medical Genetics
Professor and Chair, Department of Genetics
Director, Heflin Center for Genomic Sciences
University of Alabama at Birmingham
Alabama
USA

Third edition

WILEY-BLACKWELL
A John Wiley & Sons, Ltd., Publication

Registered office: John Wiley & Sons, Ltd, The Atrium, Southern Gate, Chichester, West Sussex, PO19 8SQ, UK

Editorial offices: 9600 Garsington Road, Oxford, OX4 2DQ, UK
The Atrium, Southern Gate, Chichester, West Sussex, PO19 8SQ, UK
111 River Street, Hoboken, NJ 07030-5774, USA

For details of our global editorial offices, for customer services and for information about how to apply for permission to reuse the copyright material in this book please see our website at www.wiley.com/wiley-blackwell.

Library of Congress Cataloging-in-Publication Data
Pritchard, D. J. (Dorian J.)
  Medical genetics at a glance / Dorian J. Pritchard, Bruce R. Korf. – 3rd ed.
        p. ; cm. – (At a glance series)
  Includes bibliographical references and index.
  ISBN 978-0-470-65654-9 (softback : alk. paper) – ISBN 978-1-118-68900-4 (mobi) –
ISBN 978-1-118-68901-1 (pub) – ISBN 978-1-118-68902-8 (pdf)
  I. Korf, Bruce R.   II. Title.   III. Series: At a glance series (Oxford, England)
  [DNLM: 1. Genetic Diseases, Inborn.   2. Chromosome Aberrations.   3. Genetics, Medical.
QZ 50]
  RB155
  616′.042–dc23
                                                2013007103

A catalogue record for this book is available from the British Library.

Cover image: Tim Vernon, LTH NHS Trust/Science Photo Library
Cover design by Meaden Creative

Set in 9 on 11.5 pt Times by Toppan Best-set Premedia Limited
Printed and bound in Malaysia by Vivar Printing Sdn Bhd

1   2013

Contents

Preface to the first edition

This book is written primarily for medical students seeking a summary of genetics and its medical applications, but it should be of value also to advanced students in the biosciences, paramedical scientists, established medical doctors and health professionals who need to extend or update their knowledge. It should be of especial value to those preparing for examinations.

Medical genetics is unusual in that, whereas its fundamentals usually form part of first-year medical teaching within basic biology, those aspects that relate to inheritance may be presented as an aspect of reproductive biology. Clinical issues usually form a part of later instruction, extending into the postgraduate years. This book is there-fore presented in three sections, which can be taken together as a single course, or separately as components of several courses. Chapters are however intended to be read in essentially the order of presentation, as concepts and specialised vocabulary are developed progressively.

There are many excellent introductory textbooks in our subject, but none, so far as we know, is at the same time so comprehensive and so succinct. We believe the relative depth of treatment of topics appropriately reflects the importance of these matters in current thinking.

Dorian Pritchard
Bruce Korf

Preface to the third edition

The first two editions have been quite successful, having been translated into Chinese, Japanese, Greek, Serbo-Croat, Korean, Italian and Russian. In keeping with this international readership, we stress clinical issues of particular relevance to the major ethnic groups, with information on relative disease allele frequencies in diverse populations. The second edition was awarded First Prize in the Medicine category of the 2008 British Medical Association Medical Book Competition Awards. In this third edition we aim to exceed previous standards.

Editions one and two presented information across all subject areas in order of the developing complexity of the whole field, so that a reader's vocabulary, knowledge and understanding could progress on a broad front. That approach was popular with student reviewers, but their teachers commented on difficulty in accessing specific subject areas. The structure of this third edition has therefore been completely revised into subject-based sections, of which there are fourteen.

Three former introductory chapters have been combined and all other chapters revised and updated. In addition we have written seventeen new chapters and five new case studies, with illustrations to accompany the latter. New features include a comprehensively illustrated treatment of cardiac developmental pathology, a radically revised outline of cancer, a much extended review of biochemical genetics and outline descriptions of some of the most recent genomic diagnostic techniques.

Dorian Pritchard
Bruce Korf

Acknowledgements

We thank thousands of students, for the motivation they provided by their enthusiastic reception of the lectures on which these chapters are based. We appreciate also the interest and support of many colleagues, but special mention should be made of constructive contributions to the first edition by Dr Paul Brennan of the Department of Human Genetics, University of Newcastle. We are most grateful also to Professor Angus Clarke of the Department of Medical Genetics, Cardiff University for his valuable comments on Chapter 61 of Edition 2 and to Dr J. Daniel Sharer, Assistant Professor of Genetics, University of Alabama at Birmingham for constructive advice on our diagram of the tandem mass spectrometer. DP wishes to pay tribute to the memory of Ian Cross for his friendship and professional support over many years and for his advice on the chapters dealing with cytogenetics.

We thank the staff of Wiley for their encouragement and tactful guidance throughout the production of the series and Jane Fallows and Graeme Chambers for their tasteful presentation of the artwork.

Dorian Pritchard
Bruce Korf

List of abbreviations

A:	adenine; blood group A.
α_1-AT:	α_1-antitrypsin.
AB:	blood group AB.
abl:	the Abelson proto-oncogene, normally on 9q, that participates in the Philadelphia derivative chromosome.
ACE:	angiotensin-1 converting enzyme.
ACo-D:	autosomal dominant.
AD:	autosomal dominant.
ADA:	adenosine deaminase.
ADH:	alcohol dehydrogenase.
AE:	acrodermatitis enteropathica.
AER:	ridge of ectoderm along the apex of the limb bud.
AFP:	α-fetoprotein.
AIP:	acute intermittent porphyria.
AIRE:	autoimmune regulator protein.
ALD:	adrenoleukodystrophy.
ALDH:	acetaldehyde dehydrogenase.
APC:	antigen presenting cell.
APKD:	adult polycystic kidney disease.
APP:	amyloid-β precursor protein.
APS:	autoimmune polyendocrinopathy syndrome.
AR:	autosomal recessive.
ARMS:	amplification refractory mutation system.
AS:	Angelman syndrome; ankylosing spondylitis.
ASD:	atrial septal defect.
ASO:	allele-specific oligonucleotide.
ATP:	adenosine triphosphate.
AVC:	atrioventricular canal.
AZF:	azoospermic factor.
B:	blood group B.
BAC:	bacterial artificial chromosome.
BCAA:	branched chain amino acid.
BCL:	bilateral cleft lip.
BCR:	the breakpoint cluster region, normally on 22q that participates in the Philadelphia chromosome.
BLS:	bare lymphocyte syndrome.
BMD:	Becker muscular dystrophy.
BMI:	body mass index.
BMP-4:	bone morphogenetic protein 4.
bp:	base pair.
BRCA1, BRCA2:	breast cancer susceptibility genes 1 and 2.
C:	cytosine; haploid number of single-strand chromosomes; number of concordant twin pairs; complement.
2C:	diploid number of single-strand chromosomes.
CAD:	coronary artery disease.
CAH:	congenital adrenal hyperplasia.
CAM:	cell adhesion molecule.
CATCH 22:	cardiac defects, abnormal facies, thymic hypoplasia, cleft palate and hypocalcemia caused by microdeletion at 22q11.2: an example of a medical acronym that can cause distress and should be avoided, now referred to as 'Chromosome 22q11.2 deletion syndrome'.
CBAVD:	congenital bilateral absence of the vas deferens.
CCD:	charge-coupled device.
cDNA:	DNA copy of a specific mRNA.
CF:	cystic fibrosis.
CFTR:	cystic fibrosis transmembrane conductance regulator; the cystic fibrosis gene.
CGD:	chronic granulomatous disease.
CGH:	comparative genome hybridization.
CGS:	contiguous gene syndrome.
CHARGE:	coloboma, heart defects, choanal atresia, retarded growth, genital abnormalities and abnormal ears.
CHD:	congenital heart disease.
CL ± P:	cleft lip with or without cleft palate.
CML:	chronic myelogenous leukaemia.
CMV:	*Cytomegalovirus.*
CNS:	central nervous system.
CNV:	copy number variation.
Co-D:	codominant.
CpG:	cytosine-(phosphate)-guanine (within one DNA strand).
CRASH:	corpus callosum hypoplasia, retardation, adducted thumbs, spastic paraparesis and hydrocephalus due to mutation in the L1 CAM cell adhesion molecule, a second example of a medical acronym that can cause distress and should be avoided.
CSF:	cerebrospinal fluid.
CT scan:	computerized technique that uses X-rays to obtain cross-sectional images of tissues.
CVS:	chorionic villus sampling.
CX26:	connexin 26.
CYP:	cytochrome P450.
D:	number of discordant twin pairs.
DA:	ductus arteriosus.
ddA (/T/C/G)TP:	dideoxynucleotide A (T,C,G).
del:	chromosome deletion.
der:	derivative chromosome.
DHPR:	dihydropteridine reductase.
DMD:	Duchenne muscular dystrophy.
DMPK:	dystrophia myotonica protein kinase.
DNA:	deoxyribonucleic acid.
dNTP:	deoxyribonucleotide.
DOCK:	dedicator of cytokinesis.
DOPA:	dihydroxyphenylalanine.
dup:	duplicated segment of a chromosome.
DZ:	dizygotic, arising from two zygotes.
ECM:	extracellular matrix.
EDD:	expected date of arrival.
EF:	elongation factor.
ELSI:	the Ethical, Legal and Social Implications Program of the Human Genome Project.
ER:	endoplasmic reticulum.
EVAS:	enlarged vestibular aqueduct syndrome.
EXT:	multiple hereditary exostosis.
F:	Wright's inbreeding coefficient.

FAD:	flavin adenine dinucleotide.
FAP(C):	familial adenomatous polyposis (coli).
FCH:	familial combined hyperlipidaemia.
Fe:	iron.
FGF:	fibroblast growth factor.
FGFR:	fibroblast growth factor receptor.
FH:	familial hypercholesterolaemia.
FISH:	fluorescence *in-situ* hybridization.
FMR:	a gene at Xq27.3 containing a CGG repeat, expansion of which causes fragile-X disease.
fra:	fragile site.
FRAX:	fragile-X syndrome.
FSH:	follicle-stimulating hormone.
G:	guanine.
G0, G1, G2:	phases of the mitotic cycle.
G6PD:	glucose-6-phosphate dehydrogenase.
Gal 1 PUT:	galactose-1-phosphate uridyltransferase.
GALC:	galactocerebrosidase.
GALT:	galactose-1-phosphate uridyltransferase.
GCDHD:	glutaryl-CoA dehydrogenase deficiency.
GF:	growth factor.
GFR:	growth factor receptor.
GI:	gastrointestinal.
GlcNAc:	*N*-acetylglucosamine.
GLI3:	a zinc finger transcription controlling protein.
GM:	ganglioside.
GSD:	glycogen storage disorder.
GVH:	graft versus host.
HA:	homogentisic acid.
HAO:	hereditary angioneurotic oedema.
HbA:	normal allele for β-globin.
HbS:	sickle cell allele of β-globin.
HFE:	High Fe: the haemochromatosis gene.
HFI:	hereditary fructose intolerance.
HGPRT/HPRT:	hypoxanthine-guanine phosphoribosyl transferase.
HIV:	human immunodeficiency virus.
HMGCoA:	hydroxymethylglutaryl coenzyme A.
HMSN:	hereditary motor and sensory neuropathy, Charcot–Marie–Tooth disease.
HNF:	hepatic nuclear factor.
HNPCC:	hereditary non-polyposis colon cancer.
hnRNA:	heterogeneous nuclear RNA.
HoxA–D:	Homeobox genes A–D.
i:	isochromosome.
ICSI:	intracytoplasmic sperm injection.
IDDM:	insulin-dependent diabetes mellitus, a term now replaced by T2D or T2DM, q.v.
Ig:	immunoglobulin.
Ig-CAM:	immunoglobulin cell adhesion molecule.
IMC:	invasion metastasis cascade.
ins:	inserted segment in a chromosome.
inv:	inverted segment of a chromosome.
IP:	incontinentia pigmenti.
IQ:	intelligent quotient.
IRT:	immunoreactive trypsin.
IVC:	inferior vena cava.
kb:	kilobase (1000 bases).
λ_s:	lambda-s, relative risk for a sib.

LA:	left atrium.
LAD:	leucocyte adhesion deficiency.
LCHAD:	long-chain hydroxyacyl coenzyme A deficiency.
LDLR:	low-density lipoprotein receptor.
LEFTA/B:	human equivalent of the gene Lefty-1/2.
LHON:	Leber hereditary optic neuropathy.
LINES:	Long interspersed nuclear elements.
LMP:	last menstrual period.
LNS:	Lesch–Nyhan syndrome.
lod:	'Log of the odds'; the logarithm ($\log_{10}$) of the ratio of the probability that a certain combination of phenotypes arose as a result of genetic linkage (of a specified degree) to the probability that it arose merely by chance.
LSD:	lipid storage disorder.
LV:	left ventricle.
M:	monosomy; mitotic phase of the cell cycle.
M1, M2:	first, second divisions of meiosis.
MAPH:	multiplex amplifiable probe hybridization.
Mb:	megabase (1 000 000 bases).
MBP:	mannan-binding protein.
MCAD:	medium-chain acyl-coenzyme A deficiency.
MD:	myotonic dystrophy.
MELAS:	mitochondrial encephalopathy, lactic acidosis and stroke-like episodes.
MEN:	multiple endocrine neoplasia.
MERRF:	myoclonic epilepsy with ragged red fibres.
MHC:	major histocompatibility complex.
miRNA:	microRNA.
MIS:	Müllerian inhibiting substance.
MND:	Menkes disease.
MPS:	mucopolysaccharidosis.
MRI:	magnetic resonance imaging.
mRNA:	messenger RNA.
MS:	mass spectrometry; multiple sclerosis.
MS/MS:	tandem mass spectrometry.
MTC:	medullary thyroid carcinoma.
mtDNA:	mitochondrial DNA.
MZ:	monozygotic, derived from one zygote.
N:	haploid number of chromosomal DNA double-helices; in humans, 23.
NAD:	nicotinamide adenine dinucleotide.
NARP:	neurodegeneration, ataxia and retinitis pigmentosa.
NF1, NF2:	neurofibromatosis types 1 and 2.
NFκB:	nuclear factor kappa B.
NHC protein:	non-histone chromosomal protein.
NIDDM:	non-insulin-dependent diabetes mellitus.
NOR:	nucleolar organizer region.
NSD-1:	nuclear SET domain 1; the gene at 5q35 responsible for Sotos syndrome.
NTD:	neural tube defect.
O:	blood group O.
OCA:	oculocutaneous albinism.
OHD:	21-hydroxylase deficiency.
p:	chromosomal short arm: symbol for allele frequency.
P:	degree of penetrance.

p53:	mitosis suppressor protein product of the gene, *TP53*.
PA:	phenylalanine.
PAH:	phenylalanine hydroxylase.
PCR:	polymerase chain reaction.
PDS:	Pendred syndrome.
PFGE:	pulsed-field gel electrophoresis.
PGD:	preimplantation genetic diagnosis.
Phe508del:	deletion of the codon for phenylalanine at position 508 in the *CFTR* gene.
PKU:	phenylketonuria.
PNP:	purine nucleoside phosphorylase.
Pol II:	RNA polymerase II.
P-WS:	Prader–Willi syndrome.
q:	chromosomal long arm; symbol for allele frequency.
r:	ring chromosome.
RA:	right atrium.
rad:	an absorbed dose of 100 ergs of radiation per gram of tissue.
ret:	a proto-oncogene that becomes rearranged during transfection, initiating tumorigenesis.
RFLP:	restriction fragment length polymorphism.
Rh:	Rhesus.
RISC:	RNA- induced silencing complex.
RNA:	ribonucleic acid.
RNAi:	RNA interference.
RNA-seq:	array sequencing of RNA.
rob:	Robertsonian translocation; centric fusion.
rRNA:	ribosomal RNA.
S:	Svedberg unit; DNA synthetic phase of the cell cycle.
SCID:	severe combined immunodeficiency disease.
Shh:	sonic hedgehog, a gene concerned with body patterning.
SINES:	short interspersed nuclear elements.
siRNA:	small interfering RNA.
SLE:	systemic lupus erythematosus.
SLO:	Smith–Lemli–Opitz syndrome.
SMA:	spinal muscular atrophy.
SNP:	single nucleotide polymorphism.
snRNA:	small nuclear RNA.
snRNP:	small nuclear ribonucleo-protein; protein–RNA complex important in recognition of intron/exon boundaries, intron excision or exon splicing, etc.
SRY:	Y-linked male sex determining gene.
SSCP:	single-strand conformation polymorphism; study of DNA polymorphism by electrophoresis of DNA denatured into single strands.

STAT:	signal transducer and activator of transcription.
STC:	signal transduction cascade.
STR:	short tandem repeat.
SVAS:	supravalvular aortic stenosis.
SVC:	superior vena cava.
t:	reciprocal translocation.
T:	thymine; trisomy.
T1D/T1DM:	type 1 diabetes mellitus.
T2D/T2DM:	type 2 diabetes mellitus.
TA:	truncus arteriosus.
TAP:	transporter associated with antigen presentation.
Taq:	*Thermus aquaticus*.
TCR:	T-cell receptor.
ter:	terminal, close to the chromosome telomere.
TFM:	testicular feminization, or androgen insensitivity syndrome.
TLR:	toll-like receptor.
TNF:	tumour necrosis factor.
TORCH:	*Toxoplasma*, other, *Rubella*, *Cytomegalovirus* and *Herpes*.
TP53:	the gene coding for protein p53.
tRNA:	transfer RNA.
ts:	tumour suppressor.
TSC:	tuberous sclerosis.
U:	uracil.
UCL:	unilateral cleft lip.
UDP:	uridine diphosphate.
VACTERL:	as for VATER with cardiac and limb defects also.
VATER:	vertebral defects, anal atresia, tracheo-oesophageal fistula and renal defects.
VCFS:	velocardiofacial syndrome.
VNTR:	variable number tandem repeat; usually applied to minisatellites.
VSD:	ventricular septal defect.
WAGR:	Wilms tumour, aniridia, genitourinary anomalies and (mental) retardation.
WES:	whole exome sequencing.
WGS:	whole genome sequencing.
XD:	X-linked dominant.
XLA:	X-linked agammaglobulinaemia.
XP:	xeroderma pigmentosum.
XR:	X-linked recessive.
YAC:	yeast artificial chromosome.
ZIC3:	a zinc finger transcription controlling protein.
ZPA:	zone of proliferating activity.
φ:	phi; coefficient of kinship.

1 The place of genetics in medicine

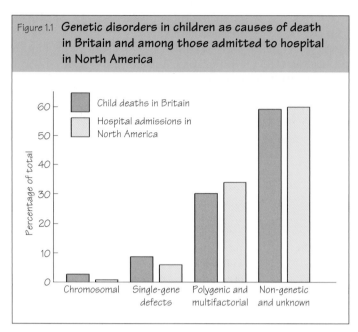

Figure 1.1 Genetic disorders in children as causes of death in Britain and among those admitted to hospital in North America

Child deaths in Britain

Hospital admissions in North America

Percentage of total

Chromosomal Single-gene defects Polygenic and multifactorial Non-genetic and unknown

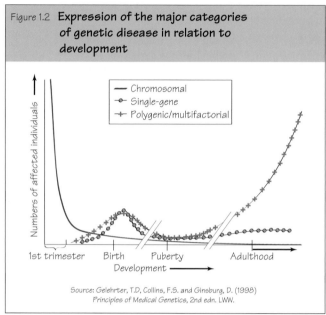

Figure 1.2 Expression of the major categories of genetic disease in relation to development

Numbers of affected individuals

— Chromosomal
—○— Single-gene
—+— Polygenic/multifactorial

1st trimester   Birth   Puberty   Adulthood
Development ⟶

Source: Gelehrter, T.D, Collins, F.S. and Ginsburg, D. (1998) Principles of Medical Genetics, 2nd edn. LWW.

The case for genetics

In recent years medicine has been in a state of transformation, created by the convergence of two major aspects of technological advance. The first is the explosion in information technology and the second, the rapidly expanding science of genetics. The likely outcome is that within the foreseeable future we will see the establishment of a new kind of medicine, **individualized medicine**, tailored uniquely to the personal needs of each patient. Some diseases, such as hypertension, have many causes for which a variety of treatments may be possible. Identification of a specific cause allows clinicians to give personal guidance on the avoidance of adverse stimuli and enable precise targeting of the disease with personally appropriate medications.

One survey of over a million consecutive births showed that at least one in 20 people under the age of 25 develops a serious disease with a major genetic component. Studies of the causes of death of more than 1200 British children suggest that about 40% died as a result of a genetic condition, while genetic factors are important in 50% of the admissions to paediatric hospitals in North America. Through variation in immune responsiveness and other host defences, genetic factors even play a role in infectious diseases.

Genetics underpins and potentially overlaps all other clinical topics, but is especially relevant to reproduction, paediatrics, epidemiology, therapeutics, internal medicine and nursing. It offers unprecedented opportunities for prevention and avoidance of disease because genetic disorders can often be predicted long before the onset of symptoms. This is known as **predictive** or **presymptomatic genetics**. Currently healthy families can be screened for persons with a particular **genotype** that might cause later trouble for them or their children.

'**Gene therapy**' is the ambitious goal of correcting errors associated with inherited deficiencies by introduction of 'normal' versions of genes into their cells. Progress along those lines has been slower than anticipated, but has now moved powerfully into related areas. Some individuals are hypersensitive to standard doses of commonly pre-scribed drugs, while others respond poorly. **Pharmacogenetics** is the study of differential responses to unusual biochemicals and the insights it provides guide physicians in the correct prescription of doses.

Genes in development

Genes do not just cause disease, they define normality and every feature of our bodies receives input from them. Typically every one of our cells contains a pair of each of our 20000–25000 genes and these are controlled and expressed in molecular terms *at the level of the cell*. During embryonic development the cells in different parts of the body become exposed to different influences and acquire divergent properties as they begin to express different combinations of the genes they each contain. Some of these genes define structural components, but most define the amino acid sequences of enzymes that catalyse biochemical processes.

Genes are in fact coded messages written within enormously long molecules of **DNA** distributed between 23 pairs of **chromosomes**. The means by which the information contained in the DNA is interpreted is so central to our understanding that the phrase: '*DNA makes RNA makes protein*'; or more correctly: '***DNA makes heterogeneous nuclear RNA, which makes messenger RNA, which makes polypeptide, which makes protein***;' has become accepted as the '**central dogma**' of molecular biology.

During the production of the gametes the 23 pairs of chromosomes are divided into 23 single sets per ovum or sperm, the normal number being restored in the **zygote** by fertilization. The zygote proliferates to become a hollow ball that implants in the maternal uterus. Prenatal development then ensues until birth, normally at around 38 weeks, but all the body organs are present in miniature by 6–8 weeks. Thereafter embryogenesis mainly involves growth and differentiation of cell types. At puberty development of the organs of reproduction is re-stimulated and the individual attains physical maturity. The period of 38 weeks is popularly considered to be 9 months, traditionally inter-

Medical Genetics at a Glance, Third Edition. Dorian J. Pritchard and Bruce R. Korf.

preted as three '**trimesters**'. The term '**mid-trimester**' refers to the period covering the 4th, 5th and 6th months of gestation.

Genotype and phenotype

Genotype is the word geneticists use for the genetic endowment a person has inherited. **Phenotype** is our word for the anatomical, physiological and psychological complex we recognize as an individual. People have diverse phenotypes partly because they inherited different genotypes, but an equally important factor is what we can loosely describe as 'environment'. A valuable concept is summarized in the equation:

Phenotype = Genotype $\times$ Environment $\times$ Time

It is very important to remember that practically every aspect of phenotype has both genetic and environmental components. Diagnosis of high liability toward 'genetic disease' is therefore not necessarily an irrevocable condemnation to ill health. In some cases optimal health can be maintained by avoidance of genotype-specific environmental hazards.

Genetics in medicine

The foundation of the science of genetics is a set of principles of heredity, discovered in the mid-19th century by an Augustinian monk called Gregor Mendel. These give rise to characteristic patterns of inheritance of variant versions of genes, called **alleles**, depending on whether the unusual allele is dominant or recessive to the common, or 'wild type' one. Any one gene may be represented in the population by many different alleles, only some of which may cause disease. Recognition of the pattern of inheritance of a disease allele is central to prediction of the risk of a couple producing an affected child. Their initial contact with the clinician therefore usually involves construction of a 'family tree' or **pedigree diagram**.

For many reasons genes are expressed differently in the sexes, but from the genetic point of view the most important relates to possession by males of only a single X-chromosome. Most sex-related inherited disease involves expression in males of recessive alleles carried on the X-chromosome.

Genetic diseases can be classed in three major categories: **monogenic, chromosomal** and **multifactorial**. Most monogenic defects reveal their presence after birth and are responsible for 6–9% of early **morbidity** and mortality. At the beginning of the 20th century, Sir Archibald Garrod coined the term '**inborn errors of metabolism**' to describe inherited disorders of physiology. Although individually most are rare, the 350 known inborn errors of metabolism account for 10% of all known single-gene disorders.

Because chromosomes on average carry about 1000 genes, too many or too few chromosomes cause gross abnormalities, most of which are incompatible with survival. Chromosomal defects can create major physiological disruption and most are incompatible with even prenatal survival. These are responsible for more than 50% of deaths in the first trimester of pregnancy and about 2.5% of childhood deaths.

'Multifactorial traits' are due to the combined action of several genes as well as environmental factors. These are of immense importance as they include most of the **common disorders of adult life**. They account for about 30% of childhood illness and in middle-to-late adult life play a major role in the common illnesses from which most of us will die.

The application of genetics

If genes reside side-by-side on the same chromosome they are '**genetically linked**'. If one is a disease gene, but cannot easily be detected, whereas its neighbour can, then alleles of the latter can be used as markers for the disease allele. This allows prenatal assessment, informing decisions about pregnancy, selection of embryos fertilized *in vitro* and presymptomatic diagnosis.

Genetically based disease varies between ethnic groups, but the term '**polymorphism**' refers to genetic variants like blood groups that occur commonly in the population, with no major health connotations. The concept of polymorphism is especially important in blood transfusion and organ transplantation.

Mutation of DNA involves a variety of changes which can be caused for example by exposure to X-rays. Repair mechanisms correct some kinds of change, but new alleles are sometimes created in the **germ cells**, which can be passed on to offspring. Damage that occurs to the DNA of somatic cells can result in **cancer**, when a cell starts to proliferate out of control. Some families have an inherited tendency toward cancer and must be given special care.

A healthy immune system eliminates possibly many thousands of potential cancer cells every day, in addition to disposing of infectious organisms. Maturation of the immune system is associated with unique rearrangements of genetic material, the study of which comes under the heading of **immunogenetics**.

The study of chromosomes is known as **cytogenetics**. This provides a broad overview of a patient's genome and depends on microscopic examination of cells. By contrast **molecular genetic** tests are each specifically for just one or a few disease alleles. The molecular approach received an enormous boost around the turn of the millennium by the detailed mapping of the human genome.

The modern application of genetics to human health is therefore complex. Because it focuses on reproduction it can impinge on deeply held ethical, religious and social convictions, which are often culture variant. At all times therefore, clinicians dealing with genetic matters must be acutely aware of the real possibility of causing personal offence and take steps to avoid that outcome.

2 Pedigree drawing

Figure 2.1 Recommended symbols for use in pedigree diagrams

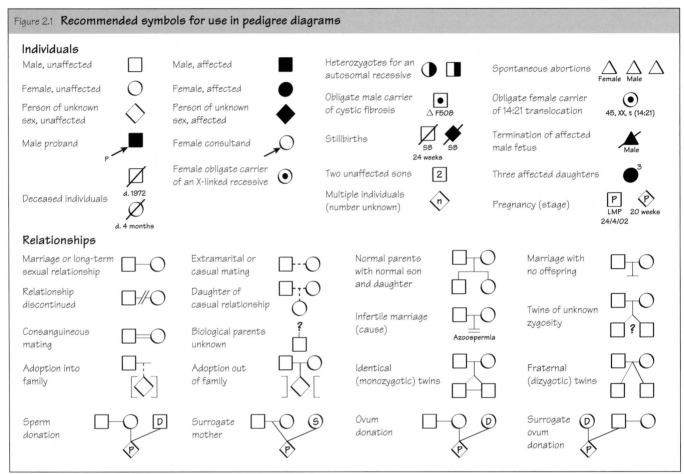

Individuals

Male, unaffected □

Male, affected ■

Female, unaffected ○

Female, affected ●

Person of unknown sex, unaffected ◇

Person of unknown sex, affected ◆

Male proband ■ (P)

Female consultand ○

Female obligate carrier of an X-linked recessive ⊙

Deceased individuals d. 1972 / d. 4 months

Heterozygotes for an autosomal recessive ◐ ◨

Obligate male carrier of cystic fibrosis ⊡ ΔF508

Stillbirths ⊘ ◈ SB 24 weeks / SB

Two unaffected sons 2

Multiple individuals (number unknown) n

Spontaneous abortions △ △ △ Female Male

Obligate female carrier of 14:21 translocation ⊙ 45, XX, t (14:21)

Termination of affected male fetus ◣ Male

Three affected daughters ●³

Pregnancy (stage) P LMP 24/4/02 / P 20 weeks

Relationships

Marriage or long-term sexual relationship □—○

Relationship discontinued □//○

Consanguineous mating □=○

Adoption into family □┄○

Sperm donation □—○—Ⓓ

Extramarital or casual mating □┄○

Daughter of casual relationship □┄○ ○?

Biological parents unknown □—○ ◇

Adoption out of family [□┄◇]

Surrogate mother □—○—Ⓢ

Normal parents with normal son and daughter □—○ □—○

Infertile marriage (cause) □—○ Azoospermia

Identical (monozygotic) twins □—○ □□

Ovum donation □—○—Ⓓ

Marriage with no offspring □—○

Twins of unknown zygosity □—○ □?□

Fraternal (dizygotic) twins □—○ □□

Surrogate ovum donation Ⓓ □—○

Figure 2.2 Sample pedigree

Consultand is II-2
Proband is II-1

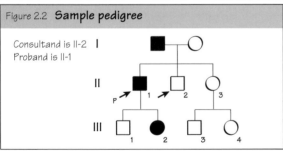

Figure 2.3 A pedigree showing an affected female homozygous for an AD condition who nevertheless had two productive marriages

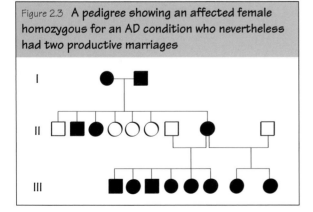

Figure 2.4 A pedigree for haemophilia showing parents who are double first cousins. The probands are affected sisters

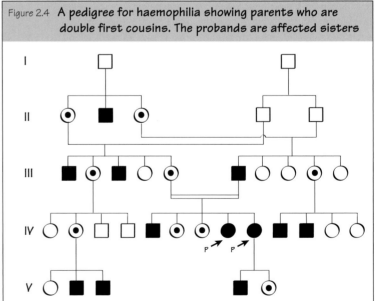

Medical Genetics at a Glance, Third Edition. Dorian J. Pritchard and Bruce R. Korf.

Overview

The collection of information about a family is the first and most important step taken by doctors, nurses or genetic counsellors when providing genetic counselling. A clear and unambiguous **pedigree diagram**, or 'family tree', provides a permanent record of the most pertinent information and is the best aid to clear thinking about family relationships.

Information is usually collected initially from the **consultand**, that is the person requesting genetic advice. If other family members need to be approached it is wise to advise them in advance of the information required. Information should be collected from both sides of the family.

The affected individual who caused the consultand(s) to seek advice is called the **propositus** (male), **proposita** (female), **proband** or **index case**. This is frequently a child or more distant relative, or the consultand may also be the proband. A standard medical history is required for the proband and all other affected family members.

The medical history

In compiling a medical history it is normal practice to carry out a **systems review** broadly along the following lines:
- **cardiovascular system**: enquire about congenital heart disease, hypertension, hyperlipidaemia, blood vessel disease, arrhythmia, heart attacks and strokes;
- **respiratory system**: asthma, bronchitis, emphysema, recurrent lung infection;
- **gastrointestinal tract**: diarrhoea, chronic constipation, polyps, atresia, fistulas and cancer;
- **genitourinary system**: ambiguous genitalia and kidney function;
- **musculoskeletal system**: muscle wasting, physical weakness;
- **neurological conditions**: developmental milestones, hearing, vision, motor coordination, fits.

Rules for pedigree diagrams

Some sample pedigrees are shown (see also Chapters 4–12). Females are symbolized by circles, males by squares, persons of unknown sex by diamonds. Affected individuals are represented by solid symbols, those unaffected, by open symbols. Marriages or matings are indicated by horizontal lines linking male and female symbols, with the male partner preferably to the left. Offspring are shown beneath the parental symbols, in birth order from left to right, linked to the mating line by a vertical, and numbered (1, 2, 3, etc.), from left to right in Arabic numerals. The generations are indicated in Roman numerals (I, II, III, etc.), from top to bottom on the left, with the earliest generation labelled I.

The proband is indicated by an arrow with the letter P, the consultand by an arrow alone. (N.B. earlier practice was to indicate the proband by an arrow without the P).

Only conventional symbols should be used, but it is admissible (and recommended) to annotate diagrams with more complex information. If there are details that could cause embarrassment (e.g. illegitimacy or extramarital paternity) these should be recorded as supplementary notes.

Include the contact address and telephone number of the consultand on supplementary notes. Add the same details for each additional individual that needs to be contacted.

The compiler of the family tree should record the date it was compiled and append his/her name or initials.

The practical approach

1 Start your drawing in the middle of the page.
2 Aim to collect details on three (or more) generations.
3 Ask specifically about:
  (a) consanguinity of partners;
  (b) miscarriages;
  (c) terminated pregnancies;
  (d) stillbirths;
  (e) neonatal and infant deaths;
  (f) handicapped or malformed children;
  (g) multiple partnerships;
  (h) deceased relatives.
4 Be aware of potentially sensitive issues such as adoption and wrongly ascribed paternity.
5 To simplify the diagram unrelated marriage partners may be omitted, but a note should be made whether their phenotype is normal or unknown.
6 Sibs of similar phenotype may be represented as one symbol, with a number to indicate how many are in that category.

The details below should be inserted beside each symbol, whether that individual is alive or dead. Personal details of normal individuals should also be specified. The ethnic background of the family should be recorded if different from that of the main population.

Details for each individual:
1 full name (including maiden name);
2 date of birth;
3 date and cause of death;
4 any specific medical diagnosis.

Use of pedigrees

A good family pedigree reveals the mode of inheritance of the disease and can be used to predict the genetic risk in several instances (see Chapter 13). These include:
1 the current pregnancy;
2 the risk for future offspring of those parents (**recurrence risk**);
3 the risk of disease among offspring of close relatives;
4 the probability of adult disease, in cases of diseases of late onset.

3 Mendel's laws

Figure 3.1 Matings between different homozygotes

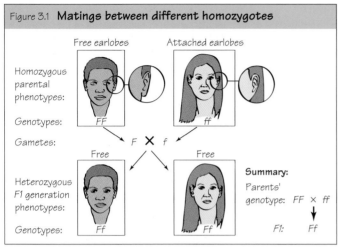

Homozygous parental phenotypes:

Free earlobes — *FF*

Attached earlobes — *ff*

Genotypes: *FF* , *ff*

Gametes: *F* × *f*

Heterozygous F1 generation phenotypes: Free, Free

Genotypes: *Ff* , *Ff*

Summary:
Parents' genotype: *FF* × *ff*

F1: *Ff*

Figure 3.2 Matings between (F1) heterozygotes

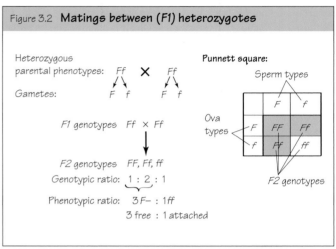

Heterozygous parental phenotypes: *Ff* × *Ff*

Gametes: *F* *f* *F* *f*

F1 genotypes *Ff* × *Ff*

F2 genotypes *FF*, *Ff*, *ff*

Genotypic ratio: 1 : 2 : 1

Phenotypic ratio: 3 *F*– : 1*ff*

3 free : 1 attached

Punnett square:

Sperm types

	F	*f*
F	*FF*	*Ff*
f	*Ff*	*ff*

Ova types

F2 genotypes

Figure 3.3 Mating of a double heterozygote with a recessive homozygote

Red hair is a homozygous recessive condition (*rr*).
Non-red is caused by *RR* or *Rr*.

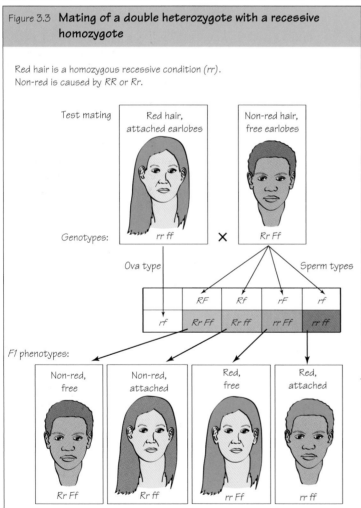

Test mating: Red hair, attached earlobes × Non-red hair, free earlobes

Genotypes: *rr ff* × *Rr Ff*

Ova type Sperm types

	RF	*Rf*	*rF*	*rf*
rf	*Rr Ff*	*Rr ff*	*rr Ff*	*rr ff*

F1 phenotypes:

Non-red, free — *Rr Ff*

Non-red, attached — *Rr ff*

Red, free — *rr Ff*

Red, attached — *rr ff*

Figure 3.4 Mating of a double heterozygote with a dominant homozygote

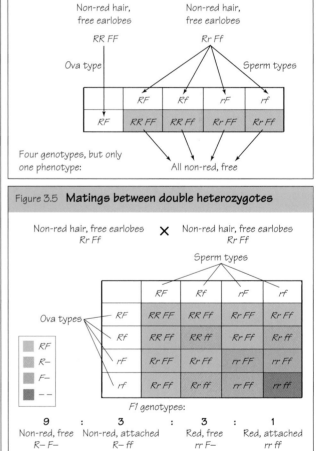

Non-red hair, free earlobes *RR FF*

Non-red hair, free earlobes *Rr Ff*

Ova type Sperm types

	RF	*Rf*	*rF*	*rf*
RF	*RR FF*	*RR Ff*	*Rr FF*	*Rr Ff*

Four genotypes, but only one phenotype: All non-red, free

Figure 3.5 Matings between double heterozygotes

Non-red hair, free earlobes *Rr Ff* × Non-red hair, free earlobes *Rr Ff*

Sperm types

	RF	*Rf*	*rF*	*rf*
RF	*RR FF*	*RR Ff*	*Rr FF*	*Rr Ff*
Rf	*RR Ff*	*RR ff*	*Rr Ff*	*Rr ff*
rF	*Rr FF*	*Rr Ff*	*rr FF*	*rr Ff*
rf	*Rr FF*	*Rr ff*	*rr FF*	*rr ff*

Ova types

Legend:
- *RF*
- *R*–
- *F*–
- – –

F1 genotypes:

9	:	3	:	3	:	1
Non-red, free *R*– *F*–		Non-red, attached *R*– *ff*		Red, free *rr F*–		Red, attached *rr ff*

Medical Genetics at a Glance, Third Edition. Dorian J. Pritchard and Bruce R. Korf.

Overview

Gregor Mendel's laws of inheritance were derived from experiments with plants, but they form the cornerstone of the whole science of genetics. Previously, heredity was considered in terms of the transmission and mixing of 'essences', as suggested by Hippocrates over 2000 years before. But, unlike fluid essences that should blend in the offspring in all proportions, Mendel showed that the instructions for contrasting characters segregate and recombine in simple mathematical proportions. He therefore suggested that the hereditary factors are particulate.

Mendel postulated four new principles concerning **unit inheritance**, **dominance**, **segregation** and **independent assortment** that apply to most genes of all diploid organisms.

The principle of unit inheritance

Hereditary characters are determined by indivisible units of information (which we now call genes). An allele is one version of a gene.

The principle of dominance

Alleles occur in pairs in each individual, but the effects of one allele may be masked by those of a dominant partner allele.

The principle of segregation

During formation of the gametes the members of each pair of alleles separate, so that each gamete carries only one allele of each pair. Allele pairs are restored at fertilization.

Example

The earlobes of some people have an elongated attachment to the neck while others are free, a distinction we can consider for the purposes of this explanation to be determined by two alleles of the same gene, *f* for **attached**, *F* for **free**. (Note: In reality some individuals have earlobes of intermediate form and in some families the genetic basis is more complex.)

Consider a man carrying two copies of *F* (i.e. *FF*), with free earlobes, married to a woman with attached earlobes and two copies of *f* (i.e. *ff*). Both can produce only one kind of gamete, *F* for the man, *f* for the woman. All their children will have one copy of each allele, i.e. are *Ff*, and it is found that all such children have free earlobes because *F is dominant to f*. The children constitute the **first filial generation** or **F1 generation** (irrespective of the symbol for the gene under consideration). Individuals with identical alleles are **homozygotes**; those with different alleles are **heterozygotes**.

The **second filial**, or **F2, generation** is composed of the grandchildren of the original couple, resulting from mating of their offspring with partners of the same genotype in this respect. In each case both parents are heterozygotes, so both produce *F* and *f* gametes in equal numbers. This creates three genotypes in the F2: *FF, Ff* (identical to *fF*) and *ff*, **in the ratio: 1:2:1**.

Due to the dominance of *F* over *f*, dominant homozygotes are phenotypically the same as heterozygotes, so there are three offspring with free earlobes to each one with attached. *The phenotypic ratio 3:1 is characteristic of the offspring of two heterozygotes.*

The principle of independent assortment

Different genes control different phenotypic characters and the alleles of different genes re-assort independently of one another.

Example

Auburn and 'red' hair occur naturally only in individuals who are homozygous for a recessive allele *r*. Non-red is dominant, with the symbol *R*. All red-haired people are therefore *rr*, while non-red are either *RR* or *Rr*.

Consider the mating between an individual with red hair and attached earlobes (*rrff*) and a partner who is heterozygous at both genetic loci (*RrFf*). The recessive homozygote can produce only one kind of gamete, of genotype *rf*, but the double heterozygote can produce gametes of four genotypes: *RF, Rf, rF* and *rf*. Offspring of four genotypes are produced: *RrFf, Rrff, rrFf* and *rrff* and *these are in the ratio 1:1:1:1*.

These offspring also have phenotypes that are all different: non-red with free earlobes, non-red with attached, red with free, and red with attached, respectively.

The test-mating

The mating described above, in which one partner is a double recessive homozygote (*rrff*), constitutes a **test-mating**, as his or her recessive alleles allow expression of all the alleles of their partner.

The value of such a test is revealed by comparison with matings in which the recessive partner is replaced by a double dominant homozygote (*RRFF*). The new partner can produce only one kind of gamete, of genotype *RF*, and four genotypically different offspring are produced, again in equal proportions: *RRFF, RRFf, RrFF* and *RrFf*. However, due to dominance all have non-red hair and free earlobes, so the genotype of the heterozygous parent remains obscure.

Matings between double heterozygotes

The triumphant mathematical proof of Mendel laws was provided by matings between pairs of double heterozygotes. Each can produce four kinds of gametes: *RF, Rf, rF* and *rf*, which combined at random produce nine different genotypic combinations. *Due to dominance there are four phenotypes, in the ratio 9:3:3:1* (total = 16). This allows us to predict the odds of producing:

1 a child with non-red hair and free earlobes (*R-F-*), as 9/16;
2 a child with non-red hair and attached earlobes (*R-ff*), as 3/16;
3 a child with red hair and free earlobes (*rrF-*), as 3/16; and
4 a child with red hair and attached earlobes (*rrff*), as 1/16.

Biological support for Mendel's laws

When published in 1866 Mendel's deductions were ignored, but in 1900 they were re-discovered and rapidly found acceptance. This was in part because the chromosomes had by then been described and the postulated behaviour of Mendel's factors coincided with the observed properties and behaviour of the chromosomes: (i) both occur in homologous pairs; (ii) at meiosis both separate, but reunite at fertilization; and (iii) the homologues of both segregate and recombine independently of one another. This coincidence is because the genes are components of the chromosomes.

Exceptions to Mendel's laws

Several patterns of inheritance deviate from those described by Gregor Mendel for which a variety of explanations has been suggested.

1. Sex-related effects

The genetic specification of sexual differentiation is described in Chapter 43. In brief, male embryos carry one short chromosome designated Y and a much longer chromosome designated X, so the male karyotype can be summarized as XY. The Y carries a small number of genes concerned with development and maturation of masculine features and also sections homologous with parts of the X. The normal female karyotype is XX, females having two X chromosomes and no Y.

A copy of the father's Y chromosome is transmitted to every son, while a copy of his X chromosome is passed to every daughter. Y-linked traits (of which there are very few) are therefore confined to males, but X-linked can show a criss-cross pattern from fathers to daughters, mothers to sons down the generations.

The most significant aspect of sex-related inheritance concerns X-linked recessive alleles, of which there are many. Those which have no counterpart on the Y are more commonly expressed in hemizygous males than in homozygous females.

2. Mitochondrial inheritance

The units of inheritance such as Mendel described are carried on the **autosomes** (non-sex chromosomes), which exist in homologous pairs. These exchange genetic material by 'crossing over' with their partners and segregate at meiosis (see Chapter 18). In addition there are multiple copies of a much smaller genome in virtually every cell of the human body, which resides in the tiny subcellular organelles called mitochondria (see Chapter 12).

The mode of inheritance of mitochondria derives from the mechanism of fertilization. Sperm are very small, light in weight and fast moving. They carry little else but a nucleus, a structure that assists penetration of the ovum and a tail powered by a battery of mitochondria. The latter are however shed before the sperm nucleus enters the ovum and so make no contribution to the mitochondrial population of the zygote. By contrast the ovum is massive and loaded with nutrients and many copies of the subcellular organelles of somatic body cells (see Chapter 14). All the genes carried in the mitochondrial genome are therefore passed on only by females, and equally to offspring of both sexes. Mitochondrial inheritance is therefore entirely from mothers, to offspring of both sexes.

3. Genetic linkage

Mendel did not know where the hereditary information resides. He was certainly unaware of the importance of chromosomes in that regard and the traits he described showed independent assortment with one another. 'Genetic linkage' refers to the observed tendency for combinations of alleles of different genes to be inherited as a group, because they reside close together on the same chromosome (see Chapter 31).

4. Polygenic conditions

Many aspects of phenotype cannot be segregated simply into positive and negative categories, but instead show a continuous range of variation. Examples are height and intelligence. The conventional explanation is that they are controlled by the joint action of many genes. In addition, environmental factors modify phenotypes, further blurring genetically based distinctions (see Chapters 50 and 51).

5. Overdominance, codominance, variable expressivity and incomplete penetrance

Mendel's concept of dominance is that expression of a dominant allele obliterates that of a recessive and that heterozygotes are phenotypically indistinguishable from dominant homozygotes, but this is not always the case. In achondroplasia, a form of short-limbed dwarfism, homozygotes for the dominant achondroplasia allele are so severely affected that they die *in utero*. This phenomenon is called **overdominance**. The consequence is that the live offspring of heterozygous achondroplastic partners occur in the ratio of two affected not three, to each unaffected recessive homozygote (see Chapter 5).

Codominance refers to the expression of *both* antigens in a heterozygote. A familiar example is the presence of both A and B antigenic determinants on the surfaces of red blood cells of AB blood group heterozygotes (see Chapter 29).

The expression of many genes is modified by alleles of other genes as well as by environmental factors. Many genetic conditions therefore show **variable expressivity**, confusing the concept of simple dominance.

In some cases an apparently dominant allele may appear to skip a generation because its expression in one carrier has been negated by other factors. Such alleles are said to show **incomplete penetrance** (see Chapter 9).

6. Genomic imprinting

A striking exception to Mendel's description is mutant alleles that confer markedly different phenotypes in relation to the parental origin of the mutant gene. For example, when a site on the long arm of the maternally derived chromosome 15 has been deleted it gives rise to Angelman syndrome in the offspring. Children with this condition show jerky movements and are severely mentally handicapped. When the equivalent site is deleted from the paternally derived chromosome 15, the child is affected in a very different way. These children have Prader–Willi syndrome, characterized by features that include compulsive consumption of food, obesity and a lesser degree of mental handicap. The explanation is in terms of differential 'imprinting' of the part of chromosome 15 concerned (see Chapter 27). Several hundred human genes receive 'imprinting'.

7. Dynamic mutation

Around 20 human genetic diseases develop with increasing severity in consecutive generations, or make their appearance in progressively younger patients. A term that relates to both features is '**dynamic mutation**', which involves progressive expansion of three-base repeats in the DNA associated with certain genes (see Chapter 28).

8. Meiotic drive

Heterozygotes produce two kinds of gametes, carrying alternative alleles at that locus and the proportions of the offspring described by Mendel indicate equal transmission of those alternatives. Rarely one allele is transmitted at greater frequency than the other, a phenomenon called **meiotic drive**. There is some evidence this may occur with myotonic dystrophy (see Chapter 28).

Conclusion

Despite being derived from simple experiments with garden plants and the existence of numerous exceptions, Mendel's laws remain the central concept in our understanding of familial patterns of inheritance in our own species, and in those of most other 'higher' organisms. Examples of simple dominant and recessive conditions of great medical significance are familial hypercholesterolaemia (Chapters 5 and 6) and cystic fibrosis (Chapter 6).

4 Principles of autosomal dominant inheritance and pharmacogenetics

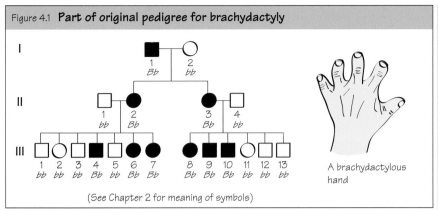

Figure 4.1 **Part of original pedigree for brachydactyly**

A brachydactylous hand

(See Chapter 2 for meaning of symbols)

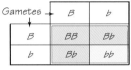

Figure 4.2 **Estimation of risk for offspring, autosomal dominant inheritance**

Heterozygote paired with a normal homozygote (*Bb* × *bb*)

Risk of *B*– : 2/4 = 50%

Heterozygote paired with another heterozygote (*Bb* × *Bb*)

Risk of *B*– : 3/4 = 75%

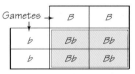

Dominant homozygote paired with a normal homozygote (*BB* × *bb*)

Risk of *B*– : 4/4 = 100%

Overview

In principle, dominant alleles are expressed when present as single copies (c.f. recessive, Chapter 6), but '**incompletely penetrant**' alleles can remain unexpressed in some circumstances (see Chapter 9). Some alleles that are especially important in medicine are revealed only when people are exposed to unusual chemicals. Some such '**pharmacogenetic traits**' are inherited as dominants, others in other ways (see below).

Rules for autosomal dominant inheritance

The following are the basic rules for simple **autosomal dominant (AD) inheritance**. These rules apply only to conditions of complete penetrance and where no novel mutation has arisen.

1 *Both males and females express the allele and can transmit it equally to sons and daughters.*

2 *Every affected person has an affected parent* ('vertical' pattern of expression in the pedigree). Direct transmission through three generations is practically diagnostic of a dominant.

3 In affected families, *the ratio of affected to unaffected children is almost always 1:1.*

4 *If both parents are unaffected, all the children are unaffected.*

Example

The first condition in humans for which the mode of inheritance was elucidated was **brachydactyly**, characterized by abnormally short phalanges.

In Mendelian symbols, dominant allele *B* causes brachydactyly and every affected individual is either a homozygote (*BB*) or a heterozygote (*Bb*). In practice most are heterozygotes, because *brachydactyly is a rare trait* (i.e. <1/5000 births), *as are almost all dominant disease alleles.* Unrelated marriage partners are therefore usually recessive homozygotes (*bb*) and the mating can be represented:

Bb × *bb*
↓
Bb,bb
  1:1

Dominant disease alleles are kept at low frequency since their carriers are less fit than normal homozygotes.

Matings between heterozygotes are the only kind that can produce homozygous offspring:

Bb × *Bb*
↓
BB, *Bb*, *bb*
1:2:1; i.e. 3 affected:1 unaffected.

Dominant disease allele homozygotes are extremely rare and with many disease alleles homozygosity is lethal or causes a more pronounced or severe phenotype.

Matings between heterozygotes may involve inbreeding (see Chapter 5), or occur when patients have met as a consequence of their disability (e.g. at a clinic for the disorder).

All offspring of affected homozygotes are affected:

BB × *bb*
↓
Bb

Unaffected members of affected families are normal homozygotes, so do not transmit the condition: *bb* × *bb* → *bb*.

Estimation of risk

In simply inherited AD conditions where the diagnosis is secure, estimation of risk for the offspring of a family member can be based simply on the predictions of Mendel's laws. For example:

1 For the offspring of a heterozygote and a normal homozygote (*Bb* × *bb* → 1 *Bb*; 1 *bb*), risk of *B*– = 1/2, or 50%.

2 For the offspring of two heterozygotes (*Bb* × *Bb* → 1 *BB*; 2 *Bb*; 1 *bb*), risk of *B*– = 3/4, or 75%.

3 For the offspring of a dominant homozygote with a normal partner (*BB* × *bb* → *Bb*), risk of *B*– = 1, or 100%.

Medical Genetics at a Glance, Third Edition. Dorian J. Pritchard and Bruce R. Korf.
© 2013 John Wiley & Sons, Ltd. Published 2013 by John Wiley & Sons, Ltd.

Table 4.1 Some important autosomal dominant inherited diseases in order of approximate frequency in Caucasians.

Condition	Frequency	Map loc.	Gene product
Dominant otosclerosis	1/300–4000	16p	
Familial hypercholesterolaemia (>900 alleles)	1/500	19p	*LDL receptor*
Dentinogenesis imperfecta	1/1000		
Adult polycystic kidney disease	1/1000	16p, etc.	*Polycystin*
Multiple exostosis	1/2000	8q, 11p	
Hereditary motor and sensory neuropathy Type I due to duplication of PMP22 gene. Slow nerve condition, exaggerated foot arch, clawing of toes.	1/3000	17p	
Neurofibromatosis Type I 80% are new mutations. Café-au-lait patches, dermal fibromas, macrocephaly, scoliosis, learning difficulties. Serious complications can be caused by compression by internal fibromas. (see Chapters 9, 57)	1/3000–1/5000	17q	*Neurofibromin t.s.*
Hereditary spherocytosis Red blood cells appear spherical leading to haemolytic anaemia.	1/5000	8p	*ankrin -1*
Osteogenesis imperfecta Highly variable, with multiple fractures and lens deformity. There are recessive forms also. Type I: blue sclerae and deafness; Type II: lethal perinatally; Type III: severe progressive deformation; Type IV: mild bone breakage, short stature, dental abnormalities.	1/5000–1/10 000	17q 7q	*Collagen – COL 1A1* *Collagen – COL 1A2*
Myotonic dystrophy Progressive muscle weakness with inability to relax muscle tone normally, cataracts, cardiac conduction defects, hypogonadism. Caused by CAG triplet expansion. (see Chapter 28)	1/9000	19p 3q	*DM kinase* *zinc finger protein*
Ehlers–Danlos syndrome Numerous types and highly variable, genetic heterogeneity suspected; skin fragility and elasticity, joint hypermobility. Type IV has high risk of early death due to vascular rupture.	1/10 000	2q, etc	*Collagen Type IV:COL 3A1*
Marfan syndrome (several hundred alleles)	1/10 000		
Achondroplasia	1/10 000–1/50 000		
Dominant blindness	1/10 000		
Dominant congenital deafness	1/10 000		
Familial adenomatous polyposis coli (see Chapter 55)	1/10 000	5q	*APC t.s.*
Tuberous sclerosis Type I Type II Highly variable, cortical brain tubers, 'ash leaf spots' and raised lesions on skin, lung lesions, severe mental handicap, epilepsy. (see Chapter 51)	1/15 000	9q 16p	*Hamartin t.s.* *Tuberin t.s.*
Adult-onset cerebellar ataxia Progressive cerebellar ataxia often associated with ophthalmoplegia and dementia.	1/20 000	6p, etc.	*Ataxin* (Spinal CA, Type I)
Huntington disease (see Chapters 28)	1/20 000	4p	*Huntingtin*
Neurofibromatosis Type II Bilateral acoustic neuromas and early cataracts. (see Chapter 56)	1/50 000	22q	*schwannomin (merlin)t.s.*
Von Hippel Lindau syndrome (see Chapter 56)	1/50 000		
Facio-scapulo-humeral dystrophy Progressive limb girdle and facial weakness particularly of the shoulder muscles.	1/50 000	4q	

Calculations involving dominant conditions can, however, be problematical as we usually do not know whether an affected offspring is homozygous or heterozygous (see Chapter 13).

Estimation of mutation rate

The frequency of dominant diseases in families with no prior cases can be used to estimate the natural frequency of new point mutations (see Chapter 26). This varies widely between genes, but averages about one mutational event in any specific gene per 500 000 zygotes. Almost all point mutations arise in sperm, each containing, at the latest estimates, 20–25 000 genes (see Chapter 19). There are therefore perhaps 25 000 mutations per 500 000 sperm, so we can expect around 5% of viable sperm (and babies) to carry a new genetic mutation. However, only a minority of these occurs within genes that produce clinically significant effects, or would behave as dominant traits.

Pharmacogenetics

Pharmacogenetic traits are inherited in a variety of ways (**AD, AR, X-linked R, ACo-D**, etc., see Abbreviations and Chapter 29).

Debrisoquine hydroxylase deficiency (AR)

Genes of the **cytochrome P450** group are of particular importance in drug deactivation (see Chapter 29). One such is **debrisoquine hydroxylase**, involved in the metabolism of the antihypertensive *debrisoquine* and other drugs. Five to 10% of Europeans show serious adverse reactions to debrisoquine.

Porphyria variegata (AD)

Skin lesions, abdominal pain, paralysis, dementia and psychosis are brought on by sulphonamides, barbiturates, etc., in about one in 500 South Africans. Death can result from concentration of haem in the liver, following induction of haem-containing Cytochrome P450 proteins.

G6PD deficiency (X-linked R) (see Chapter 11)

G6PD deficiency causes sensitivity notably to *primaquine* (used for treatment of malaria), *phenacetin*, *sulphonamides* and **fava beans** (broad beans), hence the name '**favism**' for the haemolytic crisis that occurs when they are eaten by male hemizygotes.

N-acetyl transferase deficiency (AR)

In Western populations, 50% of individuals are homozygous for a recessive allele that confers a dangerously slow rate of elimination of certain drugs, notably *isoniazid* prescribed against tuberculosis. The Japanese are predominantly rapid inactivators.

Pseudocholinesterase deficiency (AR)

One European in 3000 and 1.5% of Inuit (Eskimo) are homozygous for an enzyme deficiency that causes lethal paralysis of the diaphragm when given *succinylcholine* as a muscle relaxant during surgery.

Halothane sensitivity, malignant hyperthermia (genetically heterogeneous)

One in 10 000 patients can die in high fever when given the anaesthetic *halothane*, especially in combination with succinylcholine.

Thiopurine methyltransferase deficiency (ACo-D)

Certain drugs prescribed for leukaemia and suppression of the immune response cause serious side-effects in about 0.3% of the population with deficiency of *thiopurine methyltransferase*.

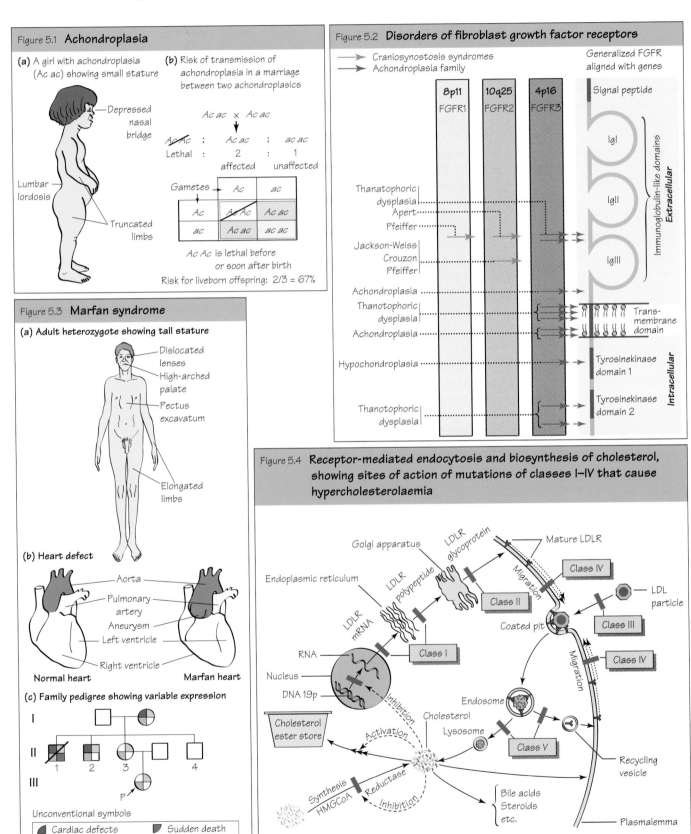

Figure 5.1 **Achondroplasia**

(a) A girl with achondroplasia (Ac ac) showing small stature

- Depressed nasal bridge
- Lumbar lordosis
- Truncated limbs

(b) Risk of transmission of achondroplasia in a marriage between two achondroplasics

$$Ac\ ac\ \times\ Ac\ ac$$

Ac Ac	:	Ac ac	:	ac ac
Lethal		2		1
		affected		unaffected

Gametes	Ac	ac
Ac	Ac Ac	Ac ac
ac	Ac ac	ac ac

Ac Ac is lethal before or soon after birth

Risk for liveborn offspring: 2/3 = 67%

Figure 5.2 **Disorders of fibroblast growth factor receptors**

⟶ Craniosynostosis syndromes
⟶ Achondroplasia family

Generalized FGFR aligned with genes

| 8p11 FGFR1 | 10q25 FGFR2 | 4p16 FGFR3 |

- Signal peptide
- IgI
- IgII
- IgIII
- Immunoglobulin-like domains / Extracellular

Thanatophoric dysplasia
Apert
Pfeiffer
Jackson-Weiss
Crouzon
Pfeiffer
Achondroplasia
Thanotophoric dysplasia
Achondroplasia
Hypochondroplasia
Thanotophoric dysplasia

- Trans-membrane domain
- Tyrosinekinase domain 1
- Tyrosinekinase domain 2
- Intracellular

Figure 5.3 **Marfan syndrome**

(a) Adult heterozygote showing tall stature

- Dislocated lenses
- High-arched palate
- Pectus excavatum
- Elongated limbs

(b) Heart defect

- Aorta
- Pulmonary artery
- Aneurysm
- Left ventricle
- Right ventricle

Normal heart   Marfan heart

(c) Family pedigree showing variable expression

I
II 1 2 3 4
III   P

Unconventional symbols

| Cardiac defects | Sudden death |
| Dislocated lenses | Elongated limbs |

Figure 5.4 **Receptor-mediated endocytosis and biosynthesis of cholesterol, showing sites of action of mutations of classes I–IV that cause hypercholesterolaemia**

- Golgi apparatus
- LDLR glycoprotein
- Mature LDLR
- Class IV
- Endoplasmic reticulum
- LDLR polypeptide
- Class II
- LDL particle
- LDLR mRNA
- Coated pit
- Class III
- RNA
- Class I
- Class IV
- Nucleus
- DNA 19p
- Migration
- Inhibition
- Endosome
- Cholesterol
- Lysosome
- Recycling vesicle
- Cholesterol ester store
- Activation
- Class V
- Synthesis HMGCoA Reductase
- Inhibition
- Bile acids Steroids etc.
- Plasmalemma
- Cholesterol precursors

Medical Genetics at a Glance, Third Edition. Dorian J. Pritchard and Bruce R. Korf.

Overview

Over 4000 autosomal dominant (AD) conditions are known, although few are more frequent than 1/5000 and deemed 'common' (see Table 4.1). The most common or most important are described here. The significant gene product in AD disease is typically a non-enzymic protein.

Disorders of the fibroblast growth factor receptors

Extracellular **fibroblast growth factor** (**FGF**) signals operate through a family of three transmembrane tyrosine kinases, the **fibroblast growth factor receptors** (**FGFR**s). Binding of FGF to their extracellular domains activates tyrosine kinase activity intracellularly.

Mutations in the genes that code for the FGFRs are implicated both in the **achondroplasia family** of skeletal dysplasias and the **craniosynostosis syndromes**. **Hypochondroplasia** is grossly similar to achondroplasia, but the head is normal; **thanatophoric dysplasia** is much more severe and invariably lethal. There is premature fusion of the cranial sutures in all the craniosynostoses, in **Apert syndrome** often associated with hand and foot abnormalities. In **Pfeiffer** the thumbs and big toes are abnormal; in **Crouzon** all limbs are normal.

Achondroplasia

Description Achondroplasia causes severe shortening of the proximal segments of the limbs, the average height of adults being only 49–51 ins (125–130 cm). The patient has a prominent forehead (**macrocephaly**), depressed nasal bridge and restricted foramen magnum that can cause cervical spinal cord compression, respiratory problems and sudden infant death. Middle ear infections are common and can lead to conductive deafness. Pelvic malformation causes a waddling gait. Lumbar **lordosis** can cause lower back pain and 'slipped disc'. Babies of women with achondroplasia are usually delivered by Caesarean section.

Aetiology FGFR3 is expressed in chondrocytes, predominantly at the growth plates of developing long bones, where the normal allele inhibits excessive growth. The achondroplasia mutation causes premature closure of growth plates due to early differentiation of chondrocytes into bone, 80% of mutations being new (see Chapter 4).

Management issues Children are often hypotonic and late in sitting and walking. Spinal cord compression due to foramen magnum restriction can cause weakness and tingling in the limbs. Breathing patterns should be monitored during childhood. Frequent attacks of otitis media must be treated quickly and there is orthopaedic treatment to lengthen limbs.

Affected individuals tend to marry affected partners and can conceive homozygotes that usually do not survive to term. Liveborn homozygotes have an extreme short-limbed, asphyxiating dysplasia causing neonatal death, so surviving offspring of achondroplasic partners have a 2/3 risk of being achondroplasic. Genetic status is determinable by DNA analysis during the first trimester (see Chapters 67 and 72).

Marfan syndrome (MFS)

Description MFS illustrates **pleiotropy**, affecting several systems, notably skeleton, heart and eyes and MFS can be confused with other conditions. For positive diagnosis the revised Ghent nosology puts most weight on the cardiovascular manifestations, with **aortic root**

aneurysm and **ectopia lentis** being cardinal features. In the absence of a family history, the presence of these two is sufficient. In the absence of either one the presence of a defined *FBN1* mutation is required, or a combination of other features such as involvement other organ systems.

Skeleton Affected individuals have joint laxity, a *span : height ratio greater than 1.05 and reduced upper-to-lower segment body ratio*. Overgrowth of bone occurs. There are unusually long, slender limbs and fingers, **pectus excavatum** (hollow chest), **pectus carinatum** (pigeon chest) and **scoliosis** that can cause cardiac and respiratory problems.

Heart Most patients develop prolapse of the mitral valve, its cusps protruding into the left atrium, allowing leakage back into the left ventricle, enlargement of which can result in congestive heart failure. More serious is **aneurysm** (widening) of the ascending aorta in 90% of patients, leading to rupture during exercise or pregnancy.

Eyes Most patients have myopia and about half **ectopia lentis** (lens displacement).

Aetiology The underlying defect is excessive elasticity of **fibrillin-1**. A dominant negative effect is created in heterozygotes by mutant protein binding to and disabling normal fibrillin. Fibrillin regulates TGF-β signalling in connective tissue: pathogenesis is believed to involve excessive signalling in the absence of functional fibrillin-1.

Management issues Clinical management includes body measurement, echocardiography, ophthalmic evaluation and lumbar MRI scan. Aortic dilatation can be prevented by β-adrenergic blockade to decrease the strength of heart contractions. Surgical replacement should be undertaken if the aortic diameter reaches 50–55 mm. Heavy exercise and contact sports should be avoided. Pregnancy is a risk factor if the aorta is dilated. Recent clinical trials suggest that treatment with **losartan** may prevent or reverse aortic dilation.

Squints may need correction. Antibiotics should be given prophylactically before minor operations to obviate **endocarditis**.

Familial hypercholesterolaemia (FH)

Description Up to 50% of deaths in many developed countries are caused by **coronary artery disease** (**CAD**). This results from **atherosclerosis**, following deposition of low density lipid (LDL; including cholesterol) in the intima of the coronary arteries. FH heterozygotes account for 1/20 of those presenting with early CAD and approximately 5% of **myocardial infarctions** (MIs) in persons under 60 years of age. FH heterozygote plasma cholesterol levels are twice as high as normal, resulting in distinctive cholesterol deposits (**xanthomas**) in tendons and skin. Approximately 75% of male FH heterozygotes develop CAD and 50% have a fatal MI by the age of 60 years. In women the equivalent figures are 45% and 15%.

Aetiology All cells require cholesterol as a component of their plasma membranes, which can be derived either by endogenous intracellular synthesis or by uptake via LDL receptors on their external surfaces.

Newly synthesized receptor protein is normally glycosylated in the Golgi apparatus before passing to the plasma membrane, where it becomes localized in **coated pits** lined with the protein **clathrin**. LDL-bound cholesterol attaches to the receptor and the coated pit sinks inwards, internalizing the LDL particle. There the lipid separates from the receptor and inhibits *de novo* cholesterol synthesis The receptor then returns to the surface to bind another LDL. Each LDLR repeats this cycle every 10 minutes. High cholesterol levels in the circulation of FH heterozygotes arise from defective LDLRs.

There are over 900 FH alleles in five classes (see Figure 5.4):

Class I: no LDLR protein is produced;

Class II: LDLR synthesis fails before glycosylation;

Class III: glycosylated LDLR reaches the coated pits, but cannot bind LDL;

Class IV: receptors reach the cell surface, but fail to congregate in coated pits;

Class V: the receptor cannot release bound LDL.

Management issues Dietary cholesterol should be restricted and bile-acid-absorbing resins can be used to sequester cholesterol from the enterohepatic circulation. Other drugs ('**statins**') block endogenous synthesis by inhibiting **HMGCoA reductase**.

Dentinogenesis imperfecta 1 (DGI)

Description DGI affects the teeth, causing them to be blue–grey or amber brown and opalescent. On dental radiographs the teeth are seen to have bulbous crowns, roots narrower than normal and chambers and root canals that are small or completely obliterated. Primary teeth are affected more than secondary.

The Shields classification recognizes three types:
- **Type 1**, associated with **osteogenesis imperfecta**;
- **Type 2**, with no associated bone defect;
- **Type 3**, less severe than Types 1 and 2, with no associated bone defects. Also known as the Brandywine form (after Brandywine, Maryland, USA).

Aetiology DGI Type1 is due to a mutation in the *DSPP* gene causing deficiency in **sialophosphoprotein** (DSPP).

Otosclerosis 1 (OTSC1)

Description Clinical otosclerosis has a prevalence of 0.2–1% among white adults, making it the single most common cause of hearing impairment. Approximately 10% of affected persons develop profound sensorineural hearing loss across all frequencies. There are seven known disease genes. Otosclerosis is nearly twice as common in females as in males, with distortion of sex ratio in patient sibships, implying prenatal selection operating against males.

Aetiology Disease is characterized by bone sclerosis of the labyrinthine capsule of the middle ear, with invasion of sclerotic foci into the 'oval window', interfering with free motion of the stapes.

Management issues The mean age of onset is in the third decade, 90% of affected persons being under 50 years at diagnosis.

Adult polycystic kidney disease (APKD, PKD)

Description Although primarily causing kidney cysts, there are also cysts in the liver, especially in females, as well as intracranial aneurysm. The kidneys can become grossly enlarged and hypertension is often an associated feature. Several genetic loci are implicated, but *PKD1*, involving protein polycystin-1 (at 16p) is the most common. Overall frequency is 1/1–4000.

There is variability in ages of onset and of reaching end-stage renal disease. Males reach the latter point 5–6 years earlier than females. Glomerular filtration efficiency and co-occurrence of hypertension are also variable. Subarachnoid haemorrhage can occur from intracranial 'berry aneurysm'.

Aetiology There is evidence of a defect in the mechanosensory function of cilia and also of reversed polarity of Na^+/K^+ ATPase in the apical luminal plasma membranes of renal tubule cells lining the renal cysts. A 'two-hit hypothesis' (see Chapter 56) suggests that in PKD heterozygotes, local homozygosity is created by somatic mutation of the normal allele at sites of cyst formation.

Management Diagnosis of cysts is generally by ultrasonography, which has permitted diagnosis prenatally, although 40% of carriers below 30 years of age do not have cysts. Renal prognosis is poorer in essential hypertensive subjects.

Multiple hereditary exostoses (EXT)

Description EXT is characterized by multiple bony projections (**exostoses**) capped by cartilage in various parts of the skeleton. There are numerous alleles of both genes *EXT1* (at 8q) and *EXT2* (at 11p) responsible for over 70% of cases. More severe disease is associated with *EXT1*, incurring additional risk of **chondrosarcoma** (cartilage cancer) in middle age. The *EXT* alleles are incompletely penetrant, affecting males and females in the ratio 1.45:1.

Typically there are protuberances at the ends and juxta-epiphyseal regions of long bones, the most frequently affected sites being the upper ends of the femurs and also the pelvis. Scapulae, vertebrae and ribs may also be affected. There can be deformity of the legs, with **genu valgum** (knock knees) and **Madelung-like deformity** of the forearms (i.e. **manus valga** – club hand with deviation to the ulnar side, and **radius curvus** – curvature of the lower extremity of the radius). Typically the metacarpals are short, with bilateral overriding of single toes. There is short stature in some (<50%) patients.

Aetiology The cause of EXT1 is loss of function of the **exostosin 1** gene, consistent with the hypothesis that the *EXT* genes have a **tumour suppressor** function (see Chapter 55).

Management issues Bilateral overriding of the toes enables diagnosis at birth. Onset is in early childhood and lesions continue to grow until closure of the epiphyseal plates. Bone overgrowth can cause peripheral nerve compression and cervical **myelopathy** (spinal cord injury).

6 Autosomal recessive inheritance, principles

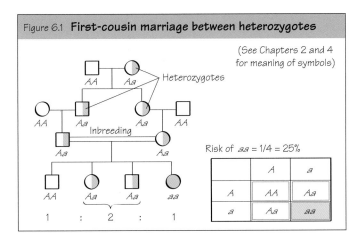

Figure 6.1 **First-cousin marriage between heterozygotes**

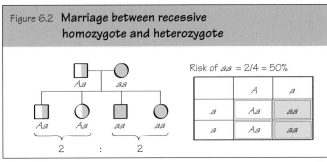

Figure 6.2 **Marriage between recessive homozygote and heterozygote**

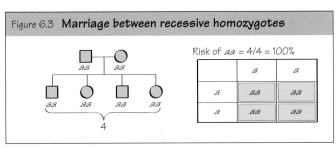

Figure 6.3 **Marriage between recessive homozygotes**

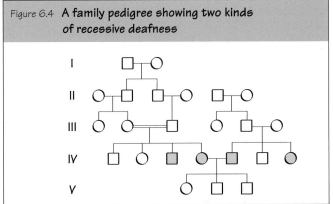

Figure 6.4 **A family pedigree showing two kinds of recessive deafness**

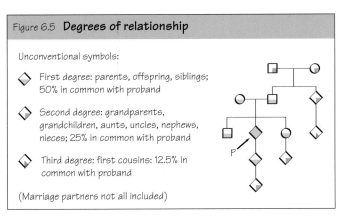

Figure 6.5 **Degrees of relationship**

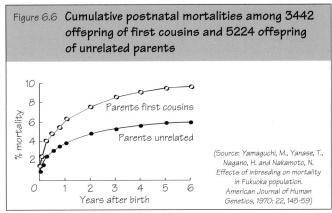

Figure 6.6 **Cumulative postnatal mortalities among 3442 offspring of first cousins and 5224 offspring of unrelated parents**

Overview

The pedigree diagram for a family in which autosomal recessive disorder is present differs markedly from those with other forms of inheritance. Recessive disorders can be relatively common, as heterozygous carriers can preserve and transmit disease alleles without adverse selection.

Rules for autosomal recessive inheritance

The following are the rules for simple **autosomal recessive inheritance**.

1 *Both males and females are affected.*
2 *There are breaks in the pedigree and typically the pattern of expression is 'horizontal'* (i.e. sibs are affected but parents are not).
3 *Affected children can be born to normal parents,* usually in the approximate ratio of one affected to three unaffected.

4 *When both parents are affected all the children are affected,* unless mimic genes are involved (see 'congenital deafness', below.)
5 *Affected individuals with normal partners usually have only normal children.*

Example: albinism

Oculocutaneous albinism (OCA; see Chapters 7 and 63) is an autosomal recessive condition, that is every affected person is a recessive homozygote (**aa**). Most are born to phenotypically normal parents, who can also produce normal homozygotes and heterozygotes in the ratio of one dominant homozygote to two pigmented heterozygotes to every one with albinism:

$Aa \times Aa \rightarrow 1\,AA : 2\,Aa : 1\,\textbf{aa}$; 3 pigmented : 1 albino

Medical Genetics at a Glance, Third Edition. Dorian J. Pritchard and Bruce R. Korf.
© 2013 John Wiley & Sons, Ltd. Published 2013 by John Wiley & Sons, Ltd.

Table 6.1 Some important autosomal recessive inherited diseases in order of approximate prevalence in Caucasians.

Condition	Freq.	Carrier freq.	Map locn.	Gene prod.
Primary haemachromatosis	1/200–1/400	1/10	6p	*HLA–H*
Iron accumulation especially in the liver, with cirrhosis, cardiomyopathy, diabetes mellitus (see Chapters 60–62)				
Recessive mental retardation	1/2000		many	
Cystic fibrosis (in Caucasians) (see Chapter 7)	1/2500	1/25	7q31	*CFTR*
Tay–Sachs disease	1/3600	1/30	15q	*hexosaminidase A*
In Ashkenazi Jews				
In American non-Jews (see Chapters 8, 62)	1/360 000	1/300		
Retinitis pigmentosa	1/4000		several	
50% of type AR, 15% AD, 5% X-linked. Night blindness, tunnel vision, pigmented areas in retina				
Albinism, oculocutaneous, type 1	1/10 000	1/100	11q	*tyrosinase*
Phenylketonuria (see Chapter 8)	1/10 000	1/50	12	*PA hydroxylase*
Spinal muscular atrophy (see Chapter 8)	1/10 000	1/50	5q13	*SMN factor,NAIP*
Recessive blindness	1/10 000			
Congenital adrenal hyperplasia	1/10 000	1/50	6	*21-hydroxylase*
Masculinization of female genitalia, precocious puberty in males, salt deficiency (see Chapter 44)				
Medium-chain acyl CoA dehydrogenase deficiency	1/10 000	1/50	1p	*MCAD*
Presents in early years with low blood glucose in response to infection or starvation, inability to produce ketones (see Chapters 60–62)				
Gaucher disease	1/25 000	1/80	1	*β-glucosidase*
In Ashkenazi Jews: (see Chapters 60–62)	1/3600	1/15		
Smith–Lemli–Opitz syndrome	1/30 000			*7-dehydrocholesterol reductase (7 DHCR)*
Type 2 is lethal neonatally, with microcephaly, heart defect, renal dysplasia, cleft palate and polydactyly; Type 1 is less severe with mental handicap, ptosis and genitourinary malformations (see Chapters 44, 60)				
Zellweger syndrome	1/50 000		several	
Peroxisome function disrupted, raised plasma levels of long chain fatty acids, severe developmental delay, hypotonia, renal and hepatic failure (see Chapter 62)				
Classical galactosaemia	1/55 000		9	*galactose-1-phosphate uridyl transferase*
Vomiting, hepatomegaly, jaundice and oedema. In later life, cataracts and mental handicap. (see Chapter 59)				
Sickle cell disease			11p	*β-globin*
In African-Americans: (see Chapter 29)	1/600	1/12		
Alpha-thalassaemia			16p	*α-globin*
In Southeast Asians, Chinese: (see Chapter 29)	1/2500	1/25		
Beta-thalassaemia			11p	*β-globin*
In Greeks, Italians: (see Chapter 29)	1/3600	1/30		
Friedreich ataxia			7q	*fraxitin*
Ataxia, pigeon chest, loss of muscle function in legs				
Adenosine deaminase deficiency	1/100 000		20q	*adenosine deaminase*
Severe immunodeficiency, recurrent infections (see Chapters 61, 65)				
Ceroid lupofuscinosis	1/150 000		1p	*PPT*
Presents in infancy or middle childhood with rapid loss of vision and dementia; early death			16p	*CLNS*

The babies produced by OCA partners all have OCA:

$$aa \times aa \to aa$$

People with OCA who have normally pigmented partners usually produce only pigmented offspring as the albinism allele is relatively rare:

$$aa \times AA \to Aa$$

On rare occasions however, a normally pigmented partner is a heterozygote and a half of the children of such matings are recessive homozygotes:

$$aa \times Aa \to Aa, aa; 1 \text{ pigmented} : 1 \text{ albino}$$

Superficially the latter pattern resembles that due to dominant heterozygotes with normal partners (see Chapter 4) and is referred to as 'pseudodominance'.

Recessive disorders can be common in reproductively closed populations and molecular tests, if available, can be used to identify unaffected carriers. The frequency of heterozygotes can be calculated from that of homozygotes by the **Hardy–Weinberg law** (see Chapter 30).

Estimation of risk

Recessive homozygotes are produced by three kinds of mating, although the first of these is by far the most common.

1 **Two heterozygotes:**

$$Aa \times Aa \to 1\ AA : 2\ Aa : 1\ aa; \text{risk} = 1/4, 0.25, \text{ or } 25\%$$

2 **Recessive homozygote and heterozygote:**

$$aa \times Aa \to 1\ Aa : 1\ aa; \text{risk} = 1/2, 0.5, \text{ or } 50\%$$

3 **Two recessive homozygotes:**

$$aa \times aa \to aa; \text{risk} = 1, \text{ or } 100\%.$$

Example: congenital deafness

There are many (>30) non-syndromic, autosomal recessive forms of congenital deafness that mimic one another at the gross phenotypic level in that all homozygotes are deaf (see Chapter 8). Such a situation is known as 'locus heterogeneity'. The frequency of heterozygotes is about 10%.

Deaf individuals frequently choose marriage partners who are also deaf and often produce offspring with normal hearing. This can occur *if the marriage partners are homozygous for mutant recessive alleles at different loci.*

If alleles *d* and *e* both cause deafness in the homozygous state, a mating between two deaf homozygotes could be represented:

ddEE × DDee
deaf deaf
↓
DdEe

all offspring have normal hearing.

Problems

1 **A man asks what is the probability he is a carrier of cystic fibrosis (AR), as his unaffected sister has had a baby with CF. What would you tell him?**

Answer His sister is an 'obligate heterozygote' (i.e. she *must* be a heterozygote) and he has a 50% chance of also being heterozygous. You could point out that the frequency of carriers is as high as 1/25 among white people, but that screening for the most common alleles that cause cystic fibrosis is available both for him and any intended partner. The affected child could also be tested to compare their disease alleles.

2 **A young woman has received a proposal of marriage from her father's brother's son. She has a sister who suffers from oculocutaneous albinism (OCA) and is concerned that if she married him, their children would have the same health problem. What would you advise her?**

Answer The mating that produced the affected sister would be *Aa × Aa*, which can also produce normal homozygotes (*AA*) and heterozygotes (*Aa*) in the ratio 1 : 2. The normally pigmented woman therefore has a 2/3 chance of being a carrier. Her father is an obligate heterozygote and the chance his brother is also a carrier is 1/2. The risk her cousin is a carrier is therefore $1/2 \times 1/2 = 1/4$ and the risk that the proposed marriage would produce offspring with OCA is: $2/3 \times 1/4 \times 1/4 = 1/24$ for each child.

7 Consanguinity and major disabling autosomal recessive conditions

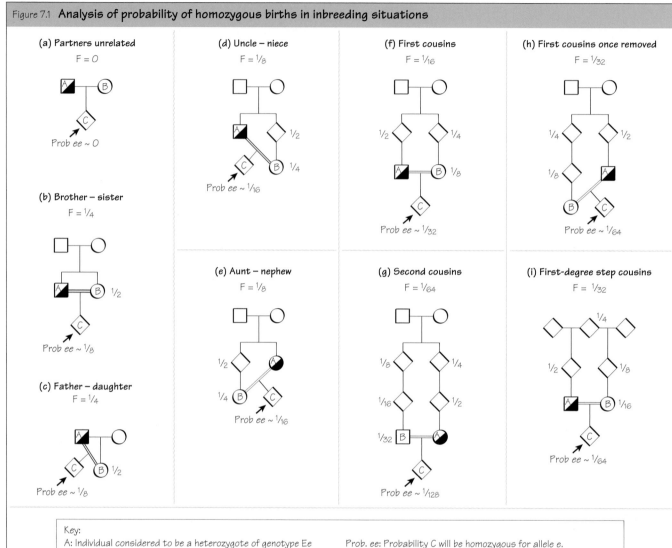

Figure 7.1 **Analysis of probability of homozygous births in inbreeding situations**

(a) Partners unrelated
F = 0
Prob ee ~ 0

(b) Brother – sister
F = 1/4
1/2
Prob ee ~ 1/8

(c) Father – daughter
F = 1/4
1/2
Prob ee ~ 1/8

(d) Uncle – niece
F = 1/8
1/2
1/4
Prob ee ~ 1/16

(e) Aunt – nephew
F = 1/8
1/2
1/4
Prob ee ~ 1/16

(f) First cousins
F = 1/16
1/2
1/4
1/8
Prob ee ~ 1/32

(g) Second cousins
F = 1/64
1/8
1/4
1/16
1/2
1/32
Prob ee ~ 1/128

(h) First cousins once removed
F = 1/32
1/4
1/2
1/8
Prob ee ~ 1/64

(i) First-degree step cousins
F = 1/32
1/4
1/2
1/8
1/16
Prob ee ~ 1/64

Key:
A: Individual considered to be a heterozygote of genotype Ee
B: Consanguineous mating partner of A
C: Offspring of consanguineous mating
F: Wright's inbreeding coefficient

Prob. ee: Probability C will be homozygous for allele e.
The annotated fractions (1/2, 1/4, etc.) indicate the probability allele e is present in the adjacent family member. This is deduced by Mendelian rules, and in each case equals 0.5F.

Overview

It has been estimated that the average person inherits several alleles for conditions lethal prenatally, plus between one and two for other harmful recessive disorders. This hidden detrimental component of the genome is called the **genetic load**. The main genetic consequence of inbreeding is to bring such recessive alleles to expression by increasing the proportion of homozygotes. Children born to incestuous (parent–offspring or brother–sister) matings include around 40% with mental defect and many with impaired hearing or vision. Offspring of marriages between first cousins are also at increased risk and are the main justification for this chapter (see Figure 6.6).

At least 1100 million people are either married to relatives as close as, or closer than, second cousins, or are the progeny of such unions. In Arab populations the most common consanguineous marriage is between first cousins who are the offspring of brothers, while in India uncle–niece liaisons constitute 10% of all marriages. In the UK double first cousins (i.e. both sets of grandparents are full siblings) are the closest relatives legally permitted to marry.

Inbred individuals typically display decreased vigour, known as **inbreeding depression**. For example, the offspring of first-cousin marriages have a slightly increased risk of multifactorial disorder, 2.5 times as many congenital malformations and 70% higher postnatal mortality than those of outbred matings.

In outbred marriages recessive diseases occur at one-quarter the square of their heterozygote frequencies (see Chapter 30) and average about 2% overall. Incidence of recessive disease is however promoted by consanguineous matings, irrespective of their rarity, so rare autosomal recessive (AR) conditions tend to occur more commonly in inbred individuals. In general, the rarer an AR disease, the higher the degree of inbreeding found in those patients. For example, in one study of **cystic fibrosis**, the most common AR disease, the frequency of cousin marriages among the parents was 1.4%. This rises to 25% for the exceedingly rare **alkaptonuria** (see Chapter 58). The combined frequency of abnormalities among offspring of first cousin marriages is almost twice the background rate faced by the average couple (Figure 6.6), but the chance that a child from such a mating will be 'normal' is still high, at 93–95% (see Chapter 71).

Management issues

To protect the welfare of babies born to incestuous matings who are to be offered for adoption it has been suggested that they be kept under observation for 6 months before the adoption is finalized, by which time many potential health problems should have become evident.

Consanguineous matings

Consanguinity, literally 'sharing of blood', means that partners share at least one ancestor, while 'relatives' are those with genes in common through descent. Strictly, all human beings are relatives, but for medical, legal and religious reasons we generally consider only members of our own, parental, grandparental, great-grandparental and descendent generations. The most remote relatives generally considered with respect to consanguinity are second cousins.

Incestuous matings are those between parent and child, or brother and sister and they involve the greatest risk. First cousins are the outbred offspring of siblings and they share two pairs of grandparents. A 'first cousin once removed' is the offspring of a first cousin. Second cousins are the offspring of two first cousins and they share two pairs of great-grandparents.

From a medical genetic viewpoint it is important to recognize the degree to which similar genetic material is shared. Three measures of this are described here, of which **Wright's inbreeding coefficient** (F) is the most widely applied. (Several other measures of consanguinity are defined and used by various authorities, but not always with consistency.)

The **coefficient of kinship, ϕ** (phi) applies to *pairs* of individuals in a family, for example mating partners A and B (see Figure 7.1), and is *the probability that an allele identified at random in A is identical by common descent to one at the same locus in B*.

Wright's inbreeding coefficient (*F*) applies to a putative homozygous individual, such as C, the offspring of A and B, and is *the probability that two alleles which C may have at a given locus are identical by descent*. F_C is numerically equal to ϕ_{AB}.

The term **coefficient of relationship** between two individuals is again subtly different, defined as: '*the proportion of genes shared by two individuals as a result of descent from a common ancestor*'. The coefficient of relationship is numerically equal to 2*F*.

All three statistics provide guidance on the probability an individual will suffer a recessive condition, as a consequence of consanguinity of his or her parents (see Figure 7.1).

Incestuous matings
Brother–sister matings

Consider how to determine the probability a child will suffer disease due to homozygosity of a rare AR allele 'e' present in one parent. The probability it has been transmitted to the first offspring, A, is 0.5. The probability it is present in the second offspring, B, is also 0.5. The coefficient of kinship, ϕ_{AB}, between the sibs (i.e. the probability it is present in *both* A and B) is the product of their independent probabilities:

$$0.5 \times 0.5 = 0.25; \text{ i.e. } \phi_{AB} = 0.25 \text{ or } 1/4$$

The inbreeding coefficient of a putative homozygous offspring produced by intercourse between brother and sister is also:

$$0.5 \times 0.5 = 0.25; \text{ i.e. } F_C = 0.25 \text{ or } 1/4$$

Parent–child matings

With a mating between father and daughter (or mother and son), we need to consider whether allele *e* present in the daughter is inherited from her father or her mother. The probability it came from the father is 0.5 and the values of both *F* and ϕ are also 0.25, or 1/4.

Risk for offspring

If every individual (e.g. A) were heterozygous for *one* harmful, but non-lethal recessive allele, *e*, the average probability of a homozygous recessive offspring (*ee*) resulting from an incestuous mating is the product of the probability *e* is present in B (=0.5) and the Mendelian probability (0.25) of producing a recessive homozygote from a mating between two heterozygotes.

i.e. risk for offspring = $0.5 \times 0.25 = 0.125$, or 1/8.

Note that the risk of a homozygous child being produced is always 0.5F (see Figure 7.1).

First cousin marriages

For matings between first cousins, the equivalent figures are:

$$F = \phi = 1/4 \times 1/4 = 1/16.$$

The probability that an allele present in one individual is shared by a first cousin by virtue of common descent is 1/8 and the chance that a homozygous baby would be produced by their mating is: $1/8 \times 1/4 = 1/32$ (3% = 0.5 *F*). This figure actually accords with the observed frequency of recessive disease among offspring of first-cousin marriages, in support of the hypothesis that on average we each carry around one harmful recessive allele in the heterozygous state. However, that analysis overlooks many prenatal losses and a mean consanguinity-associated excess of 5/1000 stillbirths. There are also 12.5/1000 extra infant deaths and 34/1000 deaths between 28 weeks and 10/12 years (Bittles, A.H. *Consanguinity in Context*, Cambridge University Press, 2012).

Mental handicap

Approximately 3% of children have significant intellectual handicap. In about 50% of cases the cause is unknown; while in around 20% there is environmental causation (see Chapter 46). In the remaining 30% the cause is genetic, and this is monogenic in half of these. Average intellectual ability is significantly lower in children from first cousin, and especially double first cousin matings, than in outbred control groups, with a decrease of about 6 IQ points per 10% in the value of the inbreeding coefficient.

AR syndromes involving mental disability include **ataxia telangiectasia** (Chapters 56 and 65), the **mucopolysaccharidoses** (Chapter 61), **phenylketonuria** (Chapters 7 and 63) and **Wilson disease** (Chapter 60).

Oculocutaneous albinism

Frequency Homozygotes: 1 / ~10 000 births.

Features They have very pale hair and skin, blue or pink irises and red pupils, and suffer from **photophobia** (avoidance of light). They also exhibit poor vision and involuntary eye movements (**nystagmus**) related to faults in the neural connections between eyes and brain.

Aetiology The biochemical defect (in OCA1) is in the enzyme **tyrosinase**, which normally converts tyrosine, through **DOPA** (dihydroxyphenylalanine), into DOPA quinone, a precursor of the dark pigment, **melanin** (see Chapter 63).

Recessive blindness

Frequency 1/10 000

Features Sightlessness can occur for many reasons, ranging from complete failure of eye formation, as in complete bilateral **anophthalmia**, degeneration of initially well-formed organs, as in **macular dystrophy**, **retinitis pigmentosa** and **optic atrophy**, to physical disruptions such as **lens dislocation** and **cataract** (lens cloudiness).

Retinitis pigmentosa (RP)

Frequency 1/4000

Features Retinitis pigmentosa is a familial degenerative condition of the retina progressing to blindness. It is the most common type of inherited retinal degenerative disorder, known also as **rod–cone dystrophy** and **pigmentary retinal degeneration**. It is genetically heterogeneous and features in several syndromes (e.g. Usher and Hunter). More than 20 causative loci are known, typically coding for proteins expressed in the retinal rods or cones. About half of these are AR.

Aetiology Vision typically deteriorates from 10–12 years of age, when diagnosis may be confirmed ophthalmoscopically, and progresses until the patient is in their fifth or sixth decade, when there is often severe visual loss. There is a relative decrease in the number of retinal photoreceptors, accompanied by clumps of pigmented tissue and degenerative changes in small blood vessels. This typically involves overall reduction in monochromatic vision, but colour vision is sometimes also affected.

Management Children may need special schooling and night vision aids. Dietary supplementation with vitamins A and E may slow progression.

Severe congenital deafness

Frequency 1/1000.

Aetiology At least half the cases of congenital deafness have a genetic basis and approximately 66% of these are AR. Over 30 different recessive loci have been identified, representing 'mimic genes' (see Chapter 6).

Connexin 26 defects (CX26)

Connexin 26 is a plasma membrane gap junction protein (see Chapter 14) responsible for K ion homeostasis in the cochlea. Mutations in the *CX26* gene probably account for up to 50% of cases of AR deafness, mutation **30delG** accounting for half of these, with a carrier frequency of 1/35.

Pendred syndrome (PDS)

Pendred syndrome accounts for up to 10% of cases of congenital deafness and in most cases also involves thyroid dysfunction. The causative gene is at 7q22-31 (see Chapter 35), coding for the transmembrane **pendrin** protein, closely related to the sulphate transporter proteins. Pathogenic lesions occur in intracellular, extracellular and transmembrane domains. Patients have **Mondini defect**, in which the cochlea has only 1.5 instead of 2.5 coils, the first two being united as an enlarged vessel especially sensitive to physical trauma. Mutations in the PDS gene also cause **enlarged vestibular aqueduct syndrome** (**EVAS**), one of the commonest forms of inner ear malformation resulting in childhood deafness.

Management Diagnosis of PDS involves the perchlorate discharge test for thyroid function, mutation detection and carrier screening.

8 Autosomal recessive inheritance, life-threatening conditions

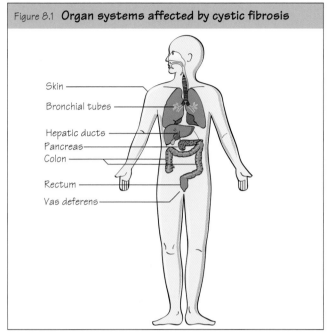

Figure 8.1 **Organ systems affected by cystic fibrosis**

Skin
Bronchial tubes
Hepatic ducts
Pancreas
Colon
Rectum
Vas deferens

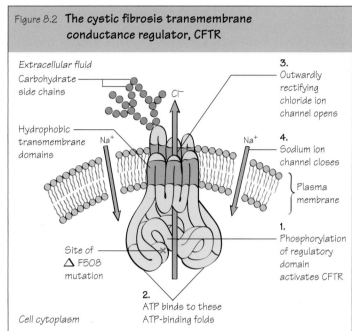

Figure 8.2 **The cystic fibrosis transmembrane conductance regulator, CFTR**

Extracellular fluid
Carbohydrate side chains
Hydrophobic transmembrane domains
Na^+
Cl^-
Na^+

3. Outwardly rectifying chloride ion channel opens
4. Sodium ion channel closes
Plasma membrane
1. Phosphorylation of regulatory domain activates CFTR

Site of Δ F508 mutation

2. ATP binds to these ATP-binding folds

Cell cytoplasm

Figure 8.3 **A phenylketonuria patient showing schneidersitz (tailor's posture) caused by muscular hypertonicity**

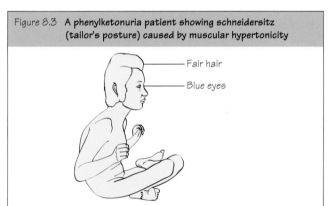

Fair hair
Blue eyes

Figure 8.4 **Transverse section of spinal cord**

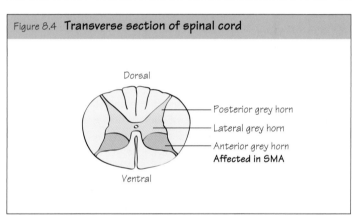

Dorsal

Posterior grey horn
Lateral grey horn
Anterior grey horn
Affected in SMA

Ventral

Figure 8.5 **Inverted duplication involved in spinal muscular atrophy**

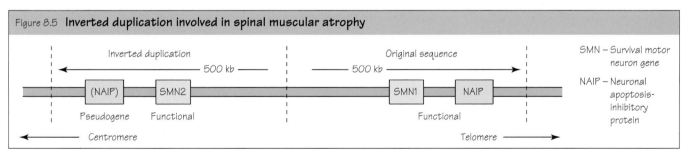

Inverted duplication
Original sequence
500 kb
500 kb
(NAIP)   SMN2
SMN1   NAIP
Pseudogene   Functional
Functional
Centromere
Telomere

SMN – Survival motor neuron gene
NAIP – Neuronal apoptosis-inhibitory protein

Medical Genetics at a Glance, Third Edition. Dorian J. Pritchard and Bruce R. Korf.
© 2013 John Wiley & Sons, Ltd. Published 2013 by John Wiley & Sons, Ltd.

Overview

We are still unable to explain the high frequencies of most common recessive diseases. High allele frequencies may arise by random 'drift', or by the 'founder effect', that is by expansion of isolated small populations. An allele could have been advantageous in the past, but now cause disease because lifestyles have changed, an example being those that promote efficient food utilization which in wealthier times predispose to diabetes mellitus (see Chapter 52). A disadvantageous allele may perhaps 'hitch-hike' along with another that is selectively advantageous, as the latter increases in frequency by natural selection. For G6PD deficiency and sickle cell disease there is good evidence for **heterozygote advantage** in resistance to malaria (see Chapter 29). In the case of cystic fibrosis the best explanation may be reproductive advantage for heterozygotes, as in highly fertile partnerships where the p.F508del allele is present, almost every baby born at high parities is a girl. This situation would preferentially promote the mutant allele and if continued over 5000 years would account for its present high frequency. This explanation is however, not generally recognized.

Cystic fibrosis (CF)

Frequency 1/~2500 Caucasians; 1/15 000 African-Americans; 1/30 000 Asian-Americans.

Genetics AR, 7q31; more than 1300 alleles, but **Phe508del** accounts for 70%.

Features Cystic fibrosis is one of the commonest serious autosomal recessive diseases in northern Europeans, in whom about one in 25 are unaffected heterozygous carriers (see Chapter 30). Among newborns 10–20% have a thick plug that blocks the colon called **meconium ileus**. Most patients have pancreatic insufficiency, leading to intestinal malabsorption, anaemia and failure to thrive, rectal prolapse and blockage of liver ducts. The sweat is very salty. Almost all males have **congenital bilateral absence of the vas deferens** (**CBAVD**). The most serious problem is chronic obstructive airway disease due to thick mucus, accompanied by bacterial infection which causes destruction of lung tissue and death in 90% of patients by 25–30 years of age. Death can also result from heat prostration.

Aetiology The basic defect is in the **cystic fibrosis transmembrane conductance regulator** (**CFTR**) protein responsible for controlled passage of chloride ions through cell membranes. CFTR forms cyclic AMP-regulated Cl^- ion channels that span the plasma membranes of specialized epithelial cells. Normally, activation of the CFTR by phosphorylation of the regulatory domain, followed by binding of ATP, opens the outwardly rectifying Cl^- ion channel and closes adjacent Na^+ channels. Defective ion transport creates salt imbalance and water depletion.

CFTR structural gene modifications include missense, frameshift, splice site, nonsense and deletion mutations (see Chapter 25). They either block or reduce CFTR synthesis, or prevent it reaching the epithelial membrane (e.g. Phe508del), or cause its malfunction.

Patients with CFTR activity of below 3% of normal have severe 'classic' CF with pancreatic insufficiency (PI); those with 3–8% have respiratory disease but pancreatic sufficiency (PS); at 8–12% male patients have CBAVD only.

Management The mainstay of treatment for lung problems is thrice-daily percussive physiotherapy and antibiotics. Inhalers and nebulizers are helpful and heart–lung transplants have been successful in very severe cases. Nutritional therapy includes pancreatic enzymes and special diets. Exercise, including swimming, is beneficial. Gene replacement therapy is still at the experimental stage and small molecule treatment to restore protein production is also being pursued.

Prenatal diagnosis is based on microvillar enzymes in amniotic fluid, or DNA analysis of amniotic fluid cells. Neonatal diagnosis includes measurement of NaCl in sweat and of immunoreactive trypsinogen (IRT) in the blood, a consequence of pancreatic duct blockage *in utero* (see Chapter 73). Population screening at birth is routine in some populations and for carriers in CF-affected families (known as 'cascade screening').

▶ Problems requiring immediate attention

Breathing tube obstruction and lung infection; sodium balance, meconium ileus.

Tay–Sachs disease, GM2 gangliosidosis

Frequency 1/3600 in Ashkenazi Jews (carrier frequency 1/30), but now reduced to 5/360 000 by genetic intervention; 1/360 000 in American non-Jews (carrier frequency 1/300).

Genetics AR; 15q

Features Tay–Sachs disease is of two overlapping main types, 'infantile' and 'late infantile' (Sandhoff disease). In the infantile form affected infants usually present with poor feeding, lethargy and hypotonia and in 90% of patients there is a cherry-red spot in the macula of the retina. In the second half of the first year there may be developmental regression, feeding becomes increasingly difficult, with progressive loss of skills. Deafness develops, or hypersensitivity to sound. Visual impairment leads to complete blindness by 1 year. In the second year head size can increase, there may be outbursts of inappropriate laughter and seizures. Hypotonia leads to spasticity, then paralysis. Death due to respiratory infection usually occurs by the age of 3 years, or in the late infantile form at 5–10 years.

Aetiology The most common mutation for Tay–Sachs disease is a four-base insertion in the gene for the α-subunit of **hexosaminidase A**. Hexosaminidase A is responsible for converting the glycosylated membrane phospholipid, or **ganglioside**, GM2 to GM3; the deficiency causing build-up of GM2 in the lysosomes (see Chapter 62). It has α and β subunits while its isozyme **hexosaminidase B** has two β subunits. In Sandhoff disease there is a defect in the β subunit and both hexosaminidases A and B are affected.

Management Management is supportive. Prenatal or preimplantation DNA-based diagnosis is possible if both parents are known to be carriers (see Chapter 62). Diagnosis in newborns is routine, on the basis of hexosaminidase A deficiency and heterozygotes are identified by intermediate levels (see Chapter 73).

▶ Problems requiring immediate attention

Confirmatory diagnosis and feeding.

Phenylketonuria (PKU)

Frequency 1/10000–1/15000 Caucasians; carriers 1/50–1/60.

Genetics AR; 12q24; >450 alleles.

Features Typically PKU homozygotes are fair-haired with blue eyes. Children have convulsions and become severely intellectually impaired, phenylalanine (PA) accumulates in the blood and related metabolites are excreted in the urine.

Aetiology The basic cause is deficiency in **phenylalanine hydroxylase (PAH)** necessary for conversion of PA into tyrosine (see Chapters 58 and 63 for details and diagnostic tests). In the early days there is severe vomiting and occasionally convulsions. There is learning disability and the baby's skin can become dry and eczematous. Untreated patients have a 'mousy' smell due to phenylacetic acid in the sweat and urine, and muscular hypertonicity. Life expectancy is reduced.

Management Physiological independence of a baby from its mother is acquired at birth and only thereafter does the homozygous infant risk trauma from PA build-up, untreated babies losing 1–2 IQ points per week. PA is essential for growth, but a PA-low diet must be introduced well before 1 month and continued for at least 10 years. Special care must be taken during pregnancy in affected females to prevent mental damage, microcephaly and congenital heart defects in offspring.

► Problems requiring immediate attention

Diet and convulsions.

Spinal muscular atrophy (SMA)

Frequency 1/10000; carrier frequency 1/50.

Genetics AR, 5q13

Features SMA includes a biochemically and genetically heterogeneous group of disorders that are among the commonest genetic causes of death in childhood.

- **Type 1 SMA (Werdnig–Hoffmann disease).** This is the most severe and most common form. Children present within the first 6 months with severe hypotonia and lack of spontaneous movement. They may have poor swallowing and respiratory function leading to death before the age of 3 years.
- **Type 2 SMA.** Muscle weakness and hypotonia are again the main features, but are less severe and onset is at 6–18 months. Children can sit unaided, but cannot achieve independent locomotion. Most survive into early adulthood.
- **Type 3 SMA (Kugelberg–Welander disease).** This form is relatively mild, with age of onset after 18 months and all patients able to walk without support. Muscle weakness is slowly progressive. There can be recurrent respiratory infection and scoliosis.

Aetiology Disability is due to degeneration of the anterior horn cells of the spinal cord, which leads to progressive muscle weakness and ultimately death.

Two relevant genes on Chromosome 5q are involved in a 500-kb inverted duplication. These are *SMN*, the **survival motor neuron gene**, and *NAIP*, which codes for **neuronal apoptosis inhibitor protein**. The duplicated section carries an alternative version of *SMN* (*SMN2*) and a non-functional pseudogene of *NAIP*. In 95% of patients there is homozygous deletion of exons 7 and 8 of the telomeric copy of *SMN* (*SMN1*).

Management DNA diagnosis, including carrier detection and prenatal diagnosis, is available. Type 3 patients need wheelchairs in early adult life. There is no effective treatment, but up-regulation of *SMN2* is an attractive future possibility (see Chapter 74).

► Problems requiring immediate attention

Respiration and feeding.

9 Aspects of dominance

Figure 9.1 Dominance and codominance in the ABO blood groups

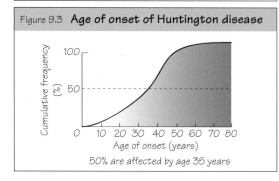

Genotypes	Description	Antigens on red cells	Blood groups
$I^A I^A$	Homozygosity	A	A
$I^A I^O$	Dominance	A	
$I^B I^B$	Homozygosity	B	B
$I^B I^O$	Dominance	B	
$I^O I^O$	Homozygosity	None	O
$I^A I^B$	Codominance	A+B	AB

Figure 9.2 A simplified pedigree for ectrodactyly, showing incomplete penetrance

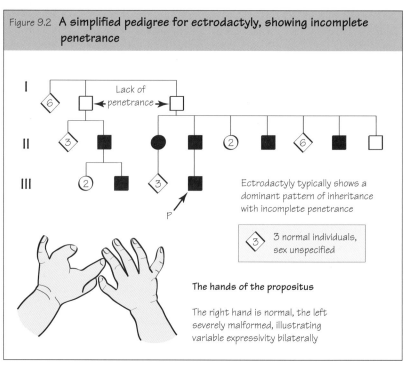

Ectrodactyly typically shows a dominant pattern of inheritance with incomplete penetrance

◇3 = 3 normal individuals, sex unspecified

The hands of the propositus

The right hand is normal, the left severely malformed, illustrating variable expressivity bilaterally

Figure 9.3 Age of onset of Huntington disease

50% are affected by age 35 years

Overview

By definition, dominant alleles reveal their presence in the heterozygous as well as the homozygous state. However, this is not always the case. Some alleles that most of the criteria of dominance are expressed only in specific circumstances, as indicated by some pharmacogenetic traits (Chapter 4) and in some cases heterozygotes do not show an equal degree of expression as the dominant homozygote. This chapter deals with such situations, including codominance and overdominance, incomplete penetrance and variable expression.

Different mutations of the same gene can show different patterns of inheritance. A mutation would be considered recessive if it only slightly reduces enzyme activity in single dose, but causes significant deficiency in double dose, while a more serious mutation of the same gene that causes disease in the heterozygous state would be classed as dominant. A useful rule is: *a dominant disease allele can produce disease in a heterozygote, whereas a recessive allele cannot*. Like achondroplasia, most 'dominant' diseases are probably more severe in the affected homozygote than in the heterozygote.

Mutations that cause abnormal gain of function at the protein level are frequently expressed as dominant (e.g. HD; see Chapter 28), while mutations that cause loss of function typically result in recessive disease (e.g. FH; see Chapter 5). 'Dominant negative' conditions often involve protein multimers in which, in heterozygotes, an abnormal polypeptide interferes with the functioning of its normal homologue (e.g. MFS; see Chapter 5).

Codominance (Co-D), the ABO blood groups

If neither of two alternative alleles is dominant over the other and both are expressed in heterozygotes, the situation is called **codominance**.

In the ABO blood group system groups A, B, AB and O are distinguished by whether the red blood cells are agglutinated by anti-A or anti-B antibody (see Chapter 29). Group O cells have a precursor glycosphingolipid embedded in their surfaces which is elaborated differentially in A, B and AB by the products of alleles I^A and I^B.

The erythrocytes of both I^B homozygotes and I^B/I^O heterozygotes are agglutinated by anti-B antibody, so both are considered Group B. Similarly Group A includes both I^A homozygotes and I^A/I^O heterozygotes. *Alleles I^A and I^B are both dominant to I^O.*

The red cells of I^O homozygotes are not agglutinated by antibodies directed against A or B. They are placed in Group O.

The red cells of Group AB individuals carry both A and B antigens. They are agglutinated by *both* anti-A and anti-B, and are therefore of Group AB. *Because both are expressed together, alleles I^A and I^B are codominant*.

The alleles of several other blood groups, the tissue antigens of the HLA system, the electrophoretic variants of many proteins and the DNA markers (see Section 13) can also be considered codominant, as their properties are assessed directly, irrespective of their derivative properties.

Incomplete dominance, overdominance and heterosis

Alpha- and β-globin, together with haem and iron, make up the **haemoglobin** of our red blood cells. The normal allele for β-globin is called HbA and the **sickle cell allele**, HbS, differs from it by one base (see Chapter 25). In HbS homozygotes the abnormal haemoglobin aggregates, causing the red cells to collapse into the shape of a sickle and to clog small blood vessels. **Sickle cell disease** is characterized

Medical Genetics at a Glance, Third Edition. Dorian J. Pritchard and Bruce R. Korf.

by anaemia, intense pain and vulnerability to infection due to loss of spleen function.

Heterozygotes have both normal (A) and abnormal (S) haemoglobin molecules in their erythrocytes, which stay undistorted most of the time, allowing them to live a normal life. At this level HbA is dominant to HbS. However, under conditions of severe oxygen stress, a proportion of cells undergoes sickling and this causes transient symptoms similar to those of homozygotes. On this basis the HbS allele can be classified as **incompletely dominant**, or because both alleles are expressed with a more varied combined outcome, as **overdominance**. HbS/HbA heterozygotes are said to possess '**sickle cell trait**'.

In early animal breeding experiments it was soon noticed that inbreeding led to deterioration in important qualities, notably in fertility and body size (see Chapter 7). By contrast, when two inbred lines were crossed the first generation (F1) hybrids were typically larger, more fertile, with improved resistance to disease. This is known as **hybrid vigour**, or **heterosis**, for which two kinds of explanation have been advanced.

Sickle cell trait provides the classic human example of heterosis based on overdominance at a single locus. The two parents transmit coding information for a single significant protein, but with somewhat different properties, both alleles are expressed and the heterozygous offspring exhibits superior functional versatility and fitness.

A second explanation of general heterosis, such as with regard to general health and vigour, is that many loci are involved, but that no population has evolved the most favourable alleles at all loci. In offspring produced by crosses between members of populations that evolved independently, heterozygosity must exist at many loci. If a significant proportion of favourable alleles is dominant over the less favourable, an improved genotype has been created.

On theoretical grounds we might expect crossing between the human races to create healthier phenotypes through heterosis. There are no known ill effects of interracial crossing with regard to perinatal or infant death, or congenital malformations. By contrast there are historical accounts of the survival of the offspring of European men and native women of Tierra del Fuego, when all pure bred Fuegan people succumbed to a measles epidemic. Heterosis possibly also contributes to the observed general increase in human stature in recent generations, but good evidence for general heterosis in humans is difficult to find.

Incomplete penetrance
Some apparently dominant alleles sometimes 'skip a generation'. **Ectrodactyly**, in which formation of the middle elements of hands and feet is variably disrupted, is caused by such a **dominant allele of reduced penetrance** (see Chapter 42).

'**Degree of penetrance**' relates to the percentage of carriers of a specific 'dominant' allele that show the relevant phenotype. For example, about 75% of women with certain mutations in the *BRCA1* gene develop breast or ovarian cancer (see Chapter 56). The joint penetrance of those mutations is 75%.

Delayed onset
Huntington disease can remain unexpressed for 30–50 years and is an example of **age-related penetrance** or a **disease of late onset**. Patients eventually undergo progressive degeneration of the nervous system, with uncontrolled movements and mental deterioration (see Chapter 28). Other examples are **haemochromatosis** (a disorder of iron absorption), **familial Alzheimer disease** (see Chapter 52) and many inherited cancers (see Chapter 56).

Variable expressivity
Sometimes a disease allele is expressed in every individual who carries it (i.e. it is dominant and fully penetrant), although its severity and expression vary considerably. This is called **variable expressivity**. The causes of variable expressivity are largely unknown, but include '**modifier genes**'. For example, a gene on Chromosome 19 seems to influence whether or not a patient with CF will develop meconium ileus (see Chapter 7). A well-studied example is neurofibromatosis type 1.

Neurofibromatosis type 1 (NF1), Von Recklinghausen disease
Frequency 1/3000–1/4000

Genetics AD; penetrance virtually 100% by the age of 5 years, variable expressivity; 50% are new mutations.

Features NF1 is highly variable in expression. In mild form it generally includes **café-au-lait spots** (pale brown spots) and axillary or inguinal freckling, benign '**Lisch nodules**' on the iris and a few non-malignant peripheral nerve tumours called **neurofibromas**. When severely expressed there may be millions of neurofibromas, **optic gliomas** (tumours of the optic nerve), disfigurement, learning disabilities, hypertension, scoliosis and malignant tumours of peripheral nerve sheath.

Identical twins with NF1 have similar symptoms, suggesting influence of co-inherited modifier genes (see Chapter 53).

► **Problems requiring immediate attention**
Sometimes high blood pressure, malignant tumours.

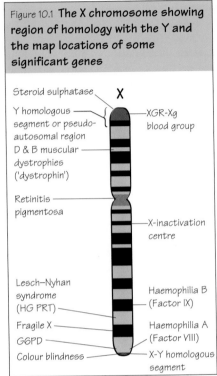

Figure 10.1 **The X chromosome showing region of homology with the Y and the map locations of some significant genes**

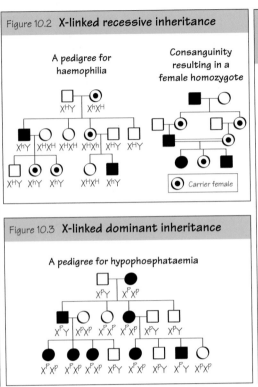

Figure 10.2 **X-linked recessive inheritance**

Figure 10.3 **X-linked dominant inheritance**

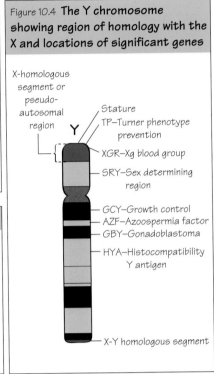

Figure 10.4 **The Y chromosome showing region of homology with the X and locations of significant genes**

Overview

With the exception of the X and the Y, all our chromosomes are normally present in two copies in each body cell nucleus. Two X chromosomes are present in female body cells, but by contrast those of males each have only one and in place of the second X is a much smaller chromosome called the Y. A small number of genes are represented on both the X and the Y, in what is called the **pseudoautosomal region**, but most X-linked genes have no counterpart on the Y. The **amelogenin** gene just outside the pseudoautosomal boundary, codes for a dental enamel ECM (extracellular matrix) protein that, being polymorphic between X and Y chromosomes, is used for forensic sexing of DNA samples (see Chapter 70).

At gross phenotypic levels females may exhibit dominant and/or recessive properties of their X-linked genes, as with autosomal genes. At the cellular level, however, some genes on the X are expressed either from one chromosome or its partner, but not from both X chromosomes in the same cell. This is because gene expression in much of one or the other X chromosome is inactivated in every female body cell line.

Most so-called '**sex-linked disorders**' are caused by X-linked recessive alleles in males. For example, because **haemophilia** is recessive, heterozygous females are normal, but males, being **hemizygous** for X-linked genes, are affected. *X-chromosome inactivation, however, can create mosaic patterns of expression in female heterozygotes, some of whom are seriously affected when the proportion inactivated is skewed* (see Chapter 43). Female homozygotes for X-linked recessive alleles generally occur at a frequency equal to the square of that of affected males (see Chapter 30).

A man (XY) receives his X chromosome from his mother (XX) and passes that X to every daughter. Both mother and daughter are there-fore **obligate carriers** of any X-linked recessive expressed by the man (unless he represents a new mutation for the gene, in which case his mother would not be a carrier).

Rules of X-linked recessive inheritance

1 *The incidence of disease is very much higher in males than in females.*
2 *The mutant allele is passed from an affected man to all of his daughters, but they do not express it.*
3 *A heterozygous 'carrier' woman passes the allele to half of her sons, who express it, and half her daughters who do not.*
4 *The mutant allele is NEVER passed from father to son.*

Examples See Chapter 11.

Estimation of risk for offspring

1 *Affected man and normal woman*

Affected man:
XY

| | XX | XY |

Normal woman: XX

| | XX | XY |

All daughters are carriers, all sons are normal.

2 *Carrier woman and normal man*

Normal man:
XY

| | XX | XY |

Carrier woman: **XX**

| | **XX** | **XY** |

Half the daughters are carriers, half the sons are affected.

Medical Genetics at a Glance, Third Edition. Dorian J. Pritchard and Bruce R. Korf.

3 *Affected man and carrier woman*

Affected man:

XY

XX   XY

Carrier woman: **XX**

XX   XY

Half the daughters are affected, half are carriers; half the sons are affected.

4 *Normal man and homozygous affected woman*

Normal man:

XY

XX   XY

Affected woman: **XX**

XX   XY

All the daughters are carriers, all the sons are affected.

X-linked dominant disorders
Rules for inheritance
1 *The condition is expressed and transmitted by BOTH sexes.*
2 *The condition occurs twice as frequently in females as in males.*
3 *An affected man passes the condition to every daughter, but never to a son.*
4 *An affected woman passes the condition to half her sons and half her daughters.*
5 *Females are usually less seriously affected than males.*

Examples See Chapter 11.

Y-linked or holandric inheritance
DNA sequencing indicates at least 20 genes on the Y chromosome, including *SRY*, which initiates male differentiation through the 'testis determining factor' (*TDF*), and the normal allele for **azoospermia** (*AZT*), which ensures production of sperm (see Chapters 43 and 44). There are genes for the male-specific tissue transplantation antigen **HYA** and for **GCY**, concerned with male stature.

Rules for inheritance
Y-linked genes are expressed in and transmitted only by males, to all their sons.

Example **Hypertrichosis** (hairiness) of ear rims.

Pseudoautosomal inheritance or 'partial sex linkage'
Crossing-over between the X and Y occurs in the pseudoautosomal region during male meiosis. Here are several 'housekeeping genes' (see Chapters 21 and 22), one that ensures non-development of **Turner syndrome** in males (see Chapter 37), others for stature and the **Xg blood group**.

Rules for inheritance
Genes in the X/Y homologous segment are transmitted by an individual woman equally to offspring of both sexes, but by an individual man predominantly to offspring of the same sex.

Example **Steroid sulphatase deficient X-linked ichthyosis**, scaly skin.

Sex limitation and sex influence
Some genes are carried on the autosomes, but are limited or influenced by sex. Sex limited traits occur in only one sex due, for instance, to anatomical differences. Penetrance and expressivity of mutant alleles may differ for recognized physiological reasons; for example, **pattern baldness** acts as AD in entire, but not castrated, males, but weakly as AR in females. Gout is largely confined to males and postmenopausal women. **Breast cancer**, **autoimmune disease** and **depressive illness** are most common in women, **haemochromatosis** (a disorder of iron accumulation) in men, women probably being protected by menstrual bleeding.

Congenital dislocation of the hip and **cleft palate** are most commonly found in girls and **pyloric stenosis**, **talipes** (clubfoot), **cleft lip and palate** and **Hirschsprung disease**, involving intestinal obstruction due to failure of innervation of the large bowel, are most commonly found in boys (see Chapter 45).

Table 10.1 X-linked recessive diseases.

	Frequency per 10 000 Caucasian male births
G6PD deficiency (geographically very variable)	0–6500
Red and green colour blindness (rhodopsin)	~800
Non-specific X-linked mental retardation	5
Duchenne muscular dystrophy (dystrophin)	3.5
Fragile X syndrome	2.5
Haemophilia A (Factor VIII)	2
Becker muscular dystrophy (dystrophin)	0.5
Haemophilia B (Factor IX)	0.3
Agammaglobulinaemia (X-linked)	0.1
Ocular albinism	<0.1
Hunter syndrome (mucopolysaccharidosis II)	<0.1
Retinitis pigmentosa	<0.1
Fabry disease (angiokeratoma)	<0.1
Anhidrotic ectodermal dysplasia	<0.1
Menkes syndrome	<0.1
Adrenoleukodystrophy	<0.1
Lesch–Nyhan syndrome (HGPRT deficiency)	<0.1
Ornithine transcarbamylase deficiency	<0.1
Chronic granulomatous disease	<0.1

Table 10.2 X-linked dominant diseases.

Hypophosphataemia (vitamin D resistant rickets)
Hereditary motor and sensory neuropathy
Incontinentia pigmenti (lethal in males)
Rett syndrome (can be lethal in males)
Oro-facio-digital syndrome

Table 10.3 Sex-influenced conditions.

Female
  Breast cancer
  Congenital dislocation of the hip
  Autoimmune disease
Male
  Pyloric stenosis
  Baldness
  Gout
  Haemochromatosis

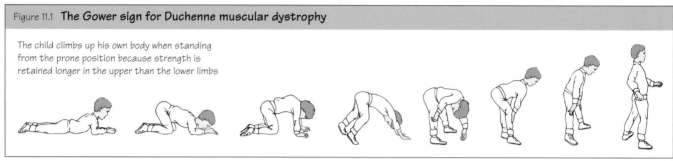

Figure 11.1 **The Gower sign for Duchenne muscular dystrophy**

The child climbs up his own body when standing from the prone position because strength is retained longer in the upper than the lower limbs

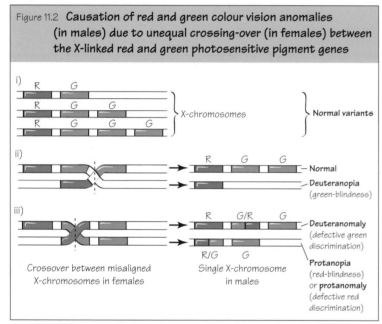

Figure 11.2 **Causation of red and green colour vision anomalies (in males) due to unequal crossing-over (in females) between the X-linked red and green photosensitive pigment genes**

i) Normal variants

ii) Normal / Deuteranopia (green-blindness)

iii) Deuteranomaly (defective green discrimination) / Protanopia (red-blindness) or protanomaly (defective red discrimination)

Crossover between misaligned X-chromosomes in females
Single X-chromosome in males

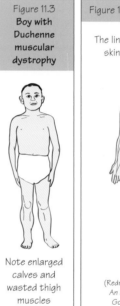

Figure 11.3 Boy with Duchenne muscular dystrophy

Note enlarged calves and wasted thigh muscles

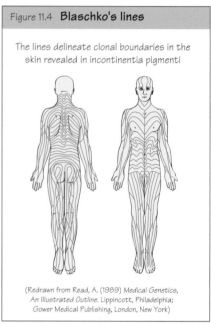

Figure 11.4 **Blaschko's lines**

The lines delineate clonal boundaries in the skin revealed in incontinentia pigmenti

(Redrawn from Read, A. (1989) *Medical Genetics, An Illustrated Outline*. Lippincott, Philadelphia; Gower Medical Publishing, London, New York)

Introduction

Most X-linked deficiencies and diseases are expressed solely or mainly in males, although due to the phenomenon of X chromosome inactivation they can also be expressed in a patchy fashion in females (see Chapter 38). The most important X-linked recessive and dominant disorders are listed in Tables 10.1 and 10.2.

Haemophilia A (HbA), classic haemophilia

Frequency 1/5000 males
Genetics XR; Xq28 (see also Chapter 25)
Gene product Blood clotting Factor VIII
Features Visible bruising, severe bleeding from large wounds. Haemorrhage into the joints (**haemarthrosis**) causes painful inflammation and diminished joint function.

Fifty per cent of patients have several bleeding episodes per month and Factor VIII levels below 1% of normal. Those with levels at 5–25% have coagulation problems only after surgery or severe trauma.
Aetiology Mutations in Factor VIII that disrupt conversion of prothrombin into thrombin include inversions, major deletions and nonsense mutations.
Management Prenatal diagnosis is by DNA testing (see Chapter 67); excessive bleeding from the umbilical cord perinatally.

Without treatment haemophilia is often fatal by the age of 20 years. Factor VIII for prophylactic use can be isolated from plasma, heat treated and screened to eliminate infection, or produced by recombinant DNA technology. It has a half-life of only 8 hours, so repeated infusions may be necessary. Ten to fifteen per cent of patients develop immunity to administered Factor VIII and require immunosuppression.

▶ Problems requiring immediate attention

Bleeding from the umbilicus, severe bleeding episodes.

Red and green colour blindness

Frequency in males Caucasians 8% (1/12); Asians 4.5%; Africans 2.5%.
Frequency in females The square of that in males, for example 0.64% in Caucasians.
Features A quarter of colour-vision-defective males are **dichromatic**, unable to perceive either red (**protanopia**) or green (**deuteranopia**) light. Most of the remainder perceive reds and greens abnormally and are termed **protanomalous** and **deuteranomalous**. (Absence of both red- and green-sensitive cones is rare and causes **blue cone monochromacy**.)
Aetiology On each X chromosome is a gene for red-sensitive **opsin** immediately adjacent to one or several green opsin genes. Their sequences are very similar, promoting a tendency for crossover errors

(see Chapters 38). Protanomaly and deuteranomaly arise when crossover creates 'hybrid' genes.

Duchenne muscular dystrophy (DMD)
Frequency in males 1/3500
Genetics XR; Xp21
Features Before 5 years of age, boys show clumsiness, muscle weakness and pseudo-hypertrophy of the calves caused by replacement of degenerate muscle with fat and connective tissue. Patients are confined to wheelchairs by the age of 11 years. Subsequent deterioration leads to lumbar lordosis, joint contractures and cardiorespiratory failure, death ensuing at a mean age of 18 years. Creatine kinase (CK) leaks into the bloodstream and can increase to over 20 times the normal levels. A third of boys have mild-to-moderate intellectual impairment. Female heterozygotes can be mildly affected.

Becker muscular dystrophy (BMD)
Frequency in males 1/18 000
Features Onset around 11 years and slower progression than DMD.
Aetiology The *DMD/BMD* gene codes for the protein **dystrophin**, with 79 exons, by far the largest gene known in humans. Dystrophin is localized on the cytoplasmic side of the muscle fibre membrane and links the internal cytoskeleton to extracellular material via glycoproteins that span the plasma membrane. Most DMD patients have serious mutations and lack dystrophin, whereas BMD patients have the protein in reduced quantity or abbreviated form.
Management Assay of dystrophin enables distinction between DMD, BMD and other limb girdle muscular dystrophies. Deletions are usually detected by multiplex polymerase chain reaction (PCR; see Chapter 69), other mutations by sequencing. Carrier females may be identified by mutation testing or by linkage to intragenic markers (allowing for an intragenic recombination rate of 12%). Diagnosis is assisted by electromyography and muscle biopsy. Physiotherapy and treatment with steroids are beneficial.

Fragile X syndrome (FRAX-A [and FRAX-E])
Frequency 1/4000 males; 1/8000 females (FRAX-E: ~1/16 000 and ~1/32 000)
Genetics The *FMR-1* gene contains a CGG triplet repeat at Xq27.3 which expands only in females, although is occasionally transmitted as a 'premutation' by **normal transmitting males** (see Chapter 28).
Features FRAX-A accounts for 40% of all males with learning difficulties. They have a high forehead and prominent lower jaw, large ears, excess joint mobility and after puberty, **macroorchidism**. There can also be mitral valve prolapse, autistic features and/or hyperactive behaviour. Speech may be halting and repetitive. Normal transmitting males sometimes suffer tremor and ataxia.
Aetiology The FRAX-A full mutation leads to methylation of the promoter and lack of expression of the gene product.
Management Diagnosis involves measurement of the length of the repeat series and its degree of methylation, by enzyme digestion, PCR and Southern blotting (see Chapters 67 and 68).

Vitamin D-resistant rickets, hypophosphataemic rickets
Genetics XD
Features Hereditary rickets when there is adequate dietary intake of vitamin D. The kidneys have impaired ability to reabsorb phosphate, resulting in abnormal ossification.

> ► **Problems requiring immediate attention**
>
> Correction of serum phosphate level.

Hereditary motor and sensory neuropathy (HMSN), Charcot–Marie–Tooth disease
Frequency of all forms 1/2500
Genetics XD, AD (the most common) and AR; classified as forms I, II, III, etc., by nerve conduction velocity.
Gene product of X-linked form Gap junction protein connexin 32 (see Chapter 14).
Features Heterogeneous, with slowly progressive distal wasting of the legs (between the ages of 10 and 30 years in HMSN I) and often later of the arms, often with ataxia and tremor. The feet develop an exaggerated arch (**pes cavus**). There is often demyelination and thickening of peripheral nerves and progressive hearing loss.
Management Monitoring of hearing and provision of hearing aids. Can be diagnosed pre-implantationally by PCR (see Chapter 69).

Incontinentia pigmenti (IP)
Frequency Rare, perhaps 1/40 000
Genetics XD, Xq28
Features Diagnosis in infants is based on reddening of a skin rash to blisters, and eventually to pigmented lesions. These follow **Blaschko's lines** (see Figure 11.4), fading during adolescence. There are conical or missing teeth, ocular and neurological abnormalities.
Aetiology The abbreviated product fails to block apoptosis by tumour necrosis factor. Since IP is lethal in male embryos, offspring in ratio 33% affected females : 33% unaffected females : 33% unaffected males.

> ► **Problems requiring immediate attention**
>
> Management of seizures in infancy.

Barth syndrome, X-linked cardioskeletal myopathy, endocardial fibroelastosis
Features Congenital generalized myopathy, cardiomyopathy and growth retardation. Tissues are deficient in cardiolipin and skeletal muscle shows a raised lipid content.
Aetiology There are mutations in the X-linked *TAZ* gene that codes for a protein in the cytochrome-C system.
Management Diagnosis requires measurement of 3-methyl glutaconic acid in urine.

Rett syndrome
Genetics XD
Frequency 1/10 000–1/15 000 females; embryonic lethality in males.
Features Autistic behaviour, deterioration in cognition, epileptic seizures breathing irregularities, gait ataxia and stereotyped hand movements, reduced life expectancy.
Aetiology Usually mutation in *MECP2*, the protein product of which fails to regulate transcription of genes concerned with brain development.
Management Monitoring of special educational needs.

> ► **Problems requiring immediate attention**
>
> Breathing irregularity, seizures.

Figure 12.1 Mitochondrial inheritance

Theoretical pedigree for a family with MERRF, showing maternal inheritance and variable expression due to heteroplasmy

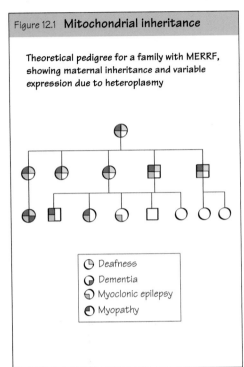

- ◔ Deafness
- ◑ Dementia
- ◕ Myoclonic epilepsy
- ● Myopathy

Figure 12.2 Mitochondrial disease gene map

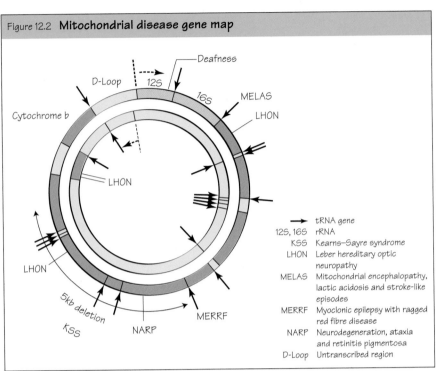

→	tRNA gene
12S, 16S	rRNA
KSS	Kearns–Sayre syndrome
LHON	Leber hereditary optic neuropathy
MELAS	Mitochondrial encephalopathy, lactic acidosis and stroke-like episodes
MERRF	Myoclonic epilepsy with ragged red fibre disease
NARP	Neurodegeneration, ataxia and retinitis pigmentosa
D-Loop	Untranscribed region

Figure 12.3 Production of mitochondrial RNA

(the bold arrows indicate the structural genes for species of mitochondrion-specific tRNAs)

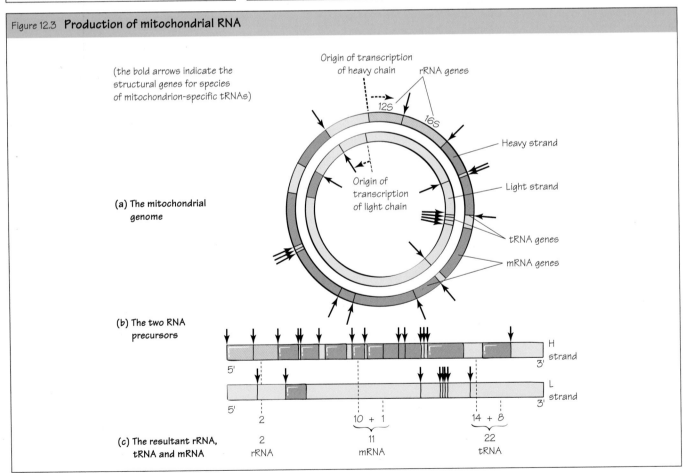

(a) The mitochondrial genome

(b) The two RNA precursors

(c) The resultant rRNA, tRNA and mRNA

Medical Genetics at a Glance, Third Edition. Dorian J. Pritchard and Bruce R. Korf.

40 © 2013 John Wiley & Sons, Ltd. Published 2013 by John Wiley & Sons, Ltd.

Overview

Mitochondria originated as aerobic bacteria that became symbiotic with anaerobic, nucleated, single-cell organisms, their partnership jointly creating the common ancestor of all 'higher' organisms. They have retained much of their ancestral independence, such as the timing of their reproduction, their own DNA (mtDNA; see Chapter 14) and many of the genes necessary for its replication. They play a major role in the generation of energy, as distinct from those encoded in the nuclear DNA.

mtDNA occurs in several copies per mitochondrion, each encoding two species of ribosomal RNA (rRNA), 22 transfer RNAs (tRNAs; see Chapter 23) and 13 polypeptides involved in oxidative phosphorylation. Another 90+ mitochondrial polypeptides are encoded in the nucleus and follow Mendelian rules of inheritance.

Altogether more than 50 mutations and over 100 mitochondrial deletions and duplications of mtDNA are known. Further accumulation of mutations throughout life probably contributes to the ageing process.

Apart from the red blood cells and lens fibres, almost every cell in the body contains thousands of mitochondria and since they play a critical role in ATP production, they are especially numerous in tissues with high energy requirement, such as muscle and brain. The mitochondria do not have DNA repair enzymes, so mtDNA has a high rate of spontaneous mutation. In most individuals the DNA is the same in all mitochondria (**homoplasmy**), but mutation can create more than one mitochondrial type in any individual, called **heteroplasmy**, when representation of the different mitochondrial populations varies between tissues and descendent individuals.

Mitochondrial disorders

The term 'mitochondrial disorder' largely applies to syndromes associated with abnormalities of the respiratory chain enzymes involved in oxidative phosphorylation. These exist as five large protein complexes on the inner surfaces of mitochondrial membranes, composed of both mitochondrial and nuclear gene products.

Mitochondrial defects typically show a combination of neurological and myopathic features. Duplications and deletions give rise to **Kearns–Sayre syndrome** (**KSS**; muscle weakness, cerebellar damage and heart failure) and **Pearson syndrome** (infantile pancreatic insufficiency, pancytopaenia (reduced blood cell count), lactic acidosis and chronic progressive external ophthalmoplegia (paralysis of eye muscles).

Sperm are each powered by a battery of mitochondria which are however considered to make no contribution to the mitochondrial population of the zygote. An embryo's mitochondria are therefore acquired solely from the cytoplasm of the ovum and mitochondrial inheritance follows a strictly maternal pattern.

Rules of mitochondrial inheritance

1 *Typically the condition is passed from a mother to ALL her children.*

2 *The condition is NEVER transmitted by men.*

Examples

Myoclonic epilepsy with ragged red fibre disease (MERRF)

Features Progressive myoclonic epilepsy, widespread degeneration in the brain with slowly progressive dementia and optic atrophy.

Aetiology There is a point mutation in the mitochondrial gene for tRNA lysine.

Mitochondrial encephalopathy, lactic acidosis and stroke-like episodes (MELAS)

Features Short stature, stroke-like episodes with vomiting, headache or visual disturbance, sometimes hemiplegia and hemianopia. Type 2 diabetes often coincides with deafness.

Aetiology Eighty per cent of patients have one of two substitutions in a mitochondrial leucine tRNA.

Neurodegeneration, ataxia and retinitis pigmentosa (NARP)

Features Night blindness, developmental delay, seizures and dementia.

Aetiology The mutation is a substitution in the ATPase gene.

Leigh disease

Genetics There are both mitochondrial and AR forms.

Features Typical spongiform brain lesions, respiratory **dyskinesia** (impairment of voluntary movement), slow recovery from anaesthesia, sometimes death in infancy. Some patients have cytochrome-C deficiency.

Leber hereditary optic neuropathy (LHON)

Genetics There are about a dozen known mutations in the mitochondrial *ND4* gene.

Features Sudden loss of central vision at age 12–30 years, especially in males.

Maternally transmitted ototoxic deafness

Ototoxicity refers to chemical damage to the inner ear, affecting hearing or balance. A form of maternally transmitted deafness is induced in susceptible families by exposure to widely used aminoglycoside antibiotics, including streptomycin, kanamycin, gentamicin and neomycin. Aminoglycoside antibiotics interfere with bacterial mRNA translation (see Chapter 24) by binding to the 50s rRNA A-site, causing misreading of the genetic code. In some human families there is a modified mitochondrial 12s rRNA sequence involving substitution of adenosine (A) by guanosine (G) at nucleotide 1555, which makes that sequence also subject to attack by these aminoglycosides. In these families medically prescribed aminoglycoside antibiotics therefore bind to the mitochondrial DNA causing irreparable inner ear damage. Furthermore, women who have been so treated can transmit the disorder to their babies, according to the mitochondrial inheritance pattern. Up to a third of patients with aminoglycoside ototoxicity carry the 1555 substitution.

The study of interactions between drugs and nucleic acids is called '**pharmacogenomics**' (see also Chapter 9).

Mitochondrial RNA

Mitochondrial DNA is in the form of a continuous loop coding for 13 polypeptides, 22 tRNAs and 2 rRNAs (one 16S, the other 23S; see Chapter 23). Most genes are on one strand, the **heavy strand**, but a few are on its complement, the **light strand** and *both strands are transcribed, as two continuous transcripts*, by a **mitochondrion-specific RNA polymerase**. The latter enzyme is coded by a nuclear gene. The two long RNA molecules are then cleaved to produce 37 separate RNA species and the mitochondrial, ribosomal and transfer RNAs join forces to translate the 13 mRNAs. Many additional proteins are imported into the mitochondria from the cytoplasm, having been transcribed from nuclear genes.

Medical issues

Maternally related members of families in which a member suffers from ototoxic deafness should not be treated with aminoglycoside antibiotics.

13 Risk assessment in Mendelian conditions

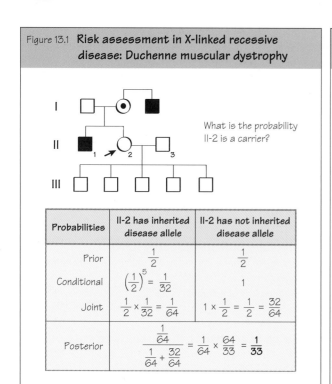

Figure 13.1 Risk assessment in X-linked recessive disease: Duchenne muscular dystrophy

What is the probability II-2 is a carrier?

Probabilities	II-2 has inherited disease allele	II-2 has not inherited disease allele
Prior	$\dfrac{1}{2}$	$\dfrac{1}{2}$
Conditional	$\left(\dfrac{1}{2}\right)^5 = \dfrac{1}{32}$	1
Joint	$\dfrac{1}{2} \times \dfrac{1}{32} = \dfrac{1}{64}$	$1 \times \dfrac{1}{2} = \dfrac{1}{2} = \dfrac{32}{64}$
Posterior	$\dfrac{\frac{1}{64}}{\frac{1}{64} + \frac{32}{64}} = \dfrac{1}{64} \times \dfrac{64}{33} = \dfrac{1}{33}$	

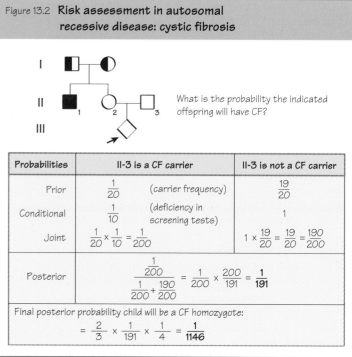

Figure 13.2 Risk assessment in autosomal recessive disease: cystic fibrosis

What is the probability the indicated offspring will have CF?

Probabilities	II-3 is a CF carrier	II-3 is not a CF carrier
Prior	$\dfrac{1}{20}$ (carrier frequency)	$\dfrac{19}{20}$
Conditional	$\dfrac{1}{10}$ (deficiency in screening tests)	1
Joint	$\dfrac{1}{20} \times \dfrac{1}{10} = \dfrac{1}{200}$	$1 \times \dfrac{19}{20} = \dfrac{19}{20} = \dfrac{190}{200}$
Posterior	$\dfrac{\frac{1}{200}}{\frac{1}{200} + \frac{190}{200}} = \dfrac{1}{200} \times \dfrac{200}{191} = \dfrac{1}{191}$	

Final posterior probability child will be a CF homozygote:
$$= \frac{2}{3} \times \frac{1}{191} \times \frac{1}{4} = \frac{1}{1146}$$

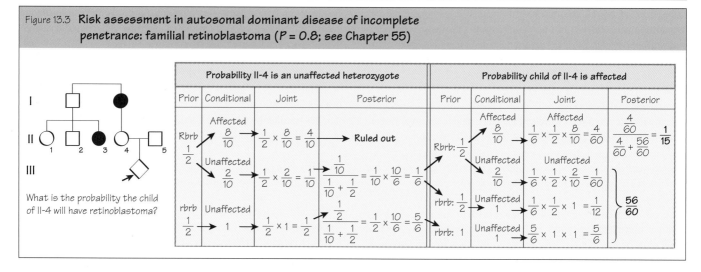

Figure 13.3 Risk assessment in autosomal dominant disease of incomplete penetrance: familial retinoblastoma ($P = 0.8$; see Chapter 55)

What is the probability the child of II-4 will have retinoblastoma?

	Probability II-4 is an unaffected heterozygote				Probability child of II-4 is affected			
	Prior	Conditional	Joint	Posterior	Prior	Conditional	Joint	Posterior
	Rbrb $\dfrac{1}{2}$	Affected $\dfrac{8}{10}$	$\dfrac{1}{2} \times \dfrac{8}{10} = \dfrac{4}{10}$ → Ruled out		Rbrb: $\dfrac{1}{2}$	Affected $\dfrac{8}{10}$	Affected $\dfrac{1}{6} \times \dfrac{1}{2} \times \dfrac{8}{10} = \dfrac{4}{60}$	$\dfrac{\frac{4}{60}}{\frac{4}{60} + \frac{56}{60}} = \dfrac{1}{15}$
		Unaffected $\dfrac{2}{10}$	$\dfrac{1}{2} \times \dfrac{2}{10} = \dfrac{1}{10}$	$\dfrac{\frac{1}{10}}{\frac{1}{10} + \frac{1}{2}} = \dfrac{1}{10} \times \dfrac{10}{6} = \dfrac{1}{6}$		Unaffected $\dfrac{2}{10}$	Unaffected $\dfrac{1}{6} \times \dfrac{1}{2} \times \dfrac{2}{10} = \dfrac{1}{60}$	
	rbrb $\dfrac{1}{2}$	Unaffected 1	$\dfrac{1}{2} \times 1 = \dfrac{1}{2}$	$\dfrac{\frac{1}{2}}{\frac{1}{10} + \frac{1}{2}} = \dfrac{1}{2} \times \dfrac{10}{6} = \dfrac{5}{6}$	rbrb: $\dfrac{1}{2}$	Unaffected 1	Unaffected $\dfrac{1}{6} \times \dfrac{1}{2} \times 1 = \dfrac{1}{12}$	$\dfrac{56}{60}$
					rbrb: 1	Unaffected 1	$\dfrac{5}{6} \times 1 \times 1 = \dfrac{5}{6}$	

Overview

A major part of the burden of a genetic disorder is the risk of recurrence in the family. A prime goal of assessment therefore is to estimate the risk of transmission by the same couple to later children and by affected and unaffected family members to their children. The simple application of Mendelian theory can often provide a rough guide, but such estimates generally need to be refined by inclusion of other considerations such as penetrance (see Chapters 9 and 53). This is most readily achieved by application of Bayes' theorem.

Risk assessment

A combination of several factors is used to determine the basic risk of transmission of a genetic disorder:

1 **Diagnosis.** A correct diagnosis is critical for the accurate assessment of genetic risks. Correct diagnosis may indicate not only the mode of inheritance, but also suggest appropriate carrier and/or prenatal diagnostic tests.

2 **Family history.** Even in the absence of a diagnosis, assessment of the family history may reveal the pattern of transmission and provide clues to penetrance (see Chapter 2).

3 **Ethnic background.** Certain ethnic groups are known to be at increased risk for specific genetic traits (see Chapters 29, 52 and Table 29.4), so providing guidance for assessment of carrier status and prenatal diagnosis.

Bayes' theorem

Bayes' theorem is a mathematical approach that allows refinement of estimates of risk by taking into account all other knowledge relating

Medical Genetics at a Glance, Third Edition. Dorian J. Pritchard and Bruce R. Korf.

to that situation. For example, the 'prior probability' of the birth of an affected child can be derived in a straightforward fashion from classic Mendelian theory. However, if that parental partnership has already produced several unaffected offspring, this allows adjustment in terms of 'conditional probability'. Multiplying the prior and conditional probabilities gives the 'joint probability' of that outcome. A parallel calculation is performed with respect to the alternative outcome of the baby being healthy. The 'relative likelihood' of a diseased child being born is then calculated as the joint probability of the first outcome, divided by the *sum* of the joint probabilities of *both* outcomes.

A benefit of using Bayes' theorem in such contexts is that it allows incorporation of a variety of modifying factors, such as age-related onset of disease, incomplete penetrance and results of genetic testing.

Application of Bayes' theorem
X-linked recessive disease
Consider a woman with both a brother and uncle with X-linked Duchenne muscular dystrophy (see Figure 13.1); because her mother is an obligate carrier she has a 50% chance also of being a carrier. This corresponds to the 'prior probability' of her being a carrier. However, if she has had five unaffected sons we can use this fact to recalculate the 'conditional probability' of her carrier status.

From the pedigree, the prior probability of this woman being a carrier is 1/2 and the conditional probability she would have five unaffected sons, given that she *is* a carrier, is $(1/2)5 = 1/32$. The prior probability of her *not* being a carrier is also 1/2, and, if so, the conditional probability of her having five normal sons would be 1. The product of the prior and conditional probabilities (i.e. the joint probabilities) are 1/64 and 1/2 respectively.

The relative likelihood (also known as the 'posterior probability') of her being a carrier, is then calculated as the joint probability of her being a carrier divided by the sum of the two joint probabilities.

In mathematical terms this is:

$$\frac{1/64}{(1/64 + 1/2)} = 1/33$$

Autosomal recessive disease
The risk of recessive disease depends on coincidence of three circumstances: mother being a carrier, father being a carrier and child inheriting both disease alleles.

Consider a phenotypically normal woman whose brother has cystic fibrosis (CF) (see Figure 13.2). She is married to a white-skinned Northern European and wishes to know the chance their planned child will have CF. The carrier risk for CF among Northern Europeans is around 1/20 and there are laboratory DNA tests for 90% of all CF mutations. The tests on him yield negative results, making his posterior probability of being a carrier 1/191 (see Figure 13.2).

In matings between two heterozygotes we expect normal homozygotes, heterozygotes and mutant homozygotes in the ratio $1:2:1$. Since this woman is unaffected, she is either a normal homozygote (CF/CF; initial probability 0.25) or a heterozygote (CF/cf; initial probability 0.5). Her probability of being a carrier is therefore $0.5/(0.5 + 0.25) = 2/3$. The relative likelihood of their having a child with CF is therefore $2/3 \times 1/191 \times 1/4 = 1/1146$.

This example is given to illustrate application of the theory: in a real situation of course the woman would usually also be tested, so reducing the range of possibilities and refining the estimate of risk.

Autosomal dominant of incomplete penetrance
Familial retinoblastoma is transmitted as a dominant of 80% penetrance (P = 0.8; see Chapter 56). As shown in Figure 13.3, the posterior probability of the child of an unaffected suspected carrier (Rb/rb) being affected is 1/15.

Isolated cases
When a disease condition occurs with no family history, discerning the pattern of inheritance is difficult. Patterns of inheritance can be obscured by small sibship size and failure of some genotypes to survive to term. There can also be diagnostic difficulties due to non-penetrance, variable gene expression or lack of accurate information on absent family members. An AD disorder could be due to a new mutation or wrongly ascribed paternity. For an isolated case of congenital deafness risk can be based on the knowledge that 70% of cases are genetic and, of these, 2/3 are recessive. On the assumption it probably is both inherited and recessive, recurrence risk is then calculated as $7/10 \times 2/3 \times 1/4 = 1/9$.

Consider the case of a single boy being born with X-linked recessive Duchenne muscular dystrophy (DMD). The parents ask what is the risk another son would have the same condition. There are three interpretations:

1 The mother is a heterozygous carrier of the disease allele; when the prior probability of recurrence would be 0.5.
2 A new mutation arose during the meiotic events that produced the ovum from which the boy is derived; recurrence risk is negligible.
3 The mother is a gonadal mosaic for a mutation that occurred during her own embryonic development; in this case recurrence risk relates to the proportion of her ova that carries the mutant X chromosome.

As a guide, among mothers of isolated DMD cases, 2/3 are carriers, in 25–30% there is a new mutation, while 5–10% are gonadal mosaics.

It is sometimes possible to deduce the probable mode of inheritance by comparison with other families with identical symptoms. However, it should be remembered that many conditions are genetically heterogeneous. In such cases ethnic background can be informative. Conversely, members of the same family may display variant manifestation of the same condition.

Empiric risks
If risks are not readily calculable, as in cases with chromosome imbalance and multifactorial disease, we refer to tables of **empiric risks**, that is observed incidences (see Chapters 51 and 52). The risk of Down syndrome is about 10% if the mother carries a 14;21 translocation, 2.5% when carried by the father. Risk of recurrence of a new translocation is low (<1%).

The relative risk of developing an HLA-associated disease can be determined from the formula:

$$\frac{\text{no. of patients with the marker allele} \times \text{no. of controls without the marker allele}}{\text{no. of controls with the marker allele} \times \text{no. of patients without the marker allele}}$$

(see Table 66.2).

14 The cell

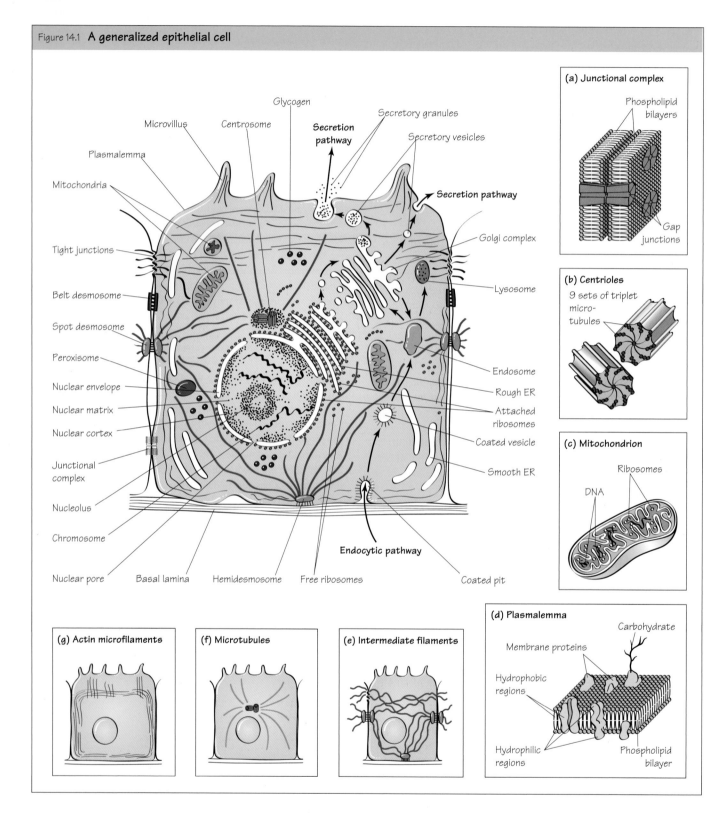

Figure 14.1 **A generalized epithelial cell**

Medical Genetics at a Glance, Third Edition. Dorian J. Pritchard and Bruce R. Korf.

Overview

The cell is the basic functional component of the body. Its **nucleus** is both the repository of the vast majority of the genetic information of that individual and the centre of activity involving its expression. There are many different types of cell (e.g. epithelial, liver, nerve, etc.) and the several kinds of **organelles** and multitudes of soluble enzymes contained within their **cytoplasms** carry out the numerous differentiated aspects of metabolism characteristic of each cell type.

The plasma membrane

The **plasma membrane**, or **plasmalemma**, is a barrier to water-soluble molecules and defines the interface between the interior and exterior of the cell. It is basically a double, side-by-side array of phospholipid molecules forming a sheet of hydrophobic lipid sandwiched between two sheets of hydrophilic phosphate groups. Within the plasmalemma are a variety of proteins positioned with their hydrophobic regions within the lipid interior and their hydrophilic regions at either surface. **Microvilli** (singular: **microvillus**) are extensions of the apical plasmalemma that provide an increased surface for molecular exchange.

The nucleus

The genetic information is carried on the **chromosomes** (see Chapter 15) suspended in the **nuclear matrix**. This is a mesh of proteinaceous material densest close to the nuclear envelope where it is called the **nuclear cortex**.

The **nucleolus** is a morphologically distinct region within the nucleus specialized for production of **ribonucleic acid** components of the **ribosomes** (**rRNA**). A typical human nucleus contains a single large nucleolus, which at interphase (see Chapter 16) contains the **nucleolar organizer regions** of the acrocentric chromosomes (see Chapters 15 and 35).

The nucleus is bounded by a double membrane called the **nuclear envelope**, perforated by **nuclear pores**.

The cytoplasm

The **cytoplasm** consists of a gel-like a material called the **cytosol**. This contains deposits of glycogen, lipid droplets and free ribosomes (see Chapter 24) and is permeated by an array of interconnected filaments and tubules that form the **cytoskeleton**. The latter has three major structural elements: **microtubules**, **microfilaments** and **intermediate filaments**.

Microtubules are straight tubes built from alternating molecules of α- and β-**tubulin**. They radiate from a structure called the **centrosome**, which contains a pair of cylindrical structures called **centrioles** with a characteristic nine-unit structure. (Similar structures occur as **basal bodies** of cilia.) The microtubular network is important in the maintenance of cell shape, separation of the chromosomes during cell division and movement of cilia and sperm.

Microfilaments are double-stranded polymers of the protein **actin** distributed mainly near the cell periphery and involved in cell movement and change of cell shape.

Intermediate filaments are tubular structures that link the desmosomes. They are composed of one of five or more different proteins, depending on cell type.

Mitochondria (singular: **mitochondrion**) are the largest and most abundant of the cytoplasmic organelles. Their main function is the production of energy through synthesis of ATP. They are semiautonomous and self-replicating, each containing ribosomes and up to 10 or more copies of a circular strand of **mitochondrial DNA** carrying the mitochondrial genes (see Chapter 12). They contain the enzymes of the tricarboxylic acid (TCA) cycle and a major fraction of those involved in the oxidation of fatty acids (see Chapter 60).

Lysosomes are cytoplasmic organelles specialized in the deconstruction of many types of complex molecules, damaged mitochondria, viruses and bacteria, etc. that arise as offshoots of the **Golgi apparatus** (or **Golgi complex**). Their development and function are outlined in Chapters 60 and 62.

Peroxisomes are partially responsible for detoxification of foreign compounds such as ethanol, but their major role is the oxidation of fatty acids (see Chapter 62).

The secretion pathway

The **endoplasmic reticulum** (**ER**) is a major site of protein and lipid synthesis and represents the beginning of the secretion pathway for proteins. It is a bulky maze of membrane-bound channels continuous with the nuclear envelope. Close to the nucleus it holds bound ribosomes and is known as '**rough ER**'. Away from the nucleus it lacks ribosomes and is called '**smooth ER**'. The ER also plays a role in neutralizing toxins.

Proteins synthesized in the ER are passed to the Golgi complex for further processing. This is a series of stacked, flattened vesicles. They are then collected in **storage vesicles** or **secretory vesicles** for **exocytosis**, that is release from the cell, in response to external stimuli (see Chapter 60).

Endocytosis

Endocytosis is the internalization and subsequent processing of constituents of the surrounding medium. Small particles are taken into vesicles by **receptor-mediated endocytosis**, which involves internalization of surface bound material through formation of a **coated pit**. Larger particles are bound to membrane receptors and engulfed as **phagocytic vacuoles**; solutes are taken in by **fluid-phase pinocytosis**. The content of both pinocytic and phagocytic vesicles is usually delivered to the lysosomes for breakdown by enzymes called **lysozymes**. During this transfer the vesicles are sometimes referred to as **endosomes** (see Chapter 60).

Cell junctions

Tight junctions create a seal between the apical environment of epithelial cells and their basolateral surfaces. **Belt desmosomes** are elongated layers of fibres that assist in the binding together of adjacent cells, together with **spot desmosomes**, which are localized points of adhesion. **Hemidesmosomes** link epithelial cells to their basal lamina, which is a specialized derivative of the **extracellular matrix**. **Gap junctions** are grouped in **junctional complexes**. Each of these contains a pore permitting molecular communication between adjacent cells.

Medical issues

Several inherited diseases result from deficiencies in specific lysozymes, including Tay–Sachs, Fabry and Gaucher diseases (see Chapter 62). Familial hypercholesterolaemia can result from failure of internalization of lipoprotein. Peroxisomes are absent in Zellweger syndrome, with malformed features, poor muscle tone, enlarged liver and renal cysts. Disorders of the mitochondria are listed in Chapter 12. A defective gap junction protein causes the X-linked form of Charcot–Marie–Tooth disease (see Chapter 11).

Many therapeutic drugs act on receptors located in the plasma membrane. Microtubule assembly is disrupted by the anticancer agents, *vincristine* and *vinblastine*, as well as *colchicine*, which is used to arrest cells at metaphase of mitosis (see Chapters 16 and 35) for examination of the chromosomes. *Clofibrate*, used clinically to lower serum lipoprotein levels, acts by inducing formation of extra peroxisomes.

15 The chromosomes

Figure 15.1 The basis of chromosome structure

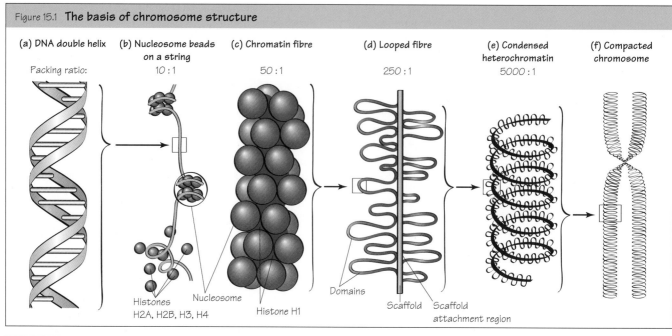

(a) DNA double helix   (b) Nucleosome beads on a string   (c) Chromatin fibre   (d) Looped fibre   (e) Condensed heterochromatin   (f) Compacted chromosome

Packing ratio:

10 : 1   50 : 1   250 : 1   5000 : 1

Histones H2A, H2B, H3, H4   Nucleosome   Histone H1   Domains   Scaffold   Scaffold attachment region

Figure 15.2 A typical chromosome at metaphase of mitosis

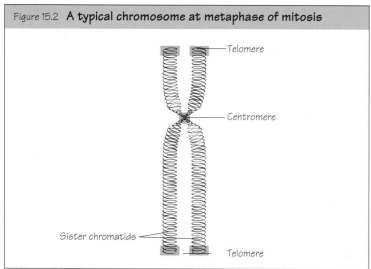

Telomere

Centromere

Sister chromatids

Telomere

Figure 15.3 The basis of chromosome banding

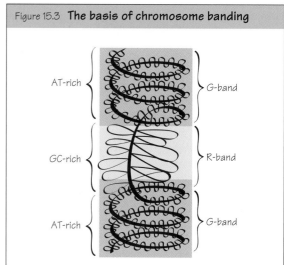

AT-rich   G-band

GC-rich   R-band

AT-rich   G-band

Medical Genetics at a Glance, Third Edition. Dorian J. Pritchard and Bruce R. Korf.

Overview

The word 'chromosome' means 'coloured body', referring to the capacity of these structures to take up certain histological stains more effectively than other cell structures. Each chromosome is composed of an extremely long molecule of DNA complexed with proteins and RNA to form a substance known as **chromatin**. They disperse throughout the nucleus during **interphase** of the cell cycle (i.e. when the cell is not dividing), but become compacted during **mitosis** and **meiosis** (see Chapters 16 and 17). DNA is packaged as chromosomes probably because packaging facilitates segregation of complete sets of genes into daughter cells at mitosis and packing into sperm heads following meiosis.

The staining properties of the chromosomes are utilized in diagnosis for their general visualization, for their individual identification and for the elucidation of chromosomal abnormalities. We can distinguish lightly staining regions designated **euchromatin**, from densely staining **heterochromatin**. Diagnostic aspects are dealt with in Chapters 35–40.

The genetic information, or **genome**, is carried in encoded form in the sequence of bases in the DNA (see Chapters 19–24). The vast majority of this information is in the nucleus, on chromosomes, but a small portion is in the form of naked loops of DNA within each mitochondrion in the cytoplasm. Nuclei are present in practically every cell of the body, the exceptions including red blood cells and the cells of the eye lens.

A typical human nucleus contains around 2 m of DNA divided between 23 pairs of chromosomes, giving an average of around 4 cm per chromosome. But prior to cell division this is reduced to less than 5 μm (0.005 mm) by intricate coiling and packing.

Chromatin structure

In each chromosome the DNA strand is wound twice around globular aggregates of eight histone proteins to form **nucleosomes**, the whole appearing as a **beaded string structure**. The proteins composing the **nucleosome core particle** are *two* molecules each of histones **H2A**, **H2B**, **H3** and **H4**. Histones are positively charged and so can make ionic bonds with negatively charged phosphate groups in the DNA. The amino acid sequences of histones show close to 100% homology across species, indicating their great importance in maintenance of chromatin structure and function. Each nucleosome accommodates about 200 base pairs of DNA and effectively reduces the length of the DNA strand to one-tenth.

The beaded string is then further coiled into a **solenoid**, or spiral coil, with five to six nucleosomes per turn, the structure being maintained by mediation of *one* molecule of histone **H1** per nucleosome. Formation of the solenoid decreases the effective length of the DNA strand by another factor of five, yielding an overall 'packing ratio' of about 50. This is the probable state of euchromatin at interphase in regions where the genes are not being expressed.

During mitosis and meiosis the chromosomes are condensed, a further 100-fold, achieving packing ratios of around 5000. The chromatin fibre is thought to be folded into a series of loops radiating from a central **scaffold** of **non-histone chromosomal proteins** (or **NHC proteins**) that bind to specific base sequences scattered along the DNA strand. Compaction of the chromosome probably involves contraction of these NHC proteins.

One of the most important of the scaffold proteins is **topoisomerase II**, a DNA-nicking-closing enzyme that permits the uncoiling of the two strands of the DNA double helix necessary for relaxation of DNA supercoils during replication or transcription (see Chapters 20 and 22). Topoisomerase II binds to **scaffold attachment regions** that are AT-rich (i.e. contain more than 65% of the bases A and T; see Chapter 19). It is believed that each loop may possibly act as an independent functional domain with respect to DNA replication or transcription.

The looped fibre is then further coiled to create the fully condensed heterochromatin of a chromosome at cell division.

Chromosome banding

Some parts of the compacted chromosome stain densely with Giemsa stain to create **G-bands**. These contain tightly packed, small loops because the scaffold attachment regions there are close together. They replicate late in S-phase (see Chapter 16) and are relatively inactive in transcription. Bands that stain lightly with Giemsa stain, **R-bands**, contain more loosely packed loops, are relatively rich in bases G and C and show most transcriptional activity. Differences between banding patterns of chromosomes allow their identification (see Chapter 35).

The centromere

When visible in early mitosis each chromosome is composed of two identical structures called **sister chromatids** connected at a **primary constriction**. This consists of a non-duplicated stretch of DNA called the **centromere** that duplicates during early anaphase of mitosis (see Chapter 16).

An organelle called the **kinetochore** becomes located on each side of each centromere in early prophase of mitosis and facilitates polymerization of **tubulin** dimers to form the **microtubules** of the **mitotic spindle**.

The telomeres

The term 'telomere' refers to the specialized end of a chromosome. Specific telomeric proteins bind to this structure to provide a cap (see Chapter 20).

The telomeres have several probable functions: preventing the abnormal end-to-end fusion of chromosomes, ensuring complete replication of chromosome extremities, assisting with chromosome pairing in **meiosis** (see Chapter 18) and helping to establish the internal structure of the nucleus during interphase by linking the chromosomes to the nuclear membrane.

Euchromatin and heterochromatin

Euchromatin is compacted during cell division, but relaxes into an open conformation during interphase. In compacted chromosomes it constitutes the palely staining R-bands and contains the majority of the structural genes.

Heterochromatin is densely compacted at cell division and remains compacted at interphase. It is largely concentrated around the nuclear periphery and nucleolus and is relatively inactive in transcription. **Constitutive heterochromatin** is common to all cells of the body, while **facultative heterochromatin** varies, representing regions of the genome that are expressed differentially in the different cell types.

16 The cell cycle

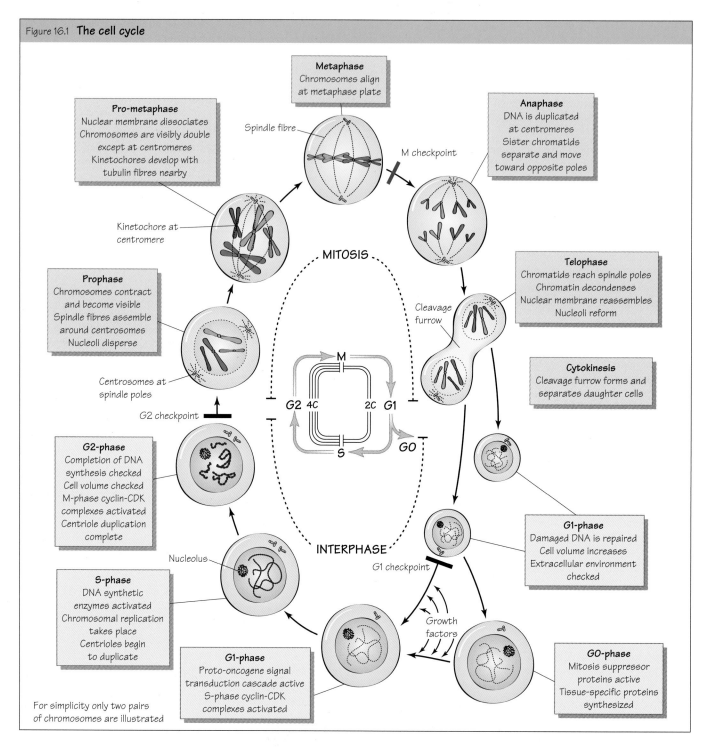

Figure 16.1 **The cell cycle**

Metaphase
Chromosomes align at metaphase plate

Anaphase
DNA is duplicated at centromeres
Sister chromatids separate and move toward opposite poles

Pro-metaphase
Nuclear membrane dissociates
Chromosomes are visibly double except at centromeres
Kinetochores develop with tubulin fibres nearby

Spindle fibre

M checkpoint

Telophase
Chromatids reach spindle poles
Chromatin decondenses
Nuclear membrane reassembles
Nucleoli reform

Kinetochore at centromere

MITOSIS

Cleavage furrow

Prophase
Chromosomes contract and become visible
Spindle fibres assemble around centrosomes
Nucleoli disperse

Cytokinesis
Cleavage furrow forms and separates daughter cells

Centrosomes at spindle poles

M
G2 4C   2C G1
G2 checkpoint
S   G0

G2-phase
Completion of DNA synthesis checked
Cell volume checked
M-phase cyclin-CDK complexes activated
Centriole duplication complete

G1-phase
Damaged DNA is repaired
Cell volume increases
Extracellular environment checked

Nucleolus

INTERPHASE

G1 checkpoint

S-phase
DNA synthetic enzymes activated
Chromosomal replication takes place
Centrioles begin to duplicate

Growth factors

G1-phase
Proto-oncogene signal transduction cascade active
S-phase cyclin-CDK complexes activated

G0-phase
Mitosis suppressor proteins active
Tissue-specific proteins synthesized

For simplicity only two pairs of chromosomes are illustrated

Overview

The body grows by increase in cell size and cell number, the latter by division, called **mitosis**. Cells proliferate in response to extracellular mitogens or '**growth factors**', passing through a repeated sequence of events known as **the cell cycle**. This has four major phases: **G1**, then **S**, **G2** and lastly the **mitotic** or **M-phase**. This is followed by division of the cytoplasm and plasma membrane to produce two identical daughter cells. G1, S and G2 together constitute **interphase**. The chromosomes are replicated during the **DNA synthetic** or **S-phase** (see Chapter 20). Most body cells are not actively dividing and are arrested at '**G0**' within G1.

Typically M-phase occupies between a half and 1 hour of a cycle time of about 20 hours. Normal (as distinct from cancer) human cells can undergo a total of about 80 mitoses.

Medical Genetics at a Glance, Third Edition. Dorian J. Pritchard and Bruce R. Korf.

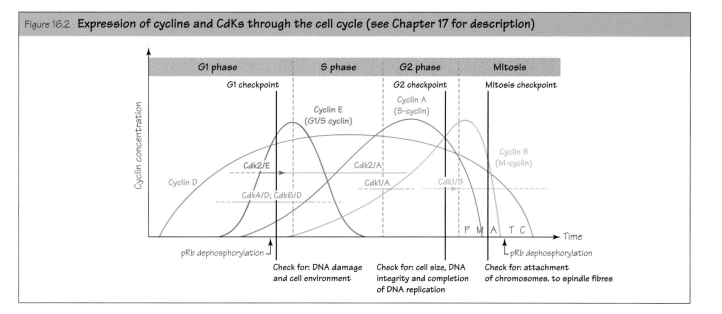

Figure 16.2 **Expression of cyclins and CdKs through the cell cycle (see Chapter 17 for description)**

G1-phase

During G1 the cytoplasm increases in volume. At the **G1 checkpoint damage to the chromosomal DNA** is repaired and the cell checks that its **environment is favourable** before committing itself to S-phase.

Non-cancerous cells are stimulated to proliferate by extracellular growth factors secreted by other cells. These operate within the target cell through the **signal transduction cascade** (see Chapter 54). If not exposed to such signals during G1 the cell diverts from the cycle and enters the mitotically inactive 'G0' state.

Some cells in G0 are merely quiescent and can rejoin the cycle for reparative growth or normal cell replacement. Others become terminally differentiated, irreversibly committed to a specialized function, as are most cells in the mature body. Such cells can still grow in size, for example neurons extend their axons during whole body growth.

S-phase

The standard number of DNA double-helices per cell, corresponding to the diploid number of single-strand chromosomes, is described as **2C**. The 2C complement is retained throughout G1 and into S-phase, when new chromosomal DNA is synthesized and the cell becomes 4C. From the end of S-phase, through G2 and into M-phase each visible chromosome contains two DNA molecules, known as **sister chromatids**, bound tightly together. In human cells therefore, from the end of S-phase to the middle of M there are 23 pairs of chromosomes (i.e. 46 observable entities), but 4C (92) nuclear DNA double-helices.

Mitosis involves sharing identical sets of chromosomes between the two daughter cells, so that each has 23 pairs and is 2C in terms of its DNA molecules. *G1 and G0 are the only phases of the cell cycle throughout which 46 chromosomes correspond to 2C DNA molecules.*

Within S-phase there are additional checkpoints at which **DNA damage prevents new origins of replication becoming active.**

The replication of DNA during S-phase is described in Chapter 20.

Mitosis or M-phase

Mitosis is traditionally considered in five or six phases.

1 Prophase. The chromosomes, each consisting of two identical chromatids, begin to contract and become visible within the nucleus. The 'spindle apparatus' of tubulin fibres begins to assemble around the centrosomes at opposite poles of the cell. The nucleoli disperse.

2 Pro-metaphase. The nuclear membrane dissociates. Proteinaceous **kinetochores** develop around the centromeres of the chromosomes. Tubulin fibres enter the nucleus and assemble around the kinetochores and linking up with those radiating from the centrosomes.

3 Metaphase. Tension in the spindle fibres causes the chromosomes to align midway between the spindle poles, so creating the **metaphase plate**.

4 Anaphase. The centromeric DNA shared by sister chromatids is duplicated, the chromatids separate and are drawn towards the spindle poles.

5 Telophase. The separated sister chromatids (now considered to be chromosomes) reach the spindle poles and a nuclear membrane assembles around each group. The condensed chromatin becomes diffuse and nucleoli reform.

6 Cytokinesis. The cell membrane contracts around the mid-region between the poles, creating a **cleavage furrow** which eventually separates the two daughter cells.

The centrosome cycle

At G1 the pair of centrioles associated with each centrosome separate. During S-phase and G2 a new daughter centriole grows at right angles to each old one. The centrosome splits at the beginning of M-phase and the two daughter centrosomes move to opposite spindle poles.

Medical issues

For karyotype analysis (see Chapters 35–38) dividing cells are artificially arrested at metaphase by use of a spindle inhibitor such as *colchicine*.

The drug *taxol* prevents spindle disassembly and is used in the treatment of cancer (see Chapter 57).

17 Biochemistry of the cell cycle

Figure 17.1 The roles of Rb protein and E2F in regulating the G1 block

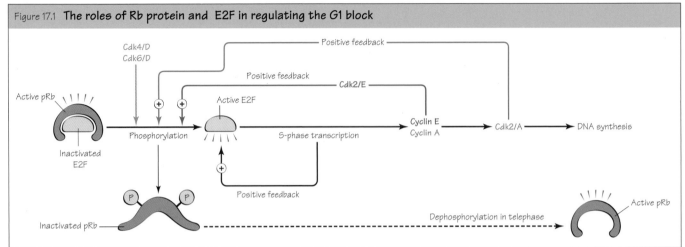

Figure 17.2 Regulation of p53 levels and mediation of p53 in protection of the genome

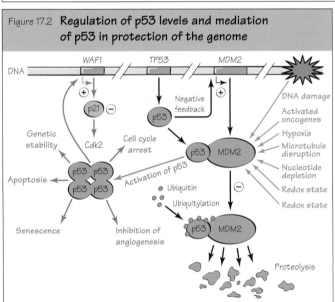

Figure 17.3 Roles of CDKN2A in reinforcement of the G1 block

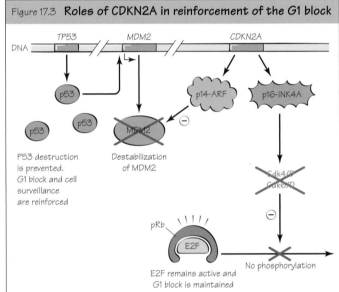

Overview

The cell cycle is driven by alternating activation and deactivation of key enzymes known as **cyclin-dependent protein kinases**, or **Cdks**, and their cofactors, the **cyclins**. This is performed by phosphorylation and dephosphorylation by other phosphokinases and phosphatases respectively, specific cyclin-Cdk complexes mediating specific phases of the cycle (see Figure 16.2). At appropriate stages the same classes of proteins cause the chromosomes to condense, the nuclear envelope to break down and the microtubules of the cytoskeleton to reorganize to form the mitotic spindle.

Cdk2 regulates entry into S-phase, that is through and after the G1 checkpoint, while Cdk1 regulates entry into mitosis, that is through and after the G2 checkpoint. Cdk concentrations are generally constant throughout the cycle, but become active only when bound by a cyclin protein. It is the cyclins that are synthesized and degraded at appropriate times and are the real regulators of the cycle.

The complex Cdk2/E is responsible for assembly of the **chromosome replication complex** and for taking the cell through the G1 checkpoint (see Figure 17.1). As the cell passes from G1 into S, Cdk2 associates instead with cyclin A, replacing Cyclin E and preventing formation of additional replication complexes. Cyclin A then takes the cell through S and G2, up to the G2 checkpoint, for the latter stage associating with Cdk1. In late G2, Cdk1 changes its affinity to Cyclin B, the latter complex supervising passage through the G2 checkpoint and mitosis, and back into G1.

The G1/S checkpoint

Three critical proteins have central roles in controlling progression from G1 into S and are especially important in ensuring normality in cell division. These are the products of the normal alleles of the retinoblastoma gene *RB1, TP53* and *CDKN2A*. Since mutation or loss of these normal alleles is a very common feature of tumourigenesis the normal proteins are commonly referred to as 'tumour suppressors'. Somatic mutations in these three coding sequences are among the most common genetic changes in cancer cells.

Medical Genetics at a Glance, Third Edition. Dorian J. Pritchard and Bruce R. Korf.

pRb/E2F

Passage from G1 into S is blocked if there is **unrepaired DNA damage** and the Rb1 protein (pRb) and protein p53, jointly cause this arrest (see below). **Irreparable DNA damage initiates cell destruction (apoptosis**; see Chapter 55).

The G1/S block is normally overcome by factors such as the specialized transcription promoter E2F and the activity of E2F is controlled by pRb. During G1, E2F is initially inactive, being bound by unmodified pRb (see Figure 17.1). At 2–4 hours before the cell enters S-phase, complexes of D cyclins and Cdk4 and/or Cdk6 phosphorylate pRb. This causes it to undergo a conformational change, conferring a much reduced affinity for E2F. E2F is therefore released and promotes transcription of mRNAs for factors necessary for S-phase, notably cyclin E, the next cyclin in the sequence, and Cyclin A. Protein pRB remains phosphorylated until telophase.

Although the *RB1* gene was identified by its default specifically in tumour cells in retinoblastoma (see Chapter 56), it helps control the cycling of all cell types. Retinoblastomas develop from retinal progenitor cells which are rapidly dividing and poorly differentiated, some of which are also unusually resistant to apoptosis. The reason why non-functionality of RB1 does not disable all cell types is probably because additional proteins of similar function are also operative in non-retinal cells. However, RB1 inactivation is also found in osteo- and other sarcomas, small cell carcinoma of the lung and carcinoma of the breast, bladder and prostate.

In cells with inherited or acquired loss of function mutations in gene *RB1*, E2F can be released inappropriately. Several viral oncoproteins also subvert normal controls by binding and sequestering, or degrading pRb; these include adenovirus E1A, SV40-T antigen, human papilloma virus E7 protein and the EBNA-5 protein of Epstein–Barr virus.

p53, 'the guardian of the genome'

If DNA damage is detected in a dividing cell the protein p53 suspends the cycle at the G1 block before that DNA can be replicated; it also activates DNA repair enzymes and if the damage is irreparable it triggers cell destruction, or **apoptosis**. Its role as master quality checker and controller of replication of our DNA inspired its affectionate title 'the guardian of the genome'.

In normal cells p53 concentrations are generally low. This is ensured by free p53 being targeted by MDM2 protein which attaches **ubiquitin** to it, thus labelling it for rapid destruction by proteases. However, transcription of MDM2 is promoted by p53, so a negative feedback loop exists that ensures p53 concentrations normally stay low. Signals from molecular sensors of DNA damage, as well as many other hazardous or inadequate conditions (see Figure 17.2) cause phosphorylation of p53, which prevents it associating with MDM2 and promotes

its tetramerization and activation for a range of functions. One of these is to increase transcription of p53 dependent genes, the products of which inhibit Cdk2 and so block the cycle (see Figure 16.2).

Loss or mutation of *TP53* is probably the commonest single genetic change in human cancer. Inherited mutations of *TP53* are characteristic of the dominantly inherited Li–Fraumeni syndrome (see Chapters 55 and 56).

CDKN2A

CDKN2A functions by reinforcing the actions of pRb and p53. It is remarkable in encoding two structurally unrelated proteins the messengers of which are transcribed from alternative promoters and translated with respect to alternative reading frames (see Chapter 24). These are p16-INK4A and p14-ARF, 'ARF' being a reference to the alternative reading frame.

Protein p16 is an inhibitor of Cdk4/6 and hence serves to keep pRb in its active, dephosphorylated state, so sequestering E2F and preventing it from stimulating progression through the G1 block. p14-ARF destabilizes MDM2, the molecule that assists in the destruction of p53. The two products of *CDKN2A* therefore assist in cycle regulation both by enhancing retention of E2F in its inactive form and by reducing destruction of p53 (see Figure 17.3).

By subverting the controls normally imposed by both pRb and p53, homozygous deletion of *CDKN2A* facilitates unrestrained progression through the G1 block and is hence a very common event in tumourigenesis.

The G2/M checkpoint

A checkpoint on **cell size, completion of DNA repair and DNA replication** occurs during G2. Passage through this checkpoint and into M depends on activation of cyclin Cdk1/B by the phosphatase Cdc25C. Incomplete DNA replication and damaged DNA generate signals that activate inhibitors of Cdc25C, preventing Cdk1 from becoming active.

The M-phase checkpoint

A significant additional checkpoint occurs also at the metaphase–anaphase transition, related to whether or not **all chromosomes are attached to the tubulin spindle**. Separation of chromatids at anaphase is triggered by an ubiquitin ligase called the **anaphase-promoting complex**, or 'cyclosome', with the responsibility of marking redundant cell cycle proteins for destruction. This includes cyclins A and B and the proteins that hold sister chromatids together.

Kinetochores that are not attached to spindle microtubules secrete a **cyclosome inhibitor** and if this signal is defective, chromatids can start to separate prematurely, leading to chromosome imbalance in daughter cells.

18 Gametogenesis

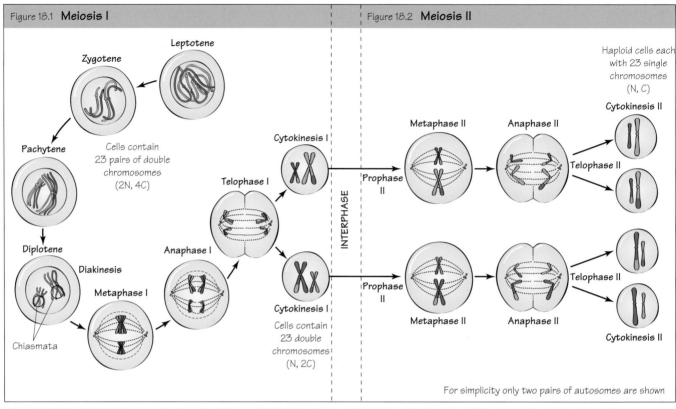

Figure 18.1 **Meiosis I**

Leptotene

Zygotene

Pachytene

Cells contain 23 pairs of double chromosomes (2N, 4C)

Diplotene

Diakinesis

Metaphase I

Anaphase I

Telophase I

Chiasmata

Cytokinesis I

Cytokinesis I

Cells contain 23 double chromosomes (N, 2C)

INTERPHASE

Figure 18.2 **Meiosis II**

Prophase II

Metaphase II

Anaphase II

Telophase II

Cytokinesis II

Haploid cells each with 23 single chromosomes (N, C)

Prophase II

Metaphase II

Anaphase II

Telophase II

Cytokinesis II

For simplicity only two pairs of autosomes are shown

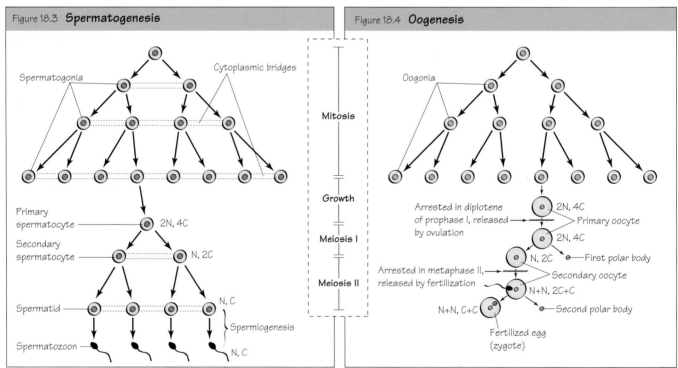

Figure 18.3 **Spermatogenesis**

Spermatogonia

Cytoplasmic bridges

Primary spermatocyte — 2N, 4C

Secondary spermatocyte — N, 2C

Spermatid — N, C

Spermiogenesis

Spermatozoon — N, C

Mitosis

Growth

Meiosis I

Meiosis II

Figure 18.4 **Oogenesis**

Oogonia

Arrested in diplotene of prophase I, released by ovulation — Primary oocyte — 2N, 4C

2N, 4C

Arrested in metaphase II, released by fertilization — Secondary oocyte — N, 2C — First polar body

N+N, 2C+C

N+N, C+C

Fertilized egg (zygote)

Second polar body

Medical Genetics at a Glance, Third Edition. Dorian J. Pritchard and Bruce R. Korf.

Overview

Each body cell contains two sets of chromosomes, one from the mother and one from the father. They are described as 2N or **diploid**. The sperm and ova contain only one set of chromosomes and are said to be 1N or **haploid**. The process by which the diploid number is reduced to haploid during the formation of the germ cells is called **meiosis**. In terms of the number of centromeres, this involves a **reductional division** followed by an **equational division** known as **Meiosis I** and **Meiosis II**. In men meiosis occurs by the pattern seen in most diploid species, but in women there are several differences.

Crossing-over between maternally and paternally derived chromosomes ensures reshuffling of the genetic information between each generation. At **fertilization**, fusion of the haploid chromosome complement of the sperm with that of the ovum restores the chromosome number to diploid in the zygote.

Meiosis I

Meiosis I has similarities with mitosis, but is much more complex and extended in time. Primary spermatocytes and primary oocytes enter meiosis following G2 of mitosis, so they each have a diploid set of chromosomes (2N), but each of these contains replicated DNA as sister chromatids (i.e. are 4C; see Chapter 16). Prophase I involves reciprocal exchange between maternal and paternal chromatids by the process of **crossing-over**.

Prophase I

1 Leptotene. The chromosomes appear as long threads attached at each end to the nuclear envelope.
2 Zygotene. The chromosomes contract, pair with and adhere closely to (or 'synapse with') their homologues. This normally involves precise registration, gene for gene throughout the entire genome. In primary spermatocytes X- and Y-chromosomes synapse at the tips of their short arms only.
3 Pachytene. Sister chromatids begin to separate, the double chromosome being known as a **bivalent**. The chromosome pair represented by four double helices is called a **tetrad**. One or both chromatids of each paternal chromosome crosses over with those from the mother in what is known as a **synaptonemal complex**. Every chromosome pair undergoes at least one crossover.
4 Diplotene. The chromatids separate except at the regions of crossover or **chiasmata** (singular: **chiasma**). This situation persists in all **primary oocytes** until they are shed at **ovulation**.
5 Diakinesis. The reorganized chromosomes begin to move apart. Each bivalent can now be seen to contain four chromatids linked by a common centromere, while non-sister chromatids are linked by chiasmata.

Metaphase I, anaphase I, telophase I, cytokinesis I

These follow a similar course to the equivalent stages in mitosis (see Chapter 16), the critical difference being that, instead of non-sister chromatids being segregated, pairs of reciprocally crossed-over sister chromatids joined at their centromeres are distributed to the daughter cells.

At the end of Meiosis I, secondary spermatocytes and secondary oocytes contain 23 chromosomes (1N), each consisting of two chromatids (i.e. 2C).

Meiosis II

There is a transient interphase, during which no chromosome replication occurs, followed by a prophase, metaphase, anaphase, telophase and cytokinesis. These resemble the equivalent phases of mitosis in that pairs of chromatids (bivalents) linked at their centromeres become aligned at the metaphase plate and are then drawn into separate daughter cells following replication of the centromeric DNA.

At the end of Meiosis II the cells contain 23 chromosomes (1N), each consisting of a single chromatid (1C).

Male meiosis

Spermatogenesis includes all the events by which spermatogonia are transformed into spermatozoa and takes about 64 days. Cytokinesis is incomplete throughout, so that each generation of cells remains linked by cytoplasmic bridges.

A diploid **primary spermatocyte** undergoes Meiosis I to form two haploid **secondary spermatocytes**. These both undergo Meiosis II to produce four haploid **spermatids**. The spermatids become elaborated into **spermatozoa** during **spermiogenesis**. This includes: (i) formation of the acrosome containing enzymes that assist with penetration of the egg; (ii) condensation of the nucleus; (iii) shedding of most of the cytoplasm; and (iv) formation of the neck, midpiece and tail.

Female meiosis

Oogenesis begins in the fetus at 12 weeks, but ceases abruptly at about 20 weeks, the **primary oocytes** remaining at diplotene of prophase I until ovulation, this suspended state being called **dictyotene**.

Ovulation begins at puberty and usually only one oocyte is shed per month. Under stimulation by hormones a primary oocyte swells, accumulating cytoplasmic materials. At completion of Meiosis I these are inherited by one daughter cell, the **secondary oocyte**. The other nucleus passes into the **first polar body**, which usually degenerates without further division. Meiosis I is completed rapidly then, after a pause, the secondary oocyte is shed into the uterine, or Fallopian, tube.

Meiosis II stops at metaphase until entry of a sperm. It then completes division, producing a large haploid **ovum** pro-nucleus, which fuses with the sperm pro-nucleus, and a very small **second polar body**, which degenerates.

The whole process takes from 12 to 50 years, depending when fertilization takes place.

The significance of meiosis

1 The diploid chromosome content of somatic cells is reduced to haploid in the gametes.
2 Paternal and maternal chromosomes become reassorted with a potential for 2^{23} (=8 388 608) different combinations, excluding recombination *within* chromosomes.
3 Reassortment of paternal and maternal alleles *within* chromosomes creates an infinite potential for genetic variation between gametes.
4 The *randomness* of reassortment of paternal and maternal alleles during meiosis (and at fertilization) ensures the applicability of probability theory to genetic ratios and the general validity of Mendel's laws (see Chapter 3).
5 The frequency of crossover between genes *within* chromosomes allows the relative positions of gene to be mapped (see Chapters 31 and 32).
6 Errors sometimes occur at chromosome pairing and crossing-over, which can produce **translocations**, as well as at their separation or **disjunction**, which can lead to **aneuploidy** (see Chapters 36–38).

19 DNA structure

Figure 19.1 A 3'–5' phosphodiester bond between two molecules of 2'-deoxyribose

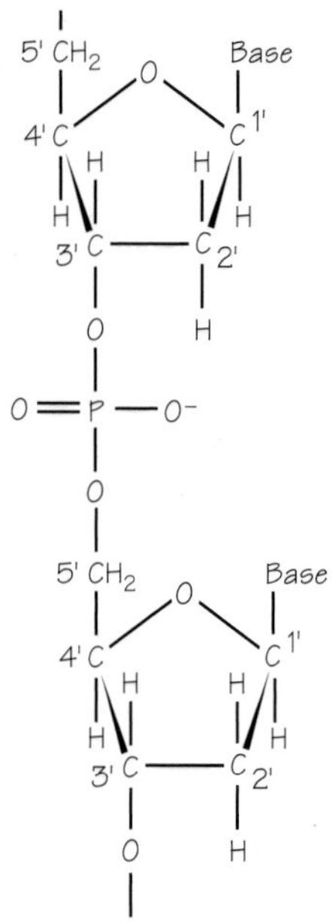

Figure 19.2 A molecule of 2'-deoxyribose

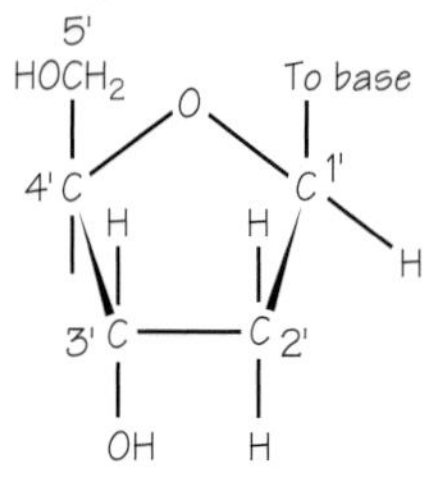

Figure 19.3 Base pair linkages

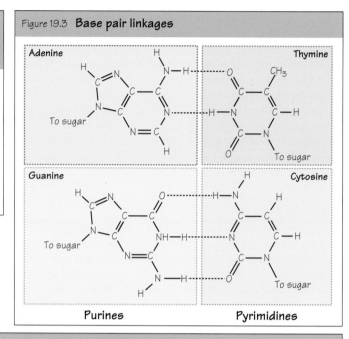

Adenine   Thymine

Guanine   Cytosine

To sugar

Purines   Pyrimidines

Figure 19.5 The DNA double helix

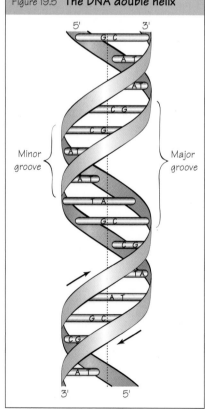

Minor groove

Major groove

Figure 19.4 Schematic diagram of a two-base-pair section of DNA

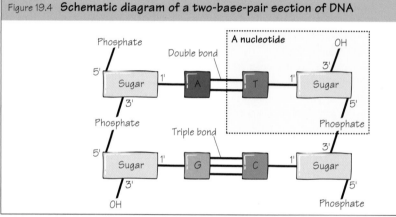

Phosphate
A nucleotide
Double bond
OH
Sugar   Sugar
Phosphate
Triple bond
Phosphate
Sugar   Sugar
OH   Phosphate

Figure 19.6 Structural classes of human DNA

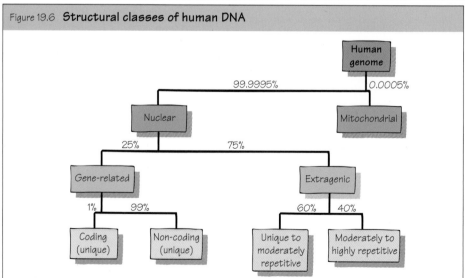

Human genome
99.9995%   0.0005%
Nuclear   Mitochondrial
25%   75%
Gene-related   Extragenic
1%   99%   60%   40%
Coding (unique)   Non-coding (unique)   Unique to moderately repetitive   Moderately to highly repetitive

Medical Genetics at a Glance, Third Edition. Dorian J. Pritchard and Bruce R. Korf.

Overview

The chromosomes are composed essentially of DNA, which contains coded instructions for synthesis of every protein in the body. DNA consists of millions of nucleotides within two interlinked, coiled chains. Each nucleotide contains one of four bases and it is the sequence of these bases that contains the coded instructions (see Chapter 24). Each base on one chain is matched by a complementary partner on the other, and each sequence provides a template for synthesis of a copy of the other. Synthesis of new DNA is called **replication** (see Chapter 20).

The unit of length of DNA is the **base pair (bp)** with 1000 bp in a **kilobase (kb)** and one million base pairs in a **megabase (Mb)**. A typical human body cell contains nearly 7000 Mb of DNA.

The structure of DNA

We can visualize DNA as an extremely long, flexible ladder that has been twisted right-handed (like a corkscrew) by coiling around a telegraph pole. Each 'upright' of the ladder is a series of **deoxyribose** sugar molecules linked together by phosphate groups attached to their 3′ ('three prime') and 5′ ('five prime') carbon atoms. At the bottom of one upright is a 3′ carbon atom carrying a free hydroxyl (–OH) group and at the top, a 5′ carbon carrying a free phosphate group. On the other upright this orientation is reversed.

The 'rungs' of the ladder are pairs of nitrogenous **bases** of two types, **purines** and **pyrimidines**. The purines are **adenine (A)** and **guanine (G)** and the pyrimidines are **cytosine (C)** and **thymine (T)**. The bases are attached to the 1′ carbon of each sugar. Each unit of purine or pyrimidine base together with one attached sugar and one phosphate group constitute a **nucleotide**. A section of double-stranded DNA is therefore essentially two linked, coiled chains of nucleotides. This **double helix** has a **major groove** corresponding to the gap between adjacent sections of the sugar–phosphate chains and a **minor groove** along the row of bases. There are 10 pairs of nucleotides per complete turn of the helix.

The pairs of bases of the 'rungs' are hydrogen-bonded together; both A and T have two sites available for bonding while C and G each have three. *A always pairs with T on the partner strand and C with G*. This **base pairing** is very specific and ensures that the strands are normally precisely complementary to one another. Thus if one strand reads 5′-CGAT-3′, the complementary strand must read 3′-GCTA-5′ in the same direction, or 5′-ATCG-3′ if we obey the normal rule of describing the sequence from 5′ to 3′. The number of A residues in a section of DNA is therefore always equal to the number of T residues; similarly, the number of C residues always equals the number of G.

The centromeres

Centromeric DNA contains short sequences of bases repeated many times 'in tandem array'. The sequences vary between chromosomes, but there are substantial regions of homology. The most important component is a 171-bp repeat called **alpha-satellite DNA**. This is AT-rich and contains a binding site for a protein contained within the **kinetochore**. The latter is responsible for assembly of the microtubules of the spindle apparatus (see Chapter 16).

The telomeres

In contrast to the centromeric repeats, telomeric sequences are the same in all human chromosomes and similar to those in other species. Human telomeric DNA consists of long arrays of tandem repeats of the sequence 5′-GGGTTA-3′ extending for several hundred bases at each chromosome end. Most of this is double-stranded, with 3′-CCCAAT-5′ on the complementary strand, but the extreme 3′ end is single-stranded and believed to loop around and invade the double helix several kilobases away (see Chapter 20).

Structural classes of human DNA

The human *haploid* genome contains around 20 000–25 000 nuclear genes, that is chromosomal coding sequences and their associated control elements, including ~6000 genes coding for RNA species other than messenger RNA, plus 37 within the mitochondrial genome (see Chapter 12). However, *the nuclear 'genome' represents no more than 3% of nuclear DNA*, the remainder having no coding function. The latter includes **introns** that interrupt the coding **exons** of most genes, plus the 75% of human nuclear DNA that is extragenic, that is outside or between the genes. Of the latter, 60% is of unique sequence or moderately repetitive, while 40% is moderately to highly repetitive.

The highly repetitive fraction includes **microsatellite** and **minisatellite DNA**, which differ in the length of the repeat. Satellite DNA is so-called because its unusual AT:GC ratio gives it a buoyant density that differs from the bulk of the DNA. This causes it to separate out as a 'satellite band' when mechanically sheared whole DNA is subjected to density gradient centrifugation.

About 10% of the nuclear DNA consists of up to 500 000 copies of repetitive sequence DNA, the average size of these repeat units being ~800 bp, called **long interspersed nuclear elements**, or **LINES**. In human and other primate DNA there are also about a million copies of a short repeat (~300 bp) known as *Alu* and ~400 000 of another of 130 bp sequence called *MIR*, constituting together ~9% of the nuclear genome. The latter are **short interspersed nuclear elements** or **SINES**.

LINES and SINES are **transposable elements, or transposons**, derived ancestrally by reverse transcription of RNA transcripts into free cDNA copies that then re-integrated into the genomic DNA. When this occurs it can have a mutagenic effect at that site.

LINES constitute about 20% of the genome and are located preferentially in the dark, AT-rich G bands (Chapter 35). They are autonomous transposons in that each still retains a gene for reverse transcriptase probably derived originally from an RNA virus, although only a small proportion retain the capacity for transposition. They reintegrate into sites such as TTTT↓T, mainly in AT-rich gene-poor regions.

Alu sequences contain their own promoter sequences, but SINES typically do not encode proteins, so are unable to act autonomously, although they can be mobilized by neighbouring LINES. SINES have a relatively high GC content and are preferentially located in the GC-rich, gene-rich R-bands (Chapter 35). They sometimes carry control elements that affect expression of neighbouring genes, but tend to be concentrated in introns and untranslated regions where some may have beneficial roles, for example one acts as a transcriptional repressor of the cellular heat shock response.

Functionally related genes often occur in clusters along the same DNA strand. Examples include the β-globin cluster on 11p (Chapter 35) and the genes of the MHC (Chapter 64).

Medical and legal issues

Microsatellite DNA is scattered throughout the genome and is useful for tracking the inheritance of disease alleles to which they are closely linked. Minisatellite DNA is concentrated near the centromeres and telomeres, so is less useful for tracking alleles, but since it is highly variable it is used for producing **DNA fingerprints** (see Chapter 70). The *Alu* sequence is used forensically for identification of primate DNA, while *MIR* characterizes mammalian DNA.

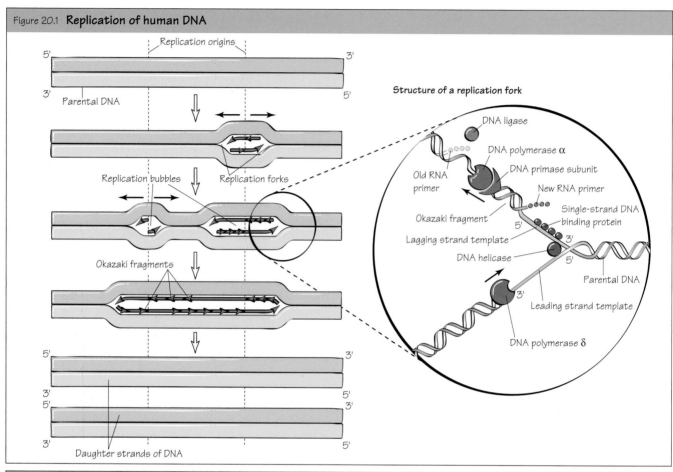

Figure 20.1 Replication of human DNA

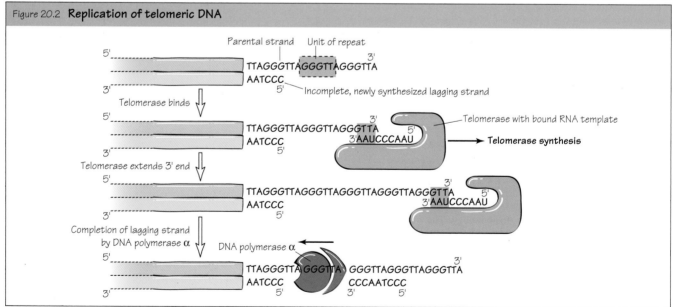

Figure 20.2 Replication of telomeric DNA

Medical Genetics at a Glance, Third Edition. Dorian J. Pritchard and Bruce R. Korf.

Overview

Cells multiply by the process of mitosis, following duplication of the nuclear genome. The latter occurs mainly during **S-phase** of the **cell cycle**, which lasts about 8 hours (see Chapter 16). The DNA at the centromeres is replicated in the middle of mitosis, just prior to chromosome segregation. Mitochondrial DNA is replicated independently and out of phase with nuclear DNA.

Although the overall sequence of events during replication of nuclear DNA in higher organisms (eukaryotes) is similar to that in bacteria (prokaryotes), the details are subtly different. In eukaryotes replication takes place while the (nuclear) DNA remains in nucleosome configuration (see Chapter 15).

Replication

GC-rich sections of the DNA, recognizable as euchromatic R-bands in condensed chromatin (see Chapter 15), contain 'housekeeping genes' that operate in every cell. These sections replicate in early S-phase. The heterochromatic AT-rich G bands (see Chapter 15) contain few genes and replicate in late S-phase. Genes in AT-rich regions that code for differentiated properties and operate only in certain cells, occur in facultative heterochromatin (see Chapter 15). This is replicated early in those cells in which the genes are expressed and late in those in which they are not.

The place on the DNA helix that first unwinds to begin replication is called the **replication origin**. Here the double strand is split open by a **helicase** enzyme to expose the base sequences. Replication proceeds along the single strands at about 40–50 nucleotides per second, simultaneously in both directions. In higher organisms there are many replication origins spaced about 50–300 kb apart. The resulting separations of the DNA strand are called **replication bubbles**, at each end of which is a **replication fork**.

New DNA is synthesized by enzymes called **DNA polymerases**, from **deoxyribonucleotide triphosphates** (**ATP**, **GTP**, etc.) which in the process are converted into monophosphate nucleotides (**AMP**, **GMP**, etc.). The release and hydrolysis of pyrophosphate from the triphosphates provides energy for the reaction and ensures it is virtually irreversible, making DNA a relatively very robust molecule.

All DNA polymerases can build new DNA only in the 5′ to 3′ direction, which means they must move along their **template strands** from 3′ to 5′. Replication can therefore occur continuously from the origin of replication along only one strand, called the **leading strand**. The other strand is called the **lagging strand** and, because of the reverse orientation of the sugars, along this strand, replication takes place only in short stretches. The new sections of DNA along the lagging strand are typically 100–200 bases long and are known as **Okazaki fragments**. Following their synthesis they are linked together by action of the enzyme **DNA ligase**. While awaiting replication the parental single-strand sequence of the lagging strand is temporarily protected by **single-strand binding protein** (or **helix destabilizing protein**).

Leading strand synthesis requires **DNA polymerase δ**; lagging strand synthesis uses a different enzyme, **DNA polymerase α**. The latter contains a **DNA primase** subunit that produces a short stretch of **RNA**, which acts as a primer for DNA synthesis.

Replication of mitochondrial DNA occurs independently of that in the nucleus and utilizes a different set of enzymes, including the mitochondria-specific **DNA polymerase γ**.

The genome contains multiple copies of the five histone genes, from which copious quantities of histones are produced, especially during S-phase. These bind immediately onto the newly replicated DNA.

Since each daughter DNA duplex contains one old strand from the parent molecule and one newly synthesized strand, the replication process is described as **semiconservative**.

Replication of the telomeres

Synthesis of DNA at the end of the lagging strand is problematical as DNA polymerase α needs to attach beyond the end of the sequence that is being replicated and work proximally, in the 5′-3′ direction. A specialized DNA synthetic enzyme called **telomerase** provides an extension of the lagging strand that enables this to happen.

Telomerase is a ribonucleoprotein that contains an RNA template with the sequence 3′-AAUCCCAAU-5′. This is complementary to one-and-a-half copies of the six-base telomeric DNA repeat, 5′-GGGTTA-3′ (see Chapter 19). The 3′-AAU of the RNA sequence of the telomerase binds to the terminal -TTA-5′ of the template lagging strand, leaving the rest of the RNA sequence exposed. Deoxyribonucleotides then assemble on this RNA template, extending the DNA repeat sequence by one unit. The telomerase then detaches and moves along to the new DNA terminal -TTA-5′, where the process is repeated. When a sufficiently long terminal repeat has been formed, DNA polymerase α attaches to the single-strand extension and assembles the complementary DNA strand in a proximal 5′-3′ direction back to the old end of the double strand, to which it becomes linked by the action of DNA ligase.

Repair systems

Occasionally a wrong base is inserted into a growing strand but, fortunately, healthy cells contain **postreplication repair enzymes** and **base mismatch proofreading systems** that correct such errors. These remove and replace the erroneously inserted bases, using the template strand as a guide. These repair systems utilize two additional DNA polymerases: **β** and **ε** (see Chapter 26).

Medical issues

Several cancer-predisposing conditions arise from defects in different aspects of the postreplication repair and mismatch repair systems. These include the chromosome breakage syndrome called **Bloom syndrome**, familial predisposition to breast cancer caused by mutations in the genes *BRCA1* and *BRCA2* and an autosomal dominant form of bowel cancer called **hereditary non-polyposis colon cancer** (**HNPCC**) (see Chapter 56).

One theory holds that telomeres are reduced in length at every round of mitosis and that the number of repeats they contain may play a role in limiting the number of times a cell can divide. On this theory, abnormally efficient, mutant telomerases may promote the indefinite growth of cancer cells by delaying telomere decay.

21 The structure of genes

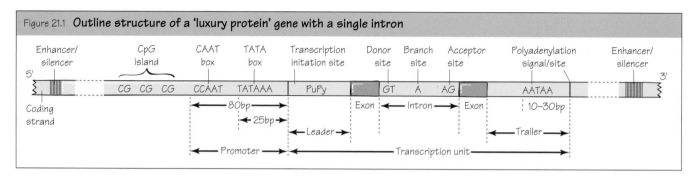

Figure 21.1 Outline structure of a 'luxury protein' gene with a single intron

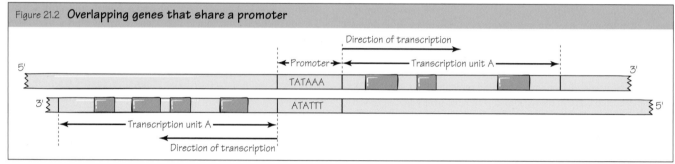

Figure 21.2 Overlapping genes that share a promoter

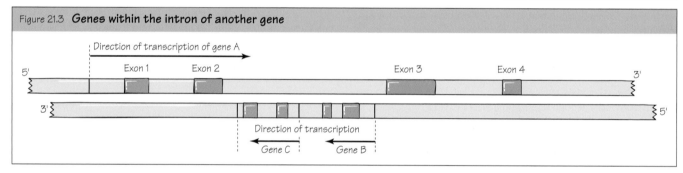

Figure 21.3 Genes within the intron of another gene

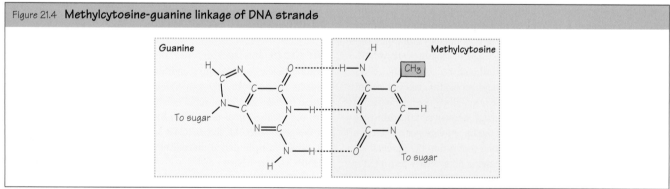

Figure 21.4 Methylcytosine-guanine linkage of DNA strands

Overview

Most metabolic processes are catalysed by proteinaceous enzymes and proteins are also the main structural components of the body. The amino acid sequences of all proteins are coded in the DNA. Conversion of the DNA-encoded information into protein involves transcription into an RNA copy, called **hnRNA (heterogeneous nuclear RNA)**, processing into **mRNA (messenger RNA)**, translation into **polypep-** tide and elaboration into protein (see Chapter 24). A 'gene' consists not only of protein-coding DNA, but also of 'upstream' controlling sequences 5′ to the coding region, non-coding sequences within the coding region and also 'downstream' sequences 3′ to the coding region concerned also with control of gene expression (Chapter 22). Some genes overlap others, or are contained within others, and the non-coding sequences of some genes act as the coding sequences of others.

Medical Genetics at a Glance, Third Edition. Dorian J. Pritchard and Bruce R. Korf.

The structure of a typical gene

Eukaryote DNA differs from that of prokaryotes in that most of its genes contain redundant DNA interrupting the coding sequences. These stretches of non-coding DNA are called **introns**, while the coding sequences are **exons**. Outside the protein-coding region are a **leader** and **trailer**, plus a variety of transcriptional control sequences.

Genes that code for protein are called 'structural genes' and their transcription is performed by RNA **polymerase II** (**Pol II**). A sequence just 'upstream' (i.e. 5′) of the coding sequence constitutes the **promoter**, which indicates where Pol II should begin its action.

Among proteins we distinguish '**housekeeping proteins**' present in all cell types and '**luxury proteins**' produced for specialized functions. The promoters of genes in the latter category and those transcribed only at certain stages of the cell cycle include a '**TATA box**', this being a variant of 5′-TATAAA-3′ (on the 'sense' or coding strand). This is located 25 bp 'upstream' (i.e. −25 bp) of the **transcription initiation site**. Mutations in the TATA box cause transcription to begin at incorrect locations.

Instead of a TATA box, genes that code for housekeeping proteins usually have one or more '**GC boxes**' in variable positions, containing a variant of 5′-GGGCGG-3′. Housekeeping proteins include DNA and RNA polymerase and the ribosomal proteins. Some genes have multiple GC boxes both upstream and downstream of the coding sequence and in either orientation. The histone genes have both TATA and GC boxes.

Another common promoter element is the '**CAAT box**' (e.g. 5′-CCAAT-3′) often at −80 bp. It is the strongest determinant of promoter efficiency and can function in either orientation. There are often also **enhancer** and **silencer** sequences some distance away, which bind controlling factors that interact with the promoter by looping of the DNA. Some 'luxury' genes have additional function-specific control elements.

'Downstream' (i.e. 3′) of the transcription initiation site is the non-coding leader sequence corresponding to the leader of the transcribed polypeptide (Chapter 24). The coding message follows, usually interrupted by several introns, followed by the non-coding trailer sequence. At the end of the trailer is the **polyadenylation site** defined by 5′-AATAA-3′ (5′-AAUAA-3′ in the RNA transcript), 10–30 bases upstream.

Introns begin with the sequence **GT**A(/G)GAGT and end with a run of Cs or Ts preceding **AG**. The first **GT** (**GU** in the hnRNA) and the last **AG**, together with an **A** residue situated within a relatively standard sequence near the downstream end, are important in intron removal (Chapter 22). The 5′ site is known as the **donor** site, the 3′ site is the **acceptor** and the A residue is the **branch site**. No general transcription termination signal has been identified in eukaryote DNA (see Chapter 22).

CpG sequences are cytosines that have guanine as a downstream neighbour (the 'p' representing the linking phosphate group). About 70% of all CpG sequences in DNA are methylated. These modified cytosines undergo base pairing with G on the opposite strand in the normal way, but the added methyl group affects chromatin structure and blocks gene expression (Chapter 22). CpG sequences are concentrated in '**CpG islands**' near the promoters of many human genes and provide scope for shutting down transcription, as in X-chromosome inactivation (Chapter 43) and gene imprinting (see Chapter 27).

Gene length

There is a general correlation between the sizes of genes and their protein products. However, the dystrophin gene is exceptionally long, 50 times that for apolipoprotein B, although the two proteins are of similar length. This difference is due to exceptionally long introns in the case of dystrophin.

Genes that share a promoter

Human genes used to be thought of as residing uniquely in one stretch of DNA, each acting as an independent transcription unit. Recently we have found this to be largely untrue: about 70% of genes are transcribed from both DNA strands and many share promoters.

In some cases two genes are transcribed from opposite strands and in opposite directions, but from the same promoter. Others are transcribed from the same strand as long, multigenic transcripts which are cleaved into multiple messengers (e.g. rRNA, Chapter 23).

In the mitochondria, the H strand is transcribed in one direction, from either of two closely spaced promoters flanking the tRNA *Phe* gene, while the L strand is transcribed in the opposite direction from a different promoter (Chapter 12). The two long primary transcripts are then both cut into separate messenger species.

The structural genes for the A and B chains of insulin are adjacent and are transcribed and translated as a single long molecule, which is cleaved at the polypeptide level to produce equal quantities of the two protein components.

Overlapping genes

About 9% of human structural genes overlap other such genes. More than 90% of overlapping genes are transcribed from opposite strands, the remainder from the same strand using different promoters and different reading frames (Chapter 24). In some cases small genes are located within the introns of large genes. Some protein-coding genes are overlapped by genes coding for non-coding RNA (Chapter 23). Some long RNA transcripts are cleaved to produce two smaller RNAs, both with controlling functions.

Chromatin conformation

The nucleosomal structure of chromatin is described in Chapter 15. Histones carry a strong positive charge, with high affinity for the negatively charged DNA, but covalent modifications of the amino acids in the histones tails, especially of H3 and H4, modulate their properties. The most common modifications are acetylation ($+COCH_3$), mono-, di- or tri-methylation ($+CH_3$), of lysines and phosphorylation ($+PO_4$) of serines. The densely packed nucleosomes of heterochromatin also contain **heterochromatin protein 1** (HP1).

Constitutive heterochromatin is largely devoid of genes, but with many nucleotide repeats and its histone H3K9 is trimethylated. Facultative heterochromatin forms reversibly during the life of a cell as a control on gene expression and its H3K9 is dimethylated.

Dimethylated and trimethylated H3K4 coincide precisely with promoter regions in euchromatin and provide a signpost recognized by TFIID in the basal transcription complex, enabling initial attachment of RNA Pol II at that site. By contrast, unmethylated H3K4 binds DNA methyltransferases that methylate cytosine in CpG sequences which 'silences' those regions. Other enzymes bind to regions signposted in this way, modifying other histones in their vicinity and reinforcing the gene expression control programmes.

Medical issues

Aberrant methylation of CpG islands, particularly those associated with 'tumour suppressor genes', is a general characteristic of cancer cells.

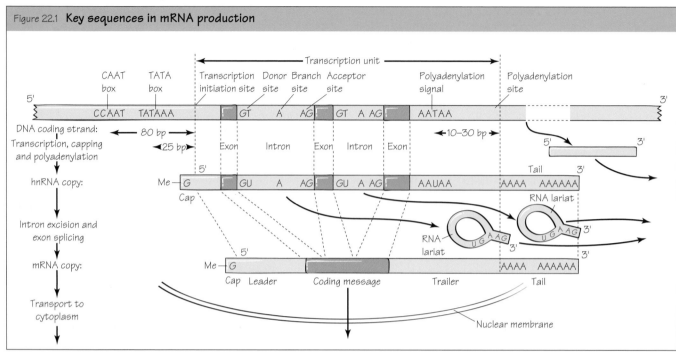

Figure 22.1 **Key sequences in mRNA production**

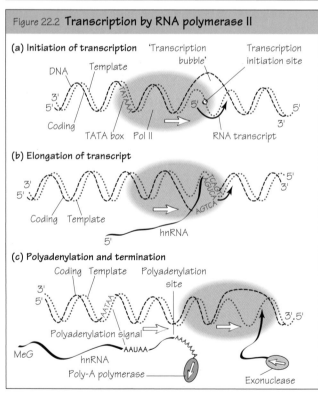

Figure 22.2 **Transcription by RNA polymerase II**

(a) Initiation of transcription

(b) Elongation of transcript

(c) Polyadenylation and termination

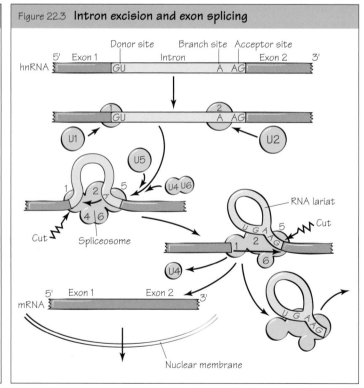

Figure 22.3 **Intron excision and exon splicing**

Overview

A typical diploid body cell contains two copies of the nuclear genome, one on each set of chromosomes. By contrast with that in the mitochondria, the nuclear genome is complex both in its structure and its transcription. Surprisingly, there are only 20 000–25 000 protein-coding genes, and not much more than 1% of human genomic DNA actually encodes proteins (see Chapter 21). This fraction is highly conserved between individuals, whereas 95% of DNA is more variable and includes highly repetitive sequences.

Despite the apparent paucity of genes, a remarkable recent finding is that at least 85% of nuclear DNA is nevertheless transcribed into RNA. Many of these transcripts have regulatory roles in protein syn-

Medical Genetics at a Glance, Third Edition. Dorian J. Pritchard and Bruce R. Korf.

thesis, or are responsible for other aspects of gene regulation (see Chapter 23). In this chapter we address the **transcription** of protein-coding genes, with production of **heterogeneous nuclear RNA (hnRNA)** and its processing into **messenger RNA (mRNA)**.

Transcription factors

Transcription factors are proteins that bind to specific sequences in the DNA and control transcription. Typically they contain an **activation domain** and a **DNA binding domain**. The latter are of four types.

1 The leucine zipper. This is an α-helical stretch of amino acids with leucine residues at every seventh position, corresponding to every second turn of the helix. This allows pairs of helices to become enmeshed, with a splayed region at the end, believed to grip the DNA like a clothes peg.

2 The helix-loop-helix. This consists of two peptide α-helices linked by a long, flexible loop that permits their packing closely parallel to one another. They are thought to exert control by blocking other gene-regulating proteins.

3 The helix-turn-helix. This motif is a feature of the homeobox (see Chapter 42). It consists of two short α-helices separated by an amino acid sequence too short for them to lie in the same plane.

4 The zinc-finger. This is a finger-like structure comprised of around 23 amino acids held by a tetravalent zinc ion, typically linked to four cysteine residues, or two cysteines and two histidines at the base of the finger.

Tissue-specific and developmentally regulated transcription factors bind to **enhancer** or **silencer** sequences in the DNA some distance from the gene. **Co-activator** and **co-repressor** proteins bind to the transcription complex itself. However, the actual selection of genes for transcription depends not so much on these molecules as on the conformation of the chromatin (see Chapter 21).

Transcription

Like translation (Chapter 24), transcription of mRNA is also best described in three phases: **initiation**, **elongation** and **termination**.

Initiation

Transcription of a typical tissue-specific, or 'luxury', protein begins with the assembly at the TATA-box promoter of 27 polypeptide sub-units, including one molecule of **RNA polymerase II (Pol II)** and five **general transcription factors (TFIIB, D, E, F and H)**, to form a **preinitiation complex**. Factor TFIID contains the **TATA-box binding protein**, plus 11 other factors. Additional tissue-restricted transcription factors may be necessary, which attach to various sites along the DNA strand and make contact with the preinitiation complex by looping of the DNA.

Elongation

When the **basal transcription complex** is fully assembled, factor TFIIH splits the double helix at the transcription initiation site 25 bases downstream of the TATA box. This is almost always at a purine (A or G) preceding a pyrimidine (C or T). TFIIH also initiates a conformational change in Pol II by phosphorylating its protruding C-terminal domain. This then allows the polymerase to begin transcription of RNA and the complex moves downstream, rather like the slider in a zip, causing local unwinding and splitting, followed by reformation of the double helix as it proceeds and creating a 17-base long **transcription bubble**.

Using the 'antisense', or **template strand**, orientated in the 3′-5′ direction (from left to right) as a reference, Pol II grabs ribonucleotides and links them one by one to produce a complementary RNA sequence, orientated with reverse polarity (i.e. 5′ to 3′). In other words, by applying the rules of base pairing to the antisense strand it creates a precise hnRNA copy of the coding strand.

Elongation of the hnRNA requires further phosphorylation of serine residues at the Pol II C-terminus and additional **elongation factors**. Transcription then proceeds at about 20 nucleotides per second through the leader sequence of the future polypeptide, the exons, introns and trailer, and indefinitely downstream.

Termination

There seems to be no specific signal for termination of transcription of most human genes. However, the RNA transcript gets cleaved 15–30 nucleotides beyond the sequence AAUAAA and this initiates the events leading to termination. The cut in the RNA is made by a protein complex containing an exonuclease tethered by the new RNA to the basal transcription complex. A race now occurs between the exonuclease chewing up the tail of the freshly created hnRNA and the transcription complex producing more RNA. When the exonuclease catches up with the transcription complex, transcription ceases.

RNA processing

As hnRNA transcripts are synthesized, they are covalently modified, which marks them as coded messages for later translation into polypeptide. The 5′ end is first capped by addition of 7-methyl GTP in reverse orientation. When the polyadenylation site appears in the hnRNA strand, it is cleaved there and **poly-A polymerase** adds on 100–200 residues of adenylic acid to form the **poly-A tail**. Both the cap and tail probably protect the molecule from degradation, contribute to the 'passport' that allows its export to the cytoplasm and later provide a recognition signal for the ribosome, indicating its availability for translation.

On average, an hnRNA molecule may have about 7000 nucleotides which are reduced to about 1200 in the mRNA by removal of as many as 50 introns. Histone genes are exceptional in having no introns.

The ribonucleoprotein complexes that remove the introns are called **spliceosomes** and they contain several snRNA species (U1–U6), each complexed with specific proteins. U1 snRNP (i.e. ribonucleoprotein containing U1 snRNA) binds to the upstream splice site **GU** in the RNA (see Chapter 21), guided by a complementary sequence in the U1 snRNA. U2 snRNP binds to the branch site, then becomes linked to the bound U1, causing a loop in the hnRNA. U2 then cuts the hnRNA immediately upstream of GU and joins that upstream cut end of the intron to the junction site, creating a **lariat** shape. The downstream end of the intron is then cut just beyond **AG**, releasing the RNA lariat, and the spliceosome brings together and joins the two exons.

The total length of a gene relates to the time taken for its transcription, very highly expressed genes generally having short introns or none. The very long dystrophin gene takes 16 hours to be transcribed. Mitochondrial genes have no introns.

Medical issues

Alternative RNA splicing occurs normally in some transcripts, but many genetic disorders involve errors in RNA splicing. In **Gilbert syndrome** jaundice relates to insertion of TA into the normal TATAA promoter of the gene for UDP-glycosyltransferase. *Alpha-amanitin* from the death cap mushroom, *Amanita phalloides*, blocks the action of Pol II. The antibiotic, *rifampicin (rifamycin)* blocks bacterial transcription by binding to the β-subunit of the bacterial RNA polymerase; *actinomycin* intercalates between G-C pairs.

㉓ Non-coding RNA

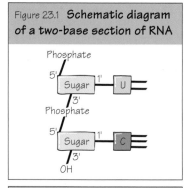

Figure 23.1 **Schematic diagram of a two-base section of RNA**

Phosphate

Phosphate

OH

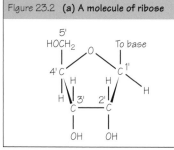

Figure 23.2 **(a) A molecule of ribose**

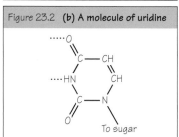

Figure 23.2 **(b) A molecule of uridine**

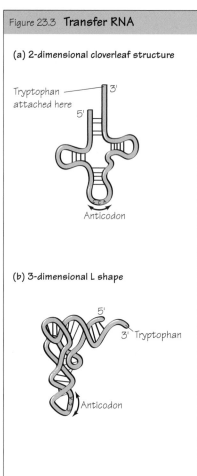

Figure 23.3 **Transfer RNA**

(a) 2-dimensional cloverleaf structure

Tryptophan attached here

Anticodon

(b) 3-dimensional L shape

Tryptophan

Anticodon

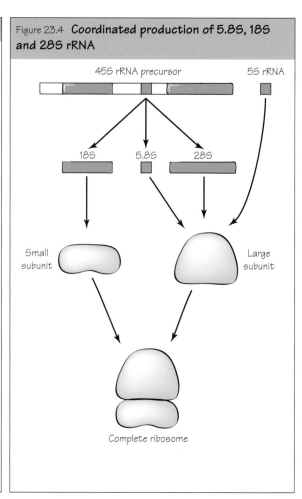

Figure 23.4 **Coordinated production of 5.8S, 18S and 28S rRNA**

45S rRNA precursor

5S rRNA

18S   5.8S   28S

Small subunit

Large subunit

Complete ribosome

Overview

In Chapter 19 we learnt that DNA is the double-stranded nucleic acid that carries the genetic information we received from our parents and which we pass on to our children. **RNA** is a similar molecule that facilitates the expression of this genetic information within our own cells. The main differences between RNA and DNA are that RNA is (usually) single-stranded, **ribose** replaces deoxyribose and **uracil** replaces thymine. In **eukaryotes** (literally organisms with a 'true nucleus', i.e. 'higher' organisms) RNA occurs as numerous types of molecule. There are **messenger RNA (mRNA)** and its precursor **heterogeneous nuclear RNA (hnRNA)**, which both carry coding information. HnRNA is characteristic of eukaryotes and is not found in **prokaryotes** (literally 'before the nucleus', e.g. bacteria and viruses). **Non-coding RNA (ncRNA)** includes **transfer RNA (tRNA)** and **ribosomal RNA (rRNA)**, both concerned with translation of mRNA-encoded data into polypeptide. **Small nuclear RNA (snRNA)** includes several species of **URNA**, so named in recognition of their high uridine content, concerned with removal of introns, **small nucleolar RNA (snoRNA)** and **small Cajal body RNA (scaRNA)** which modify bases in rRNA and spliceosomal snRNPs, respectively (see Chapter 22). The roles of **signal recognition particle RNA (srpRNA)** and **microRNA (miRNA)** are described below. Production of **mitochon-** drial RNA (mtRNA) is outlined in Chapter 12. See also the use of small interfering RNA (siRNA) in the management of genetic disease, in Chapter 74.

Heterogeneous nuclear and messenger RNA

Heterogeneous nuclear RNA and its derivative mRNA carry genetic information from the nuclear DNA into the cytoplasm.

There are as many species of hnRNA as there are functional polypeptide coding genes, hnRNA being the direct transcript of the coding sequences of the genome. It is transcribed from the DNA by the enzyme **RNA polymerase II**, or **Pol II**. Messenger RNA results from the processing of hnRNA, which includes removal of non-coding **introns** and linking together of the coding **exons** (see Chapter 22). Messenger RNA therefore carries only the coding information of the corresponding species of each hnRNA, plus the flanking leader and trailer, so is considerably shorter.

Long non-coding RNA

Long non-coding RNAs are thought to have tissue-specific regulatory roles. They include transcripts of the antisense strands of coding sequences which regulate complementary sense transcripts by base-pairing with them.

Medical Genetics at a Glance, Third Edition. Dorian J. Pritchard and Bruce R. Korf.

62 © 2013 John Wiley & Sons, Ltd. Published 2013 by John Wiley & Sons, Ltd.

Transfer RNA

Each molecule of transfer RNA consists of about 75 nucleotides linked together in a long chain which, due to internal base pairing, adopts a 'clover leaf' structure that then twists into an L shape. Transfer RNA is unusual in containing a variety of rarer bases in addition to C, G, A and U, and some of these are modified by methylation. The important feature of tRNA is that each 'charged' molecule carries an amino acid at its 3′ end, while on the middle 'leaf' of the cloverleaf structure are three characteristic bases known as the **anticodon**. The sequence of bases in the anticodon is specifically related to the species of amino acid attached to the 3′ terminus. For example, tRNA with the anticodon 5′-CCA-3′ carries the amino acid tryptophan and no other. It is this specific relationship that forms the basis of translation of the genetic message carried by mRNA (see Chapter 24).

Transfer RNA molecules are transcribed from their coding sequences in DNA by the enzyme **RNA polymerase III**, or **Pol III**. There are over 40 different tRNA subfamilies, each with several members. Mitochondrial mRNA is translated by mitochondrial tRNAs.

Ribosomal RNA

Ribosomal RNA consists of several species usually referred to by their sedimentation coefficients in Svedberg units (S), deduced by their speed of centrifugation in a dense aqueous medium.

Each **ribosome** consists of one large and one small subunit. These contain many proteins derived by translation of mRNA, plus RNA that remains untranslated. The term 'ribosomal RNA' refers to the non-translated material. The small ribosomal subunit contains **18S rRNA** and the large subunit **5S, 5.8S** and **28S rRNA**.

Ribosomal RNA is transcribed from DNA by two additional RNA polymerases. **Polymerase I (Pol I)** transcribes 5.8S, 18S and 28S, as one long **45S** transcript which is then cleaved into three sections, so ensuring they are produced in equal quantities. We each carry about 250 copies of the DNA sequence coding for the 45S transcript, per haploid genome. These are in five clusters of tandem repeats on the short arms of chromosomes 13, 14, 15, 21 and 22. These are known as the **nucleolar organizer regions**, as their transcription and the subsequent processing of the 45S transcript occurs while they are held within the nucleolus.

There are about 2000 copies of the 5S rRNA gene in at least three clusters on Chromosome 1. These are transcribed by **Pol III** outside the nucleolus and imported for **ribosome** assembly, along with ribosomal proteins.

Ribosomal RNA contains around 95 **pseudo-uridine** sites created by isomerization of uridine through the agency of snoRNA.

Small nuclear RNA

There are several categories of snRNA.
• The conversion of hnRNA into mRNA by the removal of introns occurs in the nucleus in RNA–protein complexes called **spliceosomes**. Each spliceosome has a core of three **small nuclear ribonucleoproteins** or **snRNPs** (pronounced 'snurps'). Each snRNP contains at least one snRNA and several proteins. There are several hundred different snRNAs, transcribed mainly by Pol II, which are believed to be capable of recognizing specific ribonucleic acid sequences by RNA–RNA base pairing. The most important in hnRNA processing are U1, U2, U4/U6 and U5snRNA.
• **Cajal bodies** are coiled thread-like bodies within the nucleolus. They contain **scaRNAs** involved in the maturation of spliceosomal snRNPs
• **Small nucleolar RNA** is mostly involved in directing or guiding site-specific base modifications in rRNA and snRNA, for example methylation and **pseudouridylation**.

Most snoRNAs and scaRNAs are coded within introns of protein-coding genes, so that production of mature rRNA is coupled to that of mRNA.

Signal recognition particle RNA

Signal recognition particle RNA recognizes the **signal sequence** on proteins destined for export and helps transport them across the plasma membrane (Chapter 24).

MicroRNAs

There are an estimated 200 human miRNA species, each about 22 bases long derived by ribonuclease H cleavage of double-stranded 'hairpin' RNA precursors corresponding to inverted repeats. These control translation of structural genes by binding to complementary sequences in the 3′ untranslated regions of their mRNA.

Medical issues

Patients with **systemic lupus erythematosus** have antibodies directed against their own snRNP proteins (see Chapter 66). One set of snoRNA genes on Chromosome 15q is paternally imprinted and thought to play a role in **Prader–Willi syndrome** (see Chapter 27).

24 Protein synthesis

Figure 24.1 The genetic code

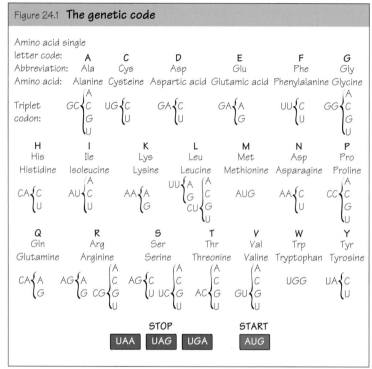

Figure 24.3 Setting of the reading frame

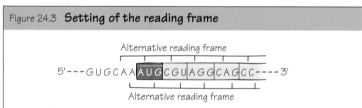

Figure 24.4 The peptidyl transferase reaction

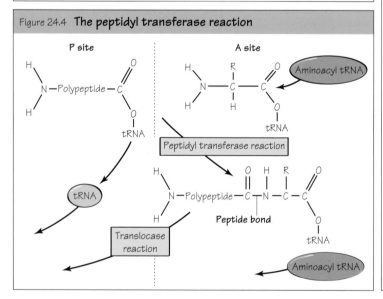

Figure 24.2 Translation

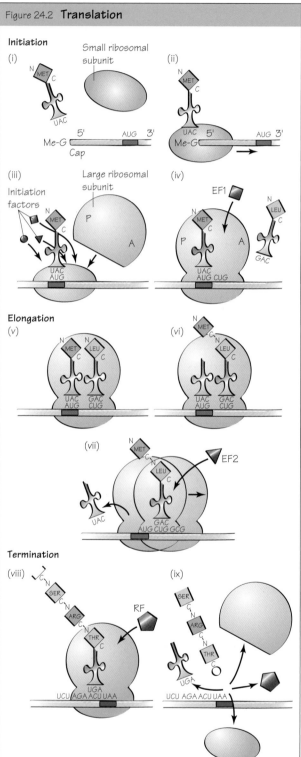

Medical Genetics at a Glance, Third Edition. Dorian J. Pritchard and Bruce R. Korf.

Overview

The main structural components of the body and most of its catalysts are **proteins**, each derived from one or more **polypeptides**. A polypeptide is a chain of amino acids, the sequence of which is determined by that of the bases in the corresponding mRNA, in accordance with 'the genetic code'. Each amino acid is represented in mRNA by one or more groups of three bases called **triplet codons**, and their interpretation as polypeptide is called **translation**. Messenger RNA is translated from the 5′ to the 3′ end within cytoplasmic **ribosomes**. The resultant polypeptides are then modified into proteins. The functional properties of proteins derive largely from the active groups they display in their tertiary and quaternary conformations.

The genetic code

Translation requires transfer RNA molecules charged with amino acids appropriate to their anticodon sequences (see Chapter 23. Some amino acids are coded by several codons, only tryptophan and methionine by one each. Three of the 64 possible threefold combinations of A, C, G and U in the mRNA represent **STOP signals**: UGA, UAG and **UAA** (see Figure 24.1). **AUG** codes for methionine and also acts as a **START signal**, simultaneously determining the amino- (or N-) terminal end of the polypeptide and selecting one of the three possible **reading frames** (see 'Setting the reading frame' in the Figure 24.3). The genetic code of mitochondria is slightly different.

Translation

Initiation

A small ribosomal subunit containing several **transcription initiation factors** and methionyl tRNA charged with methionine binds to the 5′ cap on the mRNA, then slides along until it finds and engages with the first AUG sequence. The initiation factors are then released, a large ribosomal subunit binds to the small one, and translation begins.

The large ribosomal subunit contains two sites, known as the **A site** (for aminoacyl) and the **P site** (for peptidyl). At the end of initiation the P site contains a charged met-tRNA with its anticodon engaged in the first AUG codon, while the A site is empty.

Elongation

The appropriate aminoacyl tRNA now becomes located in the A site, as dictated by the adjacent codon in the mRNA, with the help of a soluble **elongation factor** called **EF1**. The **peptidyl transferase reaction** then creates a **peptide bond** between the amino ($-NH_2$) group of the amino acid at the A site and the carboxyl ($-COOH$) group of that at the P site, while the first tRNA is released.

The **translocase reaction** next promotes expulsion of the uncharged tRNA, moves the ribosome three bases along and translocates the growing peptide from A to P. This requires **elongation factor, EF2**.

Mitochondrial mRNAs are translated by mitochondria-specific tRNAs (Chapter 12).

Termination

Elongation continues until a **STOP** codon enters the ribosome, all three being recognized by a single multivalent **release factor** **(RF)**. This modifies the specificity of peptidyl transferase so that a molecule of water is added to the peptide instead. The ribosome is then released and dissociates into its subunits, so freeing the completed polypeptide.

Synthesis of an average polypeptide of 400 amino acids takes about 20 seconds.

As each ribosome vacates the messenger cap another attaches and follows its predecessor, creating a **polyribosome** or **polysome**. The mRNA usually survives for a few hours.

Protein structure

The amino acid sequence of a polypeptide defines its **primary structure**. The **secondary structure** is the three-dimensional form of parts of the polypeptide: the **α-helix**, the **collagen pro-α helix**, or the **β-pleated sheet**.

Tertiary structure is the folded form of the whole polypeptide, composed of different secondary structures.

Quaternary structure is the final native conformation of a multimeric protein, for example **haemoglobin** is composed of two **α-globin** monomers, **two β-globin** monomers, one molecule of **haem** and an atom of ferrous iron. **Collagen fibres** are cables of many triple-helices, each formed as a rope of three pro-α helices.

Structure is frequently maintained by **disulphide bridges** between cysteine residues on adjacent strands, while enzymic properties depend on the distribution of charged groups.

Post-translational modification

Post-translational modification includes removal of the N-terminal methionine and cleavage. Association occurs between similar or different polypeptides, or with **prosthetic groups** such as haem.

Polypeptides destined for extracellular secretion are first **glycosylated** in the rough endoplasmic reticulum and Golgi apparatus. Their selection involves a **signal peptide** near the N terminus that binds to a cytoplasmic **signal recognition particle** consisting of cytoplasmic **srpRNA** and six specific proteins. This links them to a receptor in the membrane of the endoplasmic reticulum. As it is synthesized the polypeptide is transferred through the membrane; when its carboxyl terminus emerges the signal peptide is cleaved off. Polypeptides are transported to the Golgi apparatus in vesicles that bud off the endoplasmic reticulum (see Chapter 14).

Glycosylation is usually **N-linked**, involving addition of a common oligosaccharide to the side chain $-NH_2$ group of asparagine, as in the production of **antibodies** and **lysozymes**. **O-linked** oligosaccharides are attached to the -OH group on the side chain of serine, threonine or hydroxylysine, as with *secreted* ABO blood group antigens.

Other modifications include **hydroxylation** of lysine and proline, important in creation of the collagen pro-α helix, **sulphation** of tyrosine, as a signal for compartmentalization and **lipidation** of cysteine and glycine residues, necessary for anchoring them to phospholipid membranes. **Acetylation** of lysine in histone H4 modifies its binding to DNA. Protein kinases **phosphorylate** serine and tyrosine residues and can regulate enzymic properties, as in the **proto-oncogene signal transduction cascade** (see Chapter 54).

Medical issues

I-cell disease is due to deficiency in glycosylation of lysozymes. *Ricin* from castor beans blocks elongation factor EF2; diphtheria toxin blocks translocase.

Many antibiotics target translation specifically *in prokaryotes.* These include *erythromycin*, which disrupts translocase, *chloramphenicol*, which interferes with peptidyl transferase, *tetracycline*, which prevents binding of aminoacyl tRNAs, *puromycin*, which mimics an aminoacyl tRNA and *streptomycin*, which binds to the small ribosomal subunit. Human mitochondria have an evolutionary affinity with bacteria and some antibiotics interfere with mitochondrial function (see Chapter 12).

25 Types of genetic alterations

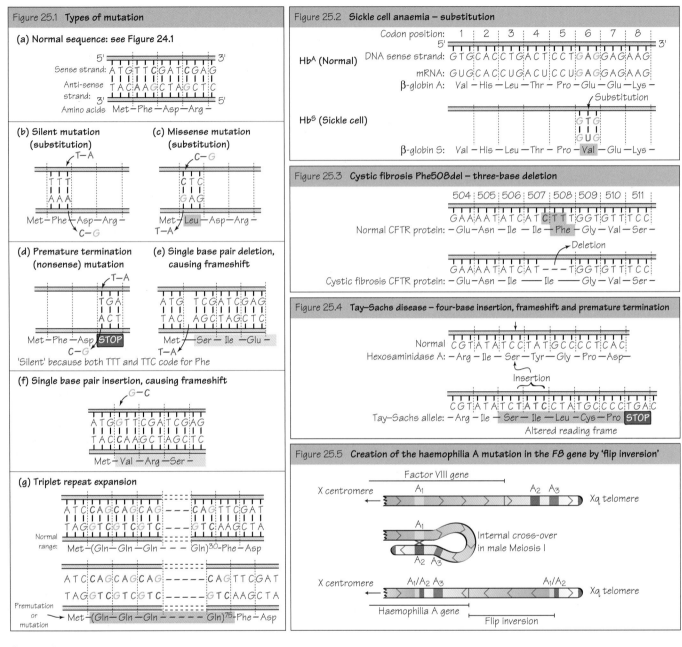

Figure 25.1 Types of mutation

(a) Normal sequence: see Figure 24.1

(b) Silent mutation (substitution)

(c) Missense mutation (substitution)

(d) Premature termination (nonsense) mutation

(e) Single base pair deletion, causing frameshift

'Silent' because both TTT and TTC code for Phe

(f) Single base pair insertion, causing frameshift

(g) Triplet repeat expansion

Figure 25.2 Sickle cell anaemia – substitution

Figure 25.3 Cystic fibrosis Phe508del – three-base deletion

Figure 25.4 Tay–Sachs disease – four-base insertion, frameshift and premature termination

Figure 25.5 Creation of the haemophilia A mutation in the F8 gene by 'flip inversion'

Overview

Mutations are permanent modifications in the base sequence of DNA. They can occur at the level of one or a few bases of DNA, as point mutations involving substitution, deletion or insertion. Substitution of a purine by another purine or of a pyrimidine by another primidine is a **transition**, exchanges of purines and pyrimidines are **transversions**. At the level of a gene, mutations involve dozens to thousands of bases. At the genomic level mutations include deletions or duplications of hundreds of thousands to millions of bases, up to chromosome rearrangements and aneuploidies (Chapter 36). **Copy number variation** (CNV) involves large deletions and insertions of various lengths created by **unequal crossing over** between misaligned segments of repetitive DNA or by non-homologous end-joining. Unequal

crossing over is the origin of X-linked anomalous colour vision (see Chapter 11).

Activation of enhancers and silencers (Chapter 21) can cause phenotypic variation in expression of the genes they control.

Dynamic mutations involve expansion of **triplet repeat sequences** (see Chapter 28), and can undergo further expansion or contraction from generation to generation.

Substitutions, deletions, insertions, frameshifts and duplications

Substitution involves replacement of a base pair. If the amino acid encoded by the new codon is the same, it is a **silent mutation**, or if different, a **missense mutation** (see Figures 25.1, 24.1). Some mis-

Medical Genetics at a Glance, Third Edition. Dorian J. Pritchard and Bruce R. Korf.

sense mutations do not alter the chemical properties of the protein (**conservative mutations**), whereas others have a deleterious effect. In some cases, though, heterozygosity of a deleterious mutation may create selective advantage. A notable example is the substitution of the sixth codon in the β-globin chain responsible for sickle cell anaemia (see Chapter 29), which in heterozygotes confers resistance to malaria.

Substitution can create a STOP codon, causing translation to come to a premature halt. This is called a **premature termination** or **nonsense** ('non-sense') **mutation**.

If a deleted or inserted segment is of other than a multiple of three bases, the translational reading frame is disrupted in a **frameshift mutation**. This causes the protein produced to be entirely erroneous 'downstream' (3′) of the deletion. The most common mutation causing **Tay–Sachs disease** (see Chapter 6) is a four-base insertion causing a frameshift and leading to premature termination, so that no functional **hexosaminidase A** is synthesized.

Duplications of whole genes can lead to disease, for example Charcot–Marie–Tooth disease. This is a peripheral nervous system disease involving progressive degeneration of peripheral nerves, leading to atrophy of distal limb muscles. It can be caused by a variety of types of mutation, but about 70% have a large duplication of chromosome 17 that includes the gene *PMP22*, encoding a peripheral myelin protein. This contributes to demyelination, whereas deletion of the same region causes a paralytic response to pressure (**hereditary neuropathy with predisposition to pressure palsies**).

Copy number variation
CNV involves amplification or deletion of a large segment of DNA. It is associated with many pathologies and sometimes distinguishes the genomes of MZ twins (Chapter 53).

Transcriptional control
Mutations in enhancer and silencer sequences can have quantitative effects by inhibiting binding of RNA polymerase or transcription factors, as in the **Factor IX** gene 5′ region, causing **haemophilia B**.

RNA processing
Splicing mutants either directly affect hnRNA donor or acceptor sites (see Chapter 22), or activate cryptic competitive splice sites in introns or exons. The acceptor sequence at the end of the first intron of β-globin is UUAGGCU (actually UUAG, plus additional 5′ bases), while within that intron is a sequence that differs by two bases: UUGGUCU. In some β-thalassaemia patients this is modified to UUAGUCU. This differs by only one base from the normal acceptor and gets misidentified as such, the hnRNA is cut in the wrong place and the resultant messenger retains some intron bases. This in turn introduces a frameshift, causing 'CUU AGG' to be read as '-CU **UAG** G-'. Translation ceases prematurely because UAG is a STOP signal, resulting in **β+ thalassaemia** (see below). Because some normal splicing may also occur, some β-globin may still be produced.

In one RNA processing mutation an A-to-C transition of the first nucleotide of the β-globin messenger inhibits capping, while in another, substitution of U by C in the trailer sequence AAUAAA inhibits polyadenylation (see Chapter 22). Both fail to suppress normal rapid degradation of the messenger RNA.

Mobile elements
SINE and Alu DNA repeats (see Chapter 19) can propagate independently and insert at other locations, causing frameshift mutations. This

has caused isolated cases of neurofibromatosis, Duchenne MD, β-thalassaemia, breast cancer, familial polyposis coli and haemophilia.

Haemoglobinopathies
The thalassaemias are collectively the most common single-gene disorder, involving reduced level of synthesis of either the α-, or β-globin chain (see Chapter 29). In the absence of a complementary chain with which to form the haemoglobin tetramer (α2β2), the chain produced at the normal rate is in relative excess and precipitates out in the red cells leading to their premature destruction.

There are at least 80 different **beta-thalassaemia** alleles, in addition to the RNA splicing error above (see Table 29.2). Most of these are point mutations and most patients are '**compound homozygotes**', with two *different* deficient alleles. Carriers of one β-thalassaemia allele have mild anaemia and are said to have **thalassaemia minor**. If no β-globin is present, the condition is **thalassaemia major**. β-globin mutations that lead to complete absence of β-globin production are referred to as β⁰ thalassaemia mutations; those compatible with some β-globin production, such as splicing mutations, are referred to as β⁺ mutations.

In **hereditary persistence of fetal haemoglobin**, the β-globin gene has been deleted and the neighbouring γ-globin gene responsible for **fetal haemoglobin** (α2γ2), remains transcriptionally active at a high level after birth.

α-Globin is coded by *two pairs* of genes per diploid genome. In the 'heterozygous' state, called **alpha-thalassaemia trait**, there are two mutant and two normal genes; either −α/−α, or − −/αα (see Table 28.1). The latter is relatively common in South-East Asia and gives rise to completely α-globin deficient homozygotes (− −/− −) with **hydrops foetalis**. The (−α) haplotype is relatively common among Melanesians, having been selected by malaria (see Chapter 29).

In **Haemoglobin Constant Spring** the UAA α-globin STOP codon is mutated to CAA, coding for glutamine, and translation continues for a further 31 frames to another STOP. The mutant mRNA is unstable, causing mild α-thalassaemia.

Haemophilia A
Fifty percent of severe cases of haemophilia A (i.e. with <1% Factor VIII activity) involve a novel mutation called a **flip inversion**. This occurs as a consequence of two unusual conditions: (1) the existence of several copies of a small gene called *A* located near the Xq telomere, plus another within intron 22 of the *F8* gene; and (2) the fact that the long arm of the X has no pairing homologue in male meiosis. As a consequence, internal recombination sometimes occurs following looping back of the end of the X. Breakage and rejoining within the *A* genes causes inversion of the intervening segment of the *F8* gene (see Figure 25.5).

Nomenclature of mutations
Mutations are named by conventional abbreviations and may be described by the change at the DNA or protein level. For example, the most common mutation responsible for cystic fibrosis (see Chapter 6) is a deletion of three bases that encode phenylalanine in the coding sequence of the gene for the '**cystic fibrosis trans-membrane regulator**' (**CFTR**), usually referred to as **Phe508del**. This is designated c.1521_1523delCTT at the cDNA level (hence the 'c.') and p.Phe508del at the protein level (hence the 'p.'). The **Gly380Arg** achondroplasia mutation denotes a substitution of glycine by arginine at amino acid 380 within the *FGFR3* gene (see Chapter 5).

26 Mutagenesis and DNA repair

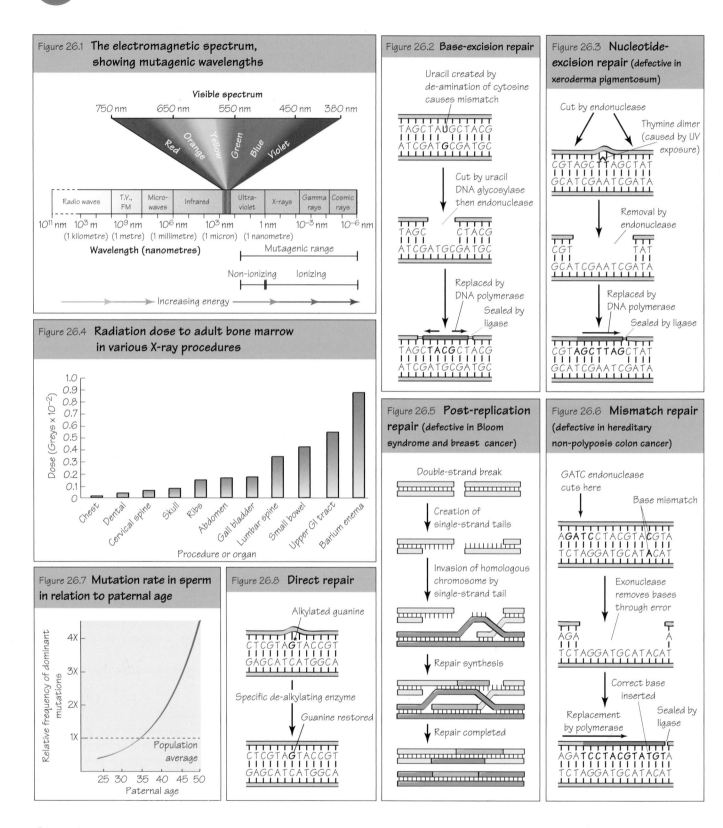

Figure 26.1 **The electromagnetic spectrum, showing mutagenic wavelengths**

Figure 26.2 **Base-excision repair**

Figure 26.3 **Nucleotide-excision repair (defective in xeroderma pigmentosum)**

Figure 26.4 **Radiation dose to adult bone marrow in various X-ray procedures**

Figure 26.5 **Post-replication repair (defective in Bloom syndrome and breast cancer)**

Figure 26.6 **Mismatch repair (defective in hereditary non-polyposis colon cancer)**

Figure 26.7 **Mutation rate in sperm in relation to paternal age**

Figure 26.8 **Direct repair**

Overview

Apart from the effects of ultraviolet (UV) light, mutagenesis of the DNA in somatic cells is no different from that in the germline. Some is **spontaneous**, caused by a base adopting a variant molecular form or **tautomer** during DNA replication; many are initiated by chemicals and 10–15% by radiation. For the **natural mutation rate**, see Chapter 4.

Medical Genetics at a Glance, Third Edition. Dorian J. Pritchard and Bruce R. Korf.

Chemical mutagenesis

Environmental **mutagens** include constituents of smoke, paints, petrochemicals, pesticides, dyes, foodstuffs, drugs, etc. Examples of the major categories are given below. The principal means of exposure are inhalation, skin absorption and ingestion. **Promutagens**, such as *nitrates* and *nitrites* are converted into mutagens by body chemistry.

1 Base analogues. *2-amino-purine* is incorporated into DNA in place of adenine, but pairs as cytosine, causing a substitution of thymine by guanine in the partner strand. *5-bromouracil* (5-BU) is incorporated as thymine, but can undergo a tautomeric shift to resemble cytosine, resulting in a transition from T-A to C-G.

2 Chemical modifiers. *Nitrous acid* converts cytosine to uracil, and adenine to hypoxanthine, a precursor of guanine. *Alkylating agents* modify bases by donating alkyl- groups.

3 Intercalating agents. The antiseptic *proflavine* and the *acridine dyes* become inserted between adjacent base pairs, producing distortions in the DNA that lead to deletions and additions.

4 Other. Cytosine adjacent to guanine (referred to as 'CpG'; see Chapter 21) is prone to methylation by methyltransferase enzymes to 5-methylcytosine which is unstable and prone to deamination to thymine. Thus CpG pairs tend to undergo transition to TpA, despite scrutiny by the DNA repair enzymes.

A wide range of chemicals cause DNA **strand breakage** and **cross-linking**.

Electromagnetic radiation

Particulate discharge from radioactive decay includes alpha-particles (helium nuclei), beta-particles (electrons) and gamma-rays. The mutagenicity of subatomic particles depends on their speed, mass and electric charge.

The energy and mutagenicity of electromagnetic radiation increases with decreasing wavelength. All radiation beyond UV causes ionization by knocking electrons out of their orbits.

Ultraviolet light

UV light is the non-visible, short wavelength fraction of sunlight responsible for tanning. It exerts a mutagenic effect by causing **dimerization** (linking) of adjacent pyrimidine residues, mainly T-T (but also T-C and C-C). It does not cause germline mutations, but is a major cause of skin cancer, especially in homozygotes for the red hair allele (see Chapter 3), who have white, freckled skin. Their phaeomelanin pigment provides a poor sun screen and releases free radicals on UV exposure.

Most UV radiation from the sun is blocked by a layer of ozone in the upper atmosphere, currently in danger of destruction by industrial *fluorocarbons*.

Atomic radiation

1 Natural background radiation. This varies with local geology. The most abundant radioisotopes are Potassium-40 and Radon-222 gas. Radon contributes 55% of all natural background radiation and may be responsible for 2500 deaths per annum in the UK.

2 Cosmic rays. These present a major theoretical hazard for aircrews, as their intensity increases with altitude. Exposure during a return flight between England and Spain is said to equal five chest X-rays.

3 Man-made radiation. This includes fallout from nuclear testing and power stations. Radiation workers are at particular risk and periosteum-seeking isotopes present a major risk of leukaemia.

4 X-rays. X-rays account for 60% of man-made and 11% of total radiation exposure. They mutagenize DNA either directly by ionizing impact, or indirectly by creating highly reactive **free radicals** that impinge on the DNA. These can be carried in the bloodstream and harm cells not directly exposed.

Biological effects of radiation

Electromagnetic radiation damages proteins and above 1 **gray** kills cells. (One gray, abbreviated **Gy**, is the amount of radiation that causes 1 kg of tissue to absorb 1 joule of energy.) At the chromosomal level it causes **major deletions**, **translocations** and **aneuploidy** (see Table 73.1). It causes **single-** and **double-strand breaks** in DNA and **base pair destruction**. X-rays damage chromosomes most readily when they are condensed, which is why they are most harmful to dividing cells, including the progenitors of sperm. The offspring of older men have a many-fold risk of genetic disease, as the DNA in their sperm has been copied many times (see Figure 26.7). The high testicular temperature caused by clothing (6°C above unclothed) also contributes to the present mutation rate in human sperm.

For the first 7 days of life the embryo is ultrasensitive to the mutagenic and lethal effects of X-rays; over weeks 2–7 teratogenic effects come to the fore. Childhood leukaemia can be induced by exposure at gestational weeks 8 to 40.

At 1 Gy, X-rays cause a 50% reduction in white blood cell count, while whole-body irradiation of 4.5 Gy kills 50% of people. Therapeutic doses of up to 10 Gy are used against cancer cells. Radiation damage is cumulative and there is no lower baseline of effect.

Safety measures when using X-rays

1 *Patients' previous X-ray exposure should be reviewed before requesting further X-rays.*

2 *The '28-day rule': a woman of child-bearing age should be X-rayed only if she has had a period within the last 28 days.*

3 *The '10-day rule': for high-radiation-dose procedures such as abdominal or pelvic computed tomography (CAT scan) and barium enema, the examination should be postponed to the first 10 days of the menstrual cycle.*

DNA repair

Apart from direct repair, all the DNA repair systems in human cells require **exonucleases**, **endonucleases** (defective in **Cocayne syndrome**), **polymerases** and **ligases**. **Ataxia telangiectasia** and **Fanconi anaemia** patients have defects in DNA damage detection and are extremely sensitive to X-rays.

1 Direct repair: A specific enzyme reverses the damage, for example by de-alkylation of alkylated guanine.

2 Base-excision repair. The damaged base, plus a few others on either side, are removed by cutting the sugar–phosphate backbone and the gap filled by re-synthesis directed by the intact strand.

3 Nucleotide excision repair. This removes **thymine dimers** and chemically modified bases over a longer stretch of DNA. Defects cause **xeroderma pigmentosum**.

4 Mismatch repair. This corrects base mismatches due to errors at DNA replication and involves nicking the faulty strand at the nearest GATC base sequence. Defects occur in **hereditary non-polyposis colon cancer**. The genes involved are sometimes called '**mutator genes**'.

5 Postreplication repair. This corrects double-strand breaks either unguided, or by using the homologous chromosome as a template. Defects include **Bloom syndrome** (a '**chromosome breakage syndrome**'), **breast cancer** and possibly **prostate cancer**.

Figure 27.1 (a) Prader–Willi syndrome

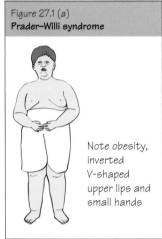

Note obesity, inverted V-shaped upper lips and small hands

Figure 27.1 (b) Angelman syndrome

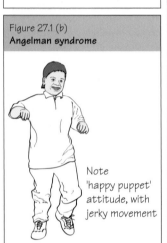

Note 'happy puppet' attitude, with jerky movement

Figure 27.2 Causation of Prader–Willi and Angelman syndromes

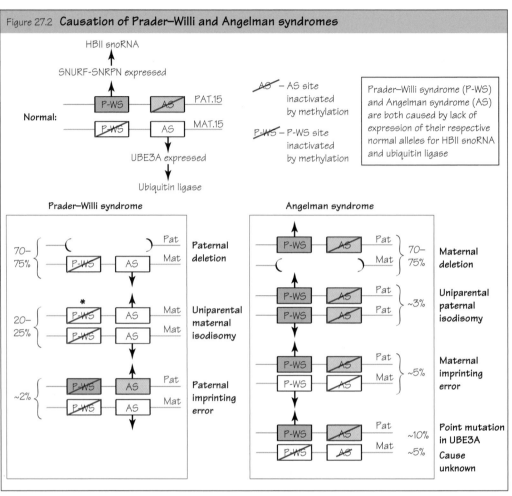

Figure 27.3 The imprinted gene cluster at 15q11-q13 deleted in some cases of Prader-Willi and Angelman syndromes

(a) PAT, MAT: paternally and maternally imprinted chromosomes in normal brain cells. The blocks represent structural genes and the vertical arrows their expression. Two genes are expressed from both chromosomes.
IC: Imprinting Control Centre.
Differential patterns of imprinting in paternal and maternal chromosomes are indicated by blue and red colouration, established by appropriate activities of the differentially activated ICs.

(b) Enlarged representation of the critical region, showing the imprinting control centre (IC), gene UBE3A and multiple exons of the SNURF-SNRPN transcription unit, with HBII sequences in its introns indicated in green.

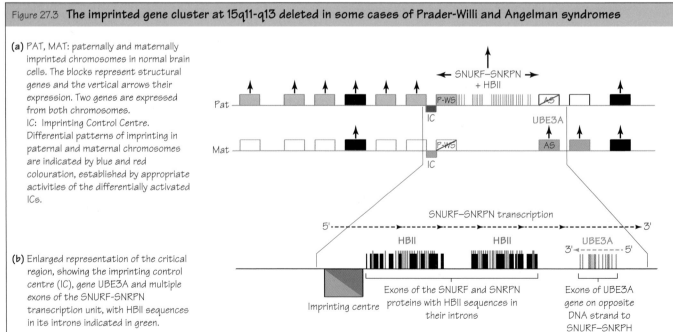

Medical Genetics at a Glance, Third Edition. Dorian J. Pritchard and Bruce R. Korf.

Overview

During gametogenesis several hundred genes receive 'genomic imprinting' that normally ensures later expression of *only one* of their two inherited alleles. In contradiction of Mendel's laws, mutations of such genes can cause dramatically different disorders depending on whether they were inherited from the mother or the father. Three conditions are of particular importance in this regard: **Angelman syndrome (AS)**, **Prader–Willi syndrome (P-WS)** and **Beckwith–Wiedemann syndrome**.

The mechanism of imprinting is probably unique for each imprinted chromosomal region. In the case of P-WS and AS there is a '**critical region**' on the long arm of Chromosome 15 that includes the Prader–Willi and Angelman sites. Here some genes are normally transcriptionally active only on the paternal chromosomal homologue, others only on the maternal. The main mechanism of this differential activation/deactivation is methylation of CpG sequences in the DNA (see Chapter 21). Imprinting is affected by pathological deletions, duplications, mutations in imprinting control elements and epigenetic modification.

Genomic imprinting has some similarities with X-chromosome inactivation, when one X-chromosome in every female body cell becomes irreversibly inactivated by CpG methylation (see Chapters 10, 38 and 43). In both cases imposed methylation patterns are maintained through mitosis by the action of **maintenance methylase**.

Genomic imprinting is a significant factor in **assisted reproduction**, as the incidence of imprinting disorders increases after use of *in vitro* **fertilization** and **intracytoplasmic sperm injection** (**ICSI**; see Chapter 71).

Prader–Willi and Angelman syndromes (P-WS and AS)

Overall frequency 1/10 000 to 1/25 000 for each disorder.

Features Prader–Willi syndrome is characterized by short stature, hypotonia, compulsive eating, obesity, small hands and feet, hypogonadism and *mild-to-moderate* neurodevelopmental delay. Angelman syndrome exhibits epilepsy, *severe* neurodevelopmental delay, uncoordinated movements and compulsive laughter.

Genetics Both conditions are associated with visible deletion or microdeletion of a region on the long arm of Chromosome 15 (15q11-q13; see Chapter 35), but in some cases, although the same chromosomal region is implicated, the cause of disease is more obscure.

Taken together, 50–60% of patients have a visible deletion and 15% a submicroscopic deletion at 15q11-13. Most of the others have no obvious damage to Chromosome 15, but instead both copies of the long arm of Chromosome 15 appear to have come from the same parent, described as **uniparental isodisomy**. A third, minor category have mutations within neighbouring DNA.

When PW-S is associated with deletion of 15q (as in 70–75% of cases)*, it is always the paternal homologue that is deleted* and when PW-S is associated with uniparental isodisomy *it is always the maternal chromosomal segment that is disomic*, the paternal copy being absent. By contrast, among AS patients, some 70% have deletion of *the maternal homologue*, while in a further 3% there is *paternal* uniparental isodisomy of 15q. Many of the non-deletion cases of AS instead have a mutation in the gene *UBE3A* and a small percentage of both AS and P-WS patients have a deletion in the so-called **imprinting centre (IC)**.

Aetiology The explanation is that during spermatogenesis and oogenesis, sequences within the IC, at around 15q12, receive differential inactivation by CpG methylation, the imprinting pattern in oocytes being opposite to that in sperm. These ICs then impose differential methylation patterns on neighbouring sequences, subsequently causing their selective activation or silencing in brain cells of the offspring. In other tissues the same sequences are expressed biallelically, that is in this case imprinting is a feature of brain cell cytodifferentiation. Mutations of the IC result in erroneous methylation patterns.

For normal brain function one copy of a long sequence called ***SNURF-SNRPN*** must be transcribed and one copy of the sequence ***UBE3A*** must be expressed as the protein **ubiquitin ligase**. The exons of the *SNURF-SNRPN* gene encode those two proteins, but further key components are within the introns. These are six different species of snoRNA (see Chapter 23) called **HB11** that are released when the primary transcript is processed to create the two mRNAs. These snoRNAs probably control RNA processing at downstream loci.

Remarkably, the *UBE3A* and *SNURF-SNRPN* sequences overlap, but are on opposite strands of the same DNA and so are transcribed in opposite directions. This complex control system probably arose as a solution to the problem of how essential products could both be supplied from genes that happened to have evolved on opposite strands of the same DNA.

The *SNURF-SNRPN* locus contains at least 148 exons, but only the first 10 encode the SNURF and SNRPN proteins. The HB11 snoRNAs are released only when the transcript is processed and it is lack of these snoRNAs that causes PW-S.

Gene *UBE3A* is transcribed from the 3′ end of the *SNURF-SNRPN* transcription unit, but from the 'antisense' strand (with respect to the SNURF and SNRPN 'sense' sequence) and only from the maternally imprinted chromosome. Lack of the *UBE3A* product, ubiquitin ligase, causes AS.

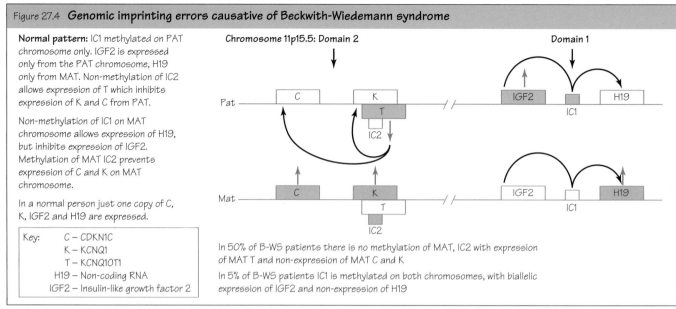

Figure 27.4 Genomic imprinting errors causative of Beckwith-Wiedemann syndrome

Normal pattern: IC1 methylated on PAT chromosome only. IGF2 is expressed only from the PAT chromosome, H19 only from MAT. Non-methylation of IC2 allows expression of T which inhibits expression of K and C from PAT.

Non-methylation of IC1 on MAT chromosome allows expression of H19, but inhibits expression of IGF2. Methylation of MAT IC2 prevents expression of C and K on MAT chromosome.

In a normal person just one copy of C, K, IGF2 and H19 are expressed.

Key:
C – CDKN1C
K – KCNQ1
T – KCNQ1OT1
H19 – Non-coding RNA
IGF2 – Insulin-like growth factor 2

Chromosome 11p15.5: Domain 2

Domain 1

In 50% of B-WS patients there is no methylation of MAT, IC2 with expression of MAT T and non-expression of MAT C and K

In 5% of B-WS patients IC1 is methylated on both chromosomes, with biallelic expression of IGF2 and non-expression of H19

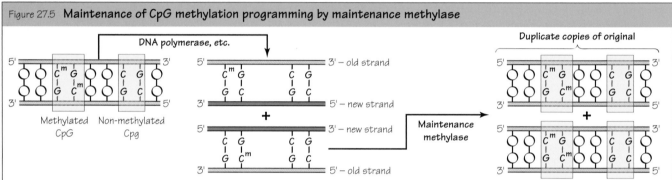

Figure 27.5 Maintenance of CpG methylation programming by maintenance methylase

Methylated CpG   Non-methylated CpG

DNA polymerase, etc.

3' – old strand
5' – new strand
+
3' – new strand
5' – old strand

Maintenance methylase

Duplicate copies of original

+

Beckwith–Wiedemann syndrome (B-WS)
Frequency 1/13 700

Genetics AD; 11p15.5. Family transmission occurs in ~15% of cases, high recurrence risks being associated with specific genetic errors. A notable feature is that discordantly affected MZ twins show a dramatic excess of females, usually showing loss of methylation of IC2.

Features Fetuses are large for gestational age, with excess amniotic fluid (**polyhydramnios**), protrusion of the umbilicus (**omphalocoele**), asymmetric limb length, prominent eyes, enlarged internal organs, facial haemangioma and a predisposition to embryonal tumours. A large, protruding tongue can cause orthodontic, breathing and speech problems.

Aetiology Imprinting Centre 1 (IC1) occurs within Domain 1 and IC2 in Domain 2. On the maternal chromosome IC1 is normally unmethylated, allowing expression of non-coding sequence *H19*, but not of **insulin-like growth factor 2** (*IGF2*); on the paternal chromosome methylation of IC1 switches *H19* off and *IGF2* on.

IC2 spans the promoter of a controlling sequence (designated T in Figure 27.4) which prevents expression of structural genes in *cis* conformation, but on the opposite strand of the same DNA (C and K in diagram). On the paternal chromosome IC2 is normally unmethylated, allowing expression of T and preventing expression of C and K, whereas the reverse applies to the maternal homologue.

In 75–80% of B-WS patients there is deregulation involving parent-of-origin-specific duplications, inversions, microdeletions, uniparental disomy, mutations in structural genes or abnormal loss or gain of methylation at IC1 or IC2. The main error involves defective imprinting of IC1, with abnormally high levels of IGF2 causing overgrowth of certain features. About 20% of patients have childhood tumours (notably Wilms kidney tumours), associated with uniparental 11p isodisomy or abnormal control of *H19* expression.

▶ Problems requiring immediate attention

Umbilical abnormalities, neonatal hypoglycaemia, breathing and feeding problems due to large tongue.

Maintenance methylase
The acquisition of tissue-related differentiated genetic programming (**cytodifferentiation**) during normal embryogenesis depends on methylation of CpG sequences at critical sites. This is accomplished by DNA methyl transferases that act on initially unmodified 5′-CpG-3′ sequences partnered to similar sequences on the opposite strand, creating symmetrical pairs of 5′-C(Me)pG-3′. Following each round of mitosis, the DNA in the daughter cells is initially methylated on only one strand. Symmetrical methylation is restored by a 'maintenance methylase' enzyme that scans the new DNA strand for hemimethylated CpGs and converts them into their fully methylated counterparts, so maintaining the correct genetic programme for that cell type.

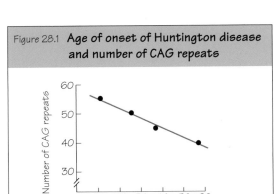

Figure 28.1 **Age of onset of Huntington disease and number of CAG repeats**

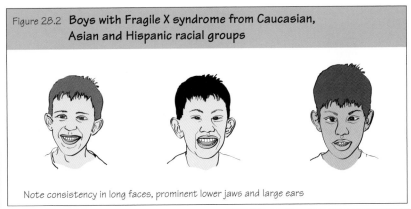

Figure 28.2 **Boys with Fragile X syndrome from Caucasian, Asian and Hispanic racial groups**

Note consistency in long faces, prominent lower jaws and large ears

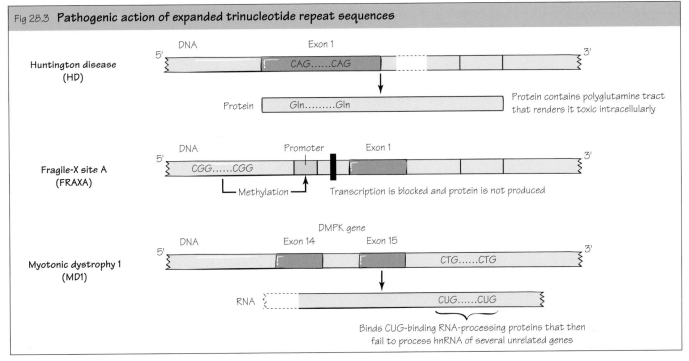

Fig 28.3 **Pathogenic action of expanded trinucleotide repeat sequences**

Overview

Dynamic mutation refers notably to the progressive expansion of 'trinucleotide repeats', or 'triplet repeats'. There are close to 20 diseases associated with mutations of this type falling into two physiological categories (Table 28.1). In these conditions symptoms often become more severe generation by generation, or appear at progressively younger ages, the latter called **anticipation**.

Trinucleotide expansion is pathogenic for different reasons, depending on where in the gene the abnormality is located. In Huntington disease it is in an exon and leads to a protein that tends to aggregate and is toxic to neurons. In fragile X-A the repeat in the upstream untranslated region (5′ UTR) triggers abnormal methylation of the promoter, blocking transcription. In myotonic dystrophy 1 a CUG repeat in the hnRNA trailer sequesters RNA processing proteins.

The triplet repeat disorders

Two of the best examples of dynamic mutation are **Huntington disease** (**HD**) and **myotonic dystrophy** (**MD**), both of which show anticipation. MD provides examples of three additional genetic principles: **pleiotropy** (see also Marfan syndrome, Chapter 5), **locus heterogeneity** and **meiotic drive**.

Huntington disease (HD); Huntington's chorea (See Table 28.2.)

Genetics AD; 4p16.3; shows anticipation *when transmitted paternally*.

Gene product huntingtin.

Frequency 1/10 000–20 000 Caucasians.

Features Slowly progressive neuronal death, characteristic 'choreic' movements (involuntary jerky movements of arms, legs, face, etc.); gait becomes unsteady and speech unclear. There is insidious impairment of intellectual function and psychiatric disturbance culminating in dementia. Advanced patients have difficulty swallowing, and generally die of pneumonia, cardiorespiratory failure, subdural haematoma after head trauma, or suicide. The average age of onset is 41 years and the mean duration of illness 15 years. Five to 10% of cases present before 20 years

Medical Genetics at a Glance, Third Edition. Dorian J. Pritchard and Bruce R. Korf.
© 2013 John Wiley & Sons, Ltd. Published 2013 by John Wiley & Sons, Ltd.

Table 28.1 Diseases caused by expansion of repeat sequences. Category 1 involves trinucleotide repeats; in Category 2 units of other numbers of nucleotides are also involved.

Disorder	Repeat unit	Normal range	Disease range	Anticipation	Parent*	Sequence
Category 1: Neurological/neuromuscular						
Huntington disease and most of the **cerebellar ataxias**, etc. (the polyglutamine tract disorders)	CAG	6–35	21–220	Yes	Father	Coding
Cleidocranial dysplasia (a polyalanine tract disorder, GC–), etc.	G – –	5–15	6–25	No	Unknown	Coding
Category 2: Neurological and muscular						
MD1, MD2, FRAX A, **FRAX E**, Friedreich ataxia, two of the cerebellar ataxias, etc.	Various	5–75	30–11 000	Yes	Mother	Non-coding

*Parent in which repeat expansion occurs.

Table 28.2 Huntington disease (HD) phenotypes.

Phenotype	No. of CAG repeats	Features
Normal	<26	Stable throughout meiosis
Normal	27–35	'Premutation' unstable in paternal meiosis
Reduced penetrance HD	36–39	Late onset or non-penetrance
Full penetrance HD	>40	Symptoms from average age 41 years
Juvenile-onset HD	>55	Symptoms before age 20 years

with rigidity, slow clumsiness and early progressive dementia, often with epileptic seizures. Eighty per cent of juvenile-onset HD cases show paternal transmission and these have especially long repeat series.

Aetiology The huntingtin gene contains a highly polymorphic **CAG** trinucleotide repeat series in an exon near the 5′ end. In most patients this is abnormally expanded, possibly due to slippage of DNA polymerase during spermatogenesis. In the mRNA, CAG codes for glutamine and the expansion is expressed in the protein as a poly-glutamine repeat. This affects the solubility of the huntingtin protein, causing it to precipitate out within and near neuronal nuclei, especially in the corpus striatum. Cleavage of the protein aggregate by the **apoptosis** enzyme **caspase** creates a toxic product that kills the cells, causing late-onset neurodegenerative disease.

HD is the prototype of a well-defined group of **polyglutamine tract diseases** which includes several of the **spinocerebellar ataxias** and **Kennedy disease**.

Management Development of HD can be monitored by magnetic resonance imaging (MRI). Treatment is with medications to control choreic movements, antipsychotic drugs and antidepressants. Caspase-specific inhibitors may be beneficial.

Fragile X disease A (FRAX-A) (Table 28.3)

FRAX-A involves repeats of **CGG** at Xq27.3, in the 5′ UTR of the *FMR-1* gene, where it triggers abnormal methylation of the promoter, blocks transcription and leads to intellectual disability, etc. (see Chapter 10). With >200 repeats the X chromosome tends to break when cells are cultured in folic acid-deficient medium, which is the origin of the name 'fragile X'.

Myotonic dystrophy type 1 (MD1) (Table 28.4)

Frequency 1/8000
Genetics AD, 19q13.3

Table 28.3 Fragile X disease A (FRAX-A) phenotypes.

	No. of repeats	Phenotypes
Male phenotype		
Normal	10–50	Normal
Premutation	50–200	Transmitting male; at risk for fragile X ataxia-tremor syndrome
Full disease	200–2000	Moderate intellectual disability
Female phenotype		
Normal	50–200	Normal, but 'premutation' unstable; may also have premature ovarian failure
Mild disease	200–2000	50% have mild learning difficulties

Table 28.4 Myotonic dystrophy type 1 (MD1) phenotypes.

Phenotype	No. of CTG repeats	Features
Normal	5–35	
Mild MD1	35–49	Mild myotonia, cataracts
Full MD1	50–1000	Classic adult-onset disease
Congenital MD1	≥2000	Severe congenital disease

Gene product **Dystrophia myotonica protein kinase (DMPK)**
Features Tonic muscle spasm with prolonged relaxation, cardiac conduction defects and arrhythmia, testicular atrophy, cataracts, disturbed gastrointestinal peristalsis, weak sphincters, increased risk of diabetes mellitus and gallstones, somnolence and frontal balding.

Aetiology The disease mutation is an expanded **CTG** trinucleotide repeat in the 3′ UTR of the *DMPK* gene. The number of repeats often increases maternally in succeeding generations, the age of onset recedes, clinical symptoms increase in severity and more body systems become involved. The repeat is represented by CUG in the trailer of the DMPK hnRNA. It causes problems by sequestering CUG binding proteins needed for mRNA processing of several other genes, causing a variety of muscular problems.

In the congenital form, newborns present with hypotonia, talipes (club foot) and respiratory distress, which can be life-threatening. Survivors tend to show lack of facial expression (**myopathic facies**), delayed motor development and learning difficulties.

Management Diagnosis is usually by DNA analysis. Regular surveillance for cardiac conduction defects is advised and education on the risks of anaesthesia.

> ► **Problems requiring immediate attention**
>
> Respiratory problems in some newborn offspring of affected females.

Pleiotropic expression

Pleiotropy is the phenomenon of one gene being responsible for diverse phenotypic effects. In a mouse model of MD1 the CTG expansion reduces production of DMPK, causing cardiac arrhythmia,, cataract, possibly by interfering with a downstream transcription factor gene, and myotonic myopathy, due to the RNA transcript blocking RNA-processing proteins.

Meiotic drive

Meiotic drive is the production by heterozygotes of unequal numbers of gametes carrying alternative alleles. This is an exception to the Mendelian rule that alternative alleles are transmitted with equal frequencies.

The relatively high population frequency of MD 'premutation' alleles may be due to healthy heterozygotes preferentially transmitting alleles with >19 CTG repeats, suggesting a means by which the disease condition could increase in frequency.

Locus heterogeneity

This refers to two or more genetic loci creating similar effects. MD2 is phenotypically similar to MD1, but associated with expansion of a different part of the genome, the four-base sequence **CCTG** at 3q21.

29 Normal polymorphism

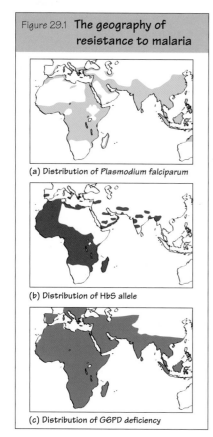

Figure 29.1 **The geography of resistance to malaria**

(a) Distribution of *Plasmodium falciparum*

(b) Distribution of HbS allele

(c) Distribution of G6PD deficiency

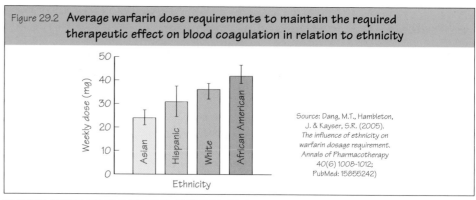

Figure 29.2 **Average warfarin dose requirements to maintain the required therapeutic effect on blood coagulation in relation to ethnicity**

Source: Dang, M.T., Hambleton, J. & Kayser, S.R. (2005). The influence of ethnicity on warfarin dosage requirement. Annals of Pharmacotherapy 40(6) 1008-1012; PubMed: 15855242)

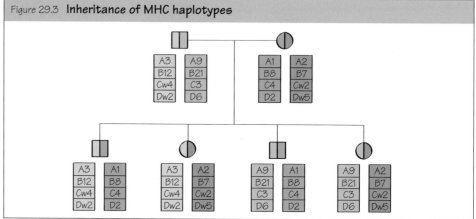

Figure 29.3 **Inheritance of MHC haplotypes**

Overview

Genetic polymorphism is the occurrence of multiple alleles at a locus, where at least two are at frequencies greater than 1%. Over 30% of the genes that code for proteins are polymorphic, many owing their high frequency to selection by environmental factors. Many previously genetically isolated human groups carry certain disease alleles at high frequency, although they may be rare in other populations (Table 29.1). Awareness of the ethnic origin of an individual can be crucial to correct prescription of drug dosage (see Figure 29.2.).

Polymorphisms can provide markers for disease alleles. At the DNA level the most useful are single nucleotide polymorphisms (SNPs), microsatellites, restriction fragment length polymorphisms (RFLPs) and minisatellites (see Section 13). **Copy number polymorphisms** consist of variations in the number of copies of segments of the genome, generally within the range 10–400 kb. They are most readily recognized by array **comparative genome hybridization** (**CGH**) (Chapter 67).

Table 29.1 Genetic isolates with high frequency of certain autosomal disorders.

Population	Disease
Old order Amish (Pennsylvania)	Chondroectodermal dysplasia
	Ellis–van Creveld syndrome
	Cartilage-hair hypoplasia
Kuna (San Blas) Indians (Panama)	Albinism
Hopi Indians (Arizona)	Albinism
Pima Indians (US Southwest)	Type 2 diabetes
Finns	Congenital chloride diarrhoea
	Aspartylglycosaminuria
	Congenital nephrotic syndrome
	Mulibrey nanism
Yupik Eskimo	Congenital adrenal hyperplasia
Afrikaners (South Africa)	Porphyria variegata
	Familial hypercholesterolaemia
	Lipoid proteinosis
	Huntington disease
	Sclereosteosis
Ashkenazi Jews	Tay–Sachs disease
	Gaucher disease
	Dysautonomia
	Canavan disease
Karaite Jews	Werdnig–Hoffmann disease
Ryukyan Islands (Japan)	Spinal muscular atrophy
Cypriots, Sardinians	β-thalassaemia

Medical Genetics at a Glance, Third Edition. Dorian J. Pritchard and Bruce R. Korf.

Environment-related polymorphism

Sunlight

Skin colour relates to the prevailing intensity of sunlight in the region of origin of a population. Sunburn, skin cancer and toxic accumulation of vitamin D select for dark skin in sunny climates. Deficiency of vitamin D selects for pale skin in less sunny regions by causing **rickets**, formerly lethal at childbirth.

Food

Worldwide, most human adults cannot tolerate **lactose**, but traditional consumption of cows' milk has selected lactose tolerance in Europeans and some North Africans. Australian aborigines readily become hypertensive if they consume common salt. See also Chapter 73.

Alcohol

Ethyl alcohol is metabolized to acetaldehyde by **alcohol dehydrogenase (ADH)**, of which there are several variants. Ninety per cent of Chinese and Japanese, and 5% of British people, have a deficient form of ADH2, making them more prone to intoxication.

Acetaldehyde is further degraded by cytosolic **acetaldehyde dehydrogenase 1 (ALDH 1)** and mitochondrial **ALDH 2**. Up to 50% of Asians are deficient in ALDH2 and experience an unpleasant '**flushing**' reaction to alcohol caused by accumulation of acetaldehyde.

Selection by malaria

Sickle cell anaemia (intermediate dominance; ID)

The *HbS* allele of β-globin causes reduced solubility of haemoglobin in homozygotes (*HbS/HbS*) and their red blood corpuscles collapse, characteristically into a sickle shape, when oxygen concentrations are low. The 'sickled cells' clog capillaries causing problems that may result in death in childhood (see Chapters 9 and 25).

Heterozygotes (*HbS/HbA*) have '**the sickle cell trait**'. In low oxygen regimes they suffer capillary blockage, but they have the '**heterozygote advantage**' (see Chapter 7) of resistance to the malaria parasite, *Plasmodium falciparum*. By eliminating normal homozygotes (*HbA/HbA*) malaria creates high population frequencies of the *HbS* allele in malarial areas (see map).

Sickle cell disease is the classic example of a **balanced polymorphism**.

Thalassaemia (AR)

Thalassaemia is a quantitative or functional deficiency of α-, or β-globin (see Chapter 25). Homozygosity of some alleles is lethal, but heterozygosity of β-thalassaemia and 'α-thalassaemia trait' afford protection in malarial areas around the Mediterranean Sea, the Middle East and South-East Asia (Tables 29.2 and 29.3).

Table 29.2 Genetic bases of α-thalassaemia.

Phenotype	Genotype	Quantity of α-globin produced (%)
Normal	αα/αα	100
'Silent carrier'	α–/αα	75
'α-thalassaemia trait'	α–/α– or ––/αα	50
Haemoglobin H (β4)	α–/––	25
Hydrops foetalis	––/––	0 (lethal)

G6PD deficiency (XR)

Deficiency of **glucose-6-phosphate dehydrogenase (G6PD)** is very common in malarial areas (see map) as it disallows growth of *Plasmodium* parasites. The advantage is confined to females because the trait is X-linked recessive.

The Duffy blood group (Co-D)

There are three alleles of the **Duffy blood group**, *FyA*, *FyB* and *FyO*, the latter reaching 100% frequency in some African populations. *FyA* and *FyB* provide an entry gate for malaria parasites into red cells, but *FyO* does not, so making homozygotes resistant.

Resistance to Human Immunodeficiency Virus, HIV

Some individuals that have slow disease progression from **HIV-1** infection to **AIDS (Acquired Immuno-Deficiency Syndrome)** have a 32-bp deletion (Δ32), in the T-cell surface receptor called **CCR5**. This causes a frameshift, inclusion of 31 novel amino acids and premature truncation of the protein. The mutant protein lacks the regions involved in intracellular signal transduction and homozygotes fail to develop disease. The Δ32 allele is highest in Finns (16%) grading south through Europe to 4% in Sardinia and 2–5% in the Middle East and India. It is virtually absent elsewhere.

Transfusion and transplantation

The ABO system

The ABO blood groups (see Chapter 9) are a vital consideration in blood transfusion and tissue transplantation because we naturally carry antibodies directed against those antigens that we do not ourselves possess (see Table 29.4).

Group O are '**universal whole blood donors**', Group AB '**universal whole blood recipients**'.

The Rhesus system

The Rhesus system is genetically complex, but can be considered as involving two alleles, *D* and *d*. *DD* and *Dd* individuals display Rhesus antigens on their red cells and are said to be **Rhesus positive (Rh+)**. Rh+ individuals can be given Rh– blood, but **Rh– (*dd*)** individuals develop an immune response if transfused with Rh+ blood.

If a Rh– woman is pregnant with a Rh+ (*Dd*) baby she can become immunized against red blood cells that leak across the placenta. Anti-Rh antibodies can then invade the body of the baby, causing **haemolytic disease of the newborn**.

Table 29.3 Genetic basis of selected cases of β-thalassaemia.

Affected population	Nature of defect	β-globin phenotype
Italian	δ/β fusion protein	β°
Sardinian	Premature termination	β°
African	RNA splicing	β°
	RNA splicing	β+
	Polyadenylation	β+
Japanese	Promoter	β+
Indian	Deletion	β°
	Frameshift + premature termination	β°
Asian	mRNA capping	β+
South-East Asian	Substitution	β+

Table 29.4 Transfusion of whole blood with respect to ABO blood groups. Donor antibodies are generally diluted to harmless levels in recipients.

Blood group	UK frequency	Antigens on RBCs	Antibodies in serum	Can receive from	Can donate to
A	0.42	A	anti-B	A or O	A or AB
B	0.09	B	anti-A	B or O	B or AB
AB	0.03	A + B	none	**everyone**	AB only
O	0.46	none	anti-A + anti-B	O only	**everyone**

The HLA system

When tissues or organs are transplanted between individuals, the ultimate success of the operation depends on close similarity between the cell surface determinants of the recipient and those of the donor. As a general rule a recipient will reject a graft from a person who possesses a cell surface antigen that is not present in the recipient. The most important of these are the molecules of the HLA (or MHC) system (see Chapter 66).

Drug metabolism

(See also 'Pharmacogenetics' section of Chapter 4.)

The **Cytochrome P450** superfamily includes genes that encode >80 different membrane-bound haemoproteins involved in drug metabolism. An example is **debrisoquine hydroxylase**, encoded by the gene **CYP2D6**. Polymorphisms of this gene variably affect the hydroxylation of >25% of all pharmaceuticals. Deficient hydroxylation of drugs occurs in ~10% of UK residents and 30% of Hong Kong Chinese, conferring high susceptibility to some drugs such as the beta-blocking effect of **propanolol**. Ultrarapid hydroxylation occurs in 20% of Saudi Arabians and ~30% of Ethiopians.

The product of the related **CYP2C9** gene hydroxylates about 16% of medicinal drugs, including the anticoagulant, **warfarin**, the anticonvulsant, **phenytoin** and the insulin-release stimulator **tolbutamide**. There are at least five polymorphic variants of **CYP2C9** that cause drug toxicity or require specific therapeutic dose rates in members of some populations.

Enzymes encoded by the **CYP3A** gene family metabolize over 50% of clinically prescribed drugs and may be the most important contributor to population-specific variant drug response. **CYP3AB** is expressed at high levels in 30% of Whites and Japanese, 40% of Chinese and 50% of African-Americans and South-East Asians.

30 Allele frequency

Figure 30.1 Diallelic autosomal system with codominance, the MN blood groups

The Hardy–Weinberg law applied to the *MN* blood group system in 100 zygotes

M-carrying cells are represented with green nuclei; *N*-carrying with pink. Frequency of *M* alleles = p = 0.6; frequency of *N* alleles = q = 0.4

Eggs
M p = 0.6   N q = 0.4

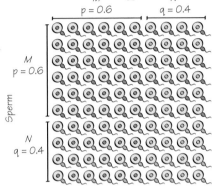

Sperm
M p = 0.6
N q = 0.4

Allele frequencies (total 1.0)

Sperm ↓ / Eggs →	M $p = 0.6$	N $q = 0.4$
M $p = 0.6$	MM $p^2 = 0.6 \times 0.6$ = 0.36 or 36% Homozygotes	MN $pq = 0.6 \times 0.4$ = 0.24 or 24% Heterozygotes
N $q = 0.4$	MN $pq = 0.6 \times 0.4$ = 0.24 or 24% Heterozygotes	NN $q^2 = 0.4 \times 0.4$ = 0.16 or 16% Homozygotes

Total $MN = 2pq = 48\%$

Figure 30.2 Diallelic autosomal system with dominance and recessivity, albinism

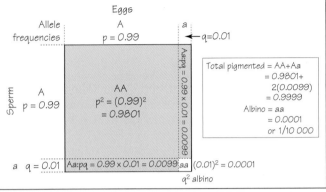

Eggs
Allele frequencies
A p = 0.99   a q=0.01

Sperm
A p = 0.99

	A $p = 0.99$	a $q = 0.01$
A $p = 0.99$	AA $p^2 = (0.99)^2$ = 0.9801	Aa:pq $0.99 \times 0.01 = 0.0099$
a $q = 0.01$	Aa:pq $0.99 \times 0.01 = 0.0099$	aa $(0.01)^2 = 0.0001$ q^2 albino

Total pigmented = AA+Aa
= 0.9801+ 2(0.0099)
= 0.9999
Albino = aa
= 0.0001
or 1/10 000

Figure 30.3 Triallelic autosomal system with codominance and dominance, the ABO blood groups

(These frequencies are imaginary, see Chapter 29 for real values)

Eggs
Allele frequencies
A p = 0.3   B q=0.2   O r = 0.5

Sperm
A p = 0.3
B q = 0.2
O r = 0.5

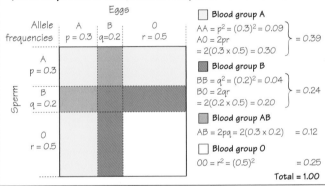

☐ Blood group A
AA = $p^2 = (0.3)^2 = 0.09$
AO = 2pr
= 2(0.3 × 0.5) = 0.30   } = 0.39

■ Blood group B
BB = $q^2 = (0.2)^2 = 0.04$
BO = 2qr
= 2(0.2 × 0.5) = 0.20   } = 0.24

■ Blood group AB
AB = 2pq = 2(0.3 × 0.2) = 0.12

☐ Blood group O
OO = $r^2 = (0.5)^2$ = 0.25

Total = 1.00

Figure 30.5 Predicted possible frequencies of a lethal AD condition of natural prevalence 1/10 000 (orange) and a lethal XR of natural prevalence 2/10 000 (blue) consequent upon medical intervention, with normal survival and reproductive capability of all mutation carriers (see chapter text)

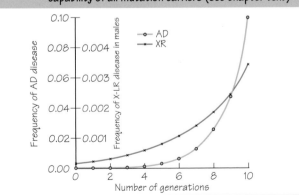

Figure 30.4 Relative frequency of recessive homozygotes and heterozygotes for some important recessive diseases

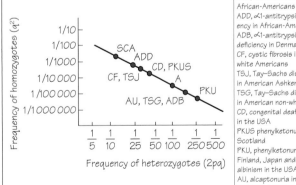

SCA, sickle cell anaemia in African-Americans
ADD, α1-antitrypsin deficiency in African-Americans
ADB, α1-antitrypsin deficiency in Denmark
CF, cystic fibrosis in white Americans
TSJ, Tay–Sachs disease in American Ashkenazi Jews
TSG, Tay–Sachs disease in American non-white Jews
CD, congenital deafness in the USA
PKUS phenylketonuria in Scotland
PKU, phenylketonuria in Finland, Japan and Jews A, albinism in the USA
AU, alcaptonuria in the USA

Medical Genetics at a Glance, Third Edition. Dorian J. Pritchard and Bruce R. Korf.
© 2013 John Wiley & Sons, Ltd. Published 2013 by John Wiley & Sons, Ltd.

Overview

Within a *randomly mating* population the relative frequencies of heterozygotes and homozygotes are mathematically related to allele frequencies by what is known as the **Hardy–Weinberg Law**. Extension of this theory reveals that *allele frequencies will remain constant from generation to generation provided none is under positive or negative selection*. This is 'Hardy–Weinberg equilibrium' (**HWE**). Some apparent exceptions are ascribed to locus heterogeneity, for example Usher syndrome (AR) can be caused by homozygosity at any of 10 or more unlinked loci.

The Hardy–Weinberg law

Diallelic autosomal system with codominance

In the **MN blood group system** alleles *M* and *N* are codominant and there are three blood groups: **M**, **MN** and **N**, M and N individuals being homozygotes. We can calculate the frequency (p) of allele *M* in a population as the proportion of group M individuals plus half the proportion of group MN. Similarly, the frequency (q) of allele *N* equals the proportion of group N people plus half the proportion of group MN. Since there are no other alleles, $p + q = 1$. If Hardy–Weinberg conditions apply the frequencies of the genotypes are given by: $(p + q)^2 = p^2 + 2pq + q^2$, that is frequency of *MM* $= p^2$; frequency of *MN* $= 2pq$ and frequency of *NN* $= q^2$.

Diallelic autosomal system with dominance and recessivity (e.g. albinism)

If the frequency of a dominant allele *A* is p and that of a recessive allele *a* at the same locus is q and there are no other alleles, then the frequencies of the genotypes are *AA*, p^2; *Aa*, $2pq$; *aa*, q^2. The frequencies of the phenotypes are **pigmented**: $p^2 + 2pq$, **albino**: q^2.

Triallelic autosomal system with codominance and dominance (e.g. the ABO blood groups)

If the population frequencies of alleles **A**, **B** and **O** are p, q and r respectively, then $p + q + r = 1$ and the frequencies of the genotypes, from $(p + q + r)^2$, are *AA*, p^2; *BB*, q^2; *OO*, r^2; *AB*, $2pq$; *AO*, $2pr$; *BO*, $2qr$. The frequencies of the blood groups are **A**, $p^2 + 2pr$; **B**, $q^2 + 2qr$; **O**, r^2; and **AB**, $2pq$.

Diallelic X-linked system with dominance and recessivity (e.g. G6PD deficiency)

If the frequency of allele *G* is p and that of allele *g* is q, then the frequency of *G* phenotype males is p and that of *g* phenotype males is q. In females the frequencies of the genotypes are: *GG*, p^2; *Gg*, $2pq$; *gg*, q^2, and the frequencies of the phenotypes are *G*, $p^2 + 2pq$; *g*, q^2.

Necessary conditions

1 Random mating. Two conditions can lead to over-representation of homozygotes: **(i) assortative mating:** usually selection of a mate on the basis of similarity with self, e.g. for deafness, stature, religion or ethnicity; and **(ii) consanguinity**, e.g. cousin marriage. Homozygosity exposes disadvantageous recessives to selection, which may alter their frequency in subsequent generations.
2 Absence of selection, i.e. no genotypic class may be less or more viable or fertile than the others. Allowance must therefore be made for disease alleles.
3 Lack of relevant mutation.

4 Large population size. In small populations random fluctuations in gene frequency (**genetic drift**) can result in **extinction** of some alleles, **fixation** of others.
5 Absence of gene flow. Both selective emigration and immigration disrupt HWE, which however is restored after just one generation of random partnerships.

Applications of the Hardy–Weinberg law

These include:
1 recognition of reduced viability of certain genotypes;
2 estimation of the probability of finding a tissue antigen match in the general population (see Chapters 29 and 66);
3 estimation of the number of potential donors of a rare blood group;
4 estimation of the frequency of carriers of autosomal recessive disease (see Chapters 6–8).

The frequency of unaffected heterozygotes is invariably very much higher than that of affected recessive homozygotes (see Figure 30.1).

Examples

Autosomal recessive conditions
Phenylketonuria

Phenylketonuria occurs in white Americans at a frequency of ~1/15 000; what is the frequency of heterozygous carriers?

Homozygote frequency, $q^2 = 1/15\,000$
Disease allele frequency, $q = \sqrt{1/15\,000} = {\sim}0.008$
Normal allele frequency, $p = 1 - q = 1 - 0.008 = 0.992$
Heterozygote frequency, $2pq = 2 \times 0.992 \times 0.008 = 0.016$
$$= 1.6\%, \text{ or } {\sim}1/60$$

Cystic fibrosis

Cystic fibrosis occurs in white Americans at a frequency of ~1/2500; what is the frequency of marriages (at random) between cystic fibrosis heterozygotes?

$q^2 = 1/2500$
$q = \sqrt{1/2500} = 1/50 = 0.02$
$p = 1 - q = 1 - 0.02 = 0.98$
Carrier frequency $= 2pq = 2 \times 0.98 \times 0.02 = 0.04$
Frequency of marriages between heterozygotes $= (2pq)^2 = (0.04)^2$
$$= 0.0016, \text{ or } 0.16\%$$

X-linked recessive conditions
Haemophilia

Haemophilia A occurs in 1/5000 male births; what is the frequency of female carriers?

$q = $ frequency of disease in males $= 1/5000 = 0.0002$
$p = 1 - q = 1 - 0.0002 = 0.9998$
Frequency of female carriers $= 2pq = 2 \times 0.9998 \times 0.0002 = 0.0004$
$$= 0.04\%, \text{ or } 1/2500$$

Colour blindness

Colour blindness is present in 8% of British males, what is the frequency of affected females?

Colour blindness allele frequency $= q = 0.08$.
Frequency of affected females $= q^2 = (0.08)^2 = 0.0064$
$$= 0.64\%, \text{ or } 1/156$$

Consequence of medical intervention

In line with Darwinian theory, when medical intervention introduces major improvements in the biological fitness of carriers of lethal or seriously disabling alleles, this has major effects on allele frequencies. For example, one-third of all copies of X-linked disease alleles are in males. A major increase in the survival or fertility of male hemizygotes can theoretically increase XL disease frequency by up to 33% *per generation*, for example in 10 generations an XL condition of natural prevalence 2/10 000 (*c.f.* haemophilia A) could show a 17-fold increase (see Figure 30.5).

Medical intervention could theoretically *double* the frequency of fully penetrant serious AD disease *at each successive generation*. In 10 generations, any AD disease that prevents reproduction could therefore increase 1000-fold over the natural mutation rate, if patients are enabled to survive and reproduce normally. The diagram shows how in 10 generations, a condition with a natural prevalence of 1 in 10 000 (*c.f.* Marfan disease), could increase until as many as 10% of the population is affected (see Figure 30.5).

Recessive disease would increase relatively slowly, but could *quadruple* in $1/q$ generations; for example if $q = 1/25$, in 25 generations.

Fortunately contemporary medicine also offers reproductive options that have the potential to ameliorate such devastating consequences (see Section 14).

Measures of disease frequency

The most commonly used measures of disease frequency are **incidence** and **prevalence**. A '**count**' enumerates the number of individuals who meet the case definition for a given condition. 'Incidence' is a count of *new cases*, 'prevalence' of the *total number* of individuals with that disease. In genetic prognosis '**risk**' describes the predictive probability that a given individual will at some time develop the disease (see Chapter 13).

31 Genetic linkage and genetic association

Figure 31.1 **Crossing over between homologous chromosomes in meiosis**

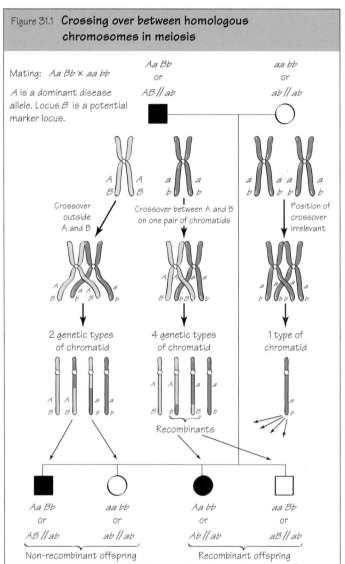

Mating: *Aa Bb* × *aa bb*

A is a dominant disease allele. Locus *B* is a potential marker locus.

Aa Bb
or
AB // ab

aa bb
or
ab // ab

Crossover outside A and B

Crossover between A and B on one pair of chromatids

Position of crossover irrelevant

2 genetic types of chromatid

4 genetic types of chromatid

1 type of chromatid

Recombinants

Aa Bb
or
AB // ab

aa bb
or
ab // ab

Aa bb
or
Ab // ab

aa Bb
or
aB // ab

Non-recombinant offspring

Recombinant offspring

Figure 31.2 **Pedigree showing linkage of the elliptocytosis locus with the rhesus factor locus. The dominant disease allele is in coupling with rhesus allele R$_1$**

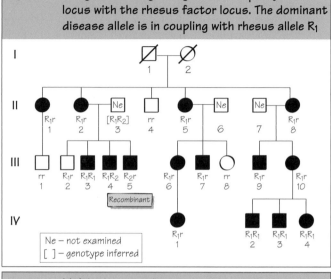

Ne – not examined
[ ] – genotype inferred

Figure 31.3 **Multipoint mapping**

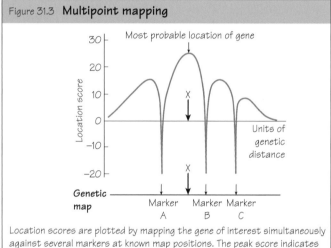

Most probable location of gene

Location score

Units of genetic distance

Genetic map

Marker A   Marker B   Marker C

Location scores are plotted by mapping the gene of interest simultaneously against several markers at known map positions. The peak score indicates the most probable location of the gene

Overview

Genes are arranged in a linear order along chromosomes that is virtually identical in all individuals. The term '**genetic linkage**' refers to the tendency for closely situated alleles to remain together through meiosis, as a **haplotype**. **Genetic linkage studies** determine the frequency with which genetic recombination occurs between any pair of loci and can be used for **gene mapping**. In some cases, a specific allele may be found to be 'associated' with a specific medical condition, either because that allele is directly causative, or else is closely linked to another locus that is intrinsically involved. **Genetic association** is particularly valuable in elucidating the genetic contribution to common multifactorial disorders.

Genetic linkage

Assume two loci, *A* and *B*, are close together on the same chromosome and we observe 'test matings' of type (i) ***AB//ab*** × ***ab//ab***, or type (ii) ***Ab//aB*** × ***ab//ab***, where '/' represents a chromosome. In type (i)

matings, dominant alleles *A* and *B* are on the same chromosome and recessive alleles *a* and *b* on its homologue. The dominants and recessives are said to be '**in coupling**', or *cis* to one another, and constitute a **haplotype**. In matings of type (ii) the dominant and recessive alleles on opposite chromosomes are '**in repulsion**', or *trans* to one another.

Since loci A and B are close, chiasmata rarely occur between them and the parental combinations *AB* and *ab*, or *Ab* and *aB*, will be more frequently represented among offspring than the recombinant combinations *Ab* and *aB*, or *AB*, *ab*, respectively.

Gregor Mendel was unaware of linkage and according to his principle of independent assortment (see Chapter 3), all four types of offspring: ***AaBb***, ***Aabb***, ***aaBb*** and ***aabb*** should be equally represented. When they are not, this is evidence of linkage.

If an allele of gene *A* causes disease, but is otherwise undetectable, whereas the alleles of gene *B* can be easily detected and distinguished, gene *B* can be used as a marker for the inherited disease. This is not completely reliable, as crossover occasionally occurs between them.

Medical Genetics at a Glance, Third Edition. Dorian J. Pritchard and Bruce R. Korf.

82   © 2013 John Wiley & Sons, Ltd. Published 2013 by John Wiley & Sons, Ltd.

For accurate prediction we need to know the **crossover frequency**, that is we need to 'map' their relative positions. A marker locus five **map units** from a disease gene segregates from it in 5% of meioses, so predictions based on that marker are accurate in 95% of cases.

Historically important linkages are of ABO to **nail–patella syndrome** and of **elliptocytosis** to **rhesus factor**. Currently the most useful markers are various types of DNA variant (see Section 13).

Genetic mapping

The genetic **map distance** between loci *A* and *B* can be deduced from the frequency of recombination between them, by the formula:

$$\frac{\text{Number of recombinant offspring} \times 100}{\text{Total number of offspring}}$$

i.e. in type (i) matings: $\dfrac{(Aabb + aaBb) \times 100}{Aabb + aaBb + AaBb + aabb}$

or, in type(ii): $\dfrac{(AaBb + aabb) \times 100}{Aabb + aaBb + AaBb + aabb}$

The unit of map distance is the **centiMorgan (cM)** and *map distances never exceed 50 cM*, as this corresponds to independent assortment, that is non-linkage. Longer distances can be mapped by adding together the map distances between intermediate loci. Since human families are relatively small, such estimates are imprecise. Instead, linkage in humans is usually calculated by '**LOD score analysis**' of family pedigrees. The LOD ('log of the odds') is the logarithm ($\log_{10}$) of the ratio of the probability that the observed ratio of offspring arose as a result of genetic linkage (of specified degree) to the probability that it arose merely by chance.

The **maximum LOD score** is the total value of the combined LODs, usually for a group of families, calculated at the most probable degree of linkage. *A value that exceeds +3 is accepted as evidence for autosomal linkage (or of +2 on the X); one of less than −2, for non-linkage.*

When many loci are involved, advanced computer programs integrate linkage data in '**multipoint maps**' to produce '**location scores**'.

A gene map constructed from male crossovers gives the same gene order as one constructed from females, but the calculated 'distances' between them are often different. This is because chiasmata occur at different frequencies in the formation of ova and sperm. There are also 'hot spots' of high recombination frequency on some chromosomes.

The total map length of the genome, estimated from visible chiasmata in primary germ cells, is ~3000 cM in males and ~4200 cM in females. Since the haploid *physical* length of the genome is about 3000 million bp, 1 cM corresponds to about a million bp in males and 700 000 in females.

Other techniques of gene mapping and its diagnostic applications are discussed in Chapters 32 and 34.

The Human Genome Project (HGP)

A fundamentally different approach is **physical mapping**, which deals with the assignment of genes to specific physical locations on chromosomes (see Chapter 32). The HGP, initiated in October 1990, had three major goals: to create (i) a complete physical map of each chromosome; (ii) a fine-scale physical map of molecular markers throughout the genome; and (iii) the complete 3000 million bp sequence.

The marker map is largely founded on the sites of **restriction fragment length polymorphisms** (**RFLPs**; see Chapter 67), **variable number tandem repeats** (**VNTRs**; see Chapter 70), and simple sequence repeats, and they are spaced an average of 1 cM apart. This provides at least one molecular marker closely linked to every disease gene. In addition, many million **single nucleotide polymorphisms** (**SNPs**) were identified and located, which are especially useful in automated genome analysis (see Chapter 70). **Sequence tagged sites** (**STSs**) are DNA sequences flanked by PCR primers, that enable amplification of unique segments of DNA (see Chapters 69 and 70). These were invaluable for working on specific segments of the genome, such sites being found at intervals averaging around 100 kb.

Sequencing involved two simultaneous projects. A publicly funded effort used large fragments of cloned DNA, determined how they overlapped one another, and sequenced them. Identification of STSs within sequenced sections then enabled each detailed sequence to be positioned on the larger map. Simultaneously, a privately funded effort fragmented the DNA of one person, sequenced the fragments, and assembled them by identification of areas of overlap. Copies of expressed genes (cDNA) were also derived by reverse transcription of mRNA and mapped by correspondence of sequence. The complete map and sequence were revealed on April 14, 2003, exactly 50 years after Watson and Crick first proposed the accepted structure of DNA.

Possession of the gene map and entire human DNA sequence has greatly increased accuracy and speed of diagnosis, and enhanced the prospect of therapeutic applications. This work laid the foundations for the new discipline of **genomics**, which places powerful new tools in the hands of physicians and permits new approaches to personalized prevention, diagnosis and treatment of disease.

The HGP has reduced the estimated number of protein-coding genes in our species from 100 000 to around 20 000. However, we now appreciate that many of these have multiple functions and that much 'intergenic' DNA is actually transcribed as RNA with controlling functions (see Chapters 19 and 23).

Genetic association

Genetic association studies have proved valuable for investigation of multifactorial traits (Chapters 50–52). Typically, groups of affected and non-affected individuals are genotyped for one or more SNPs. If a particular SNP allele occurs in the 'cases' group at higher frequency than in 'controls', this suggests the allele is either directly involved in the aetiology of the condition, or is closely linked to and in '**linkage disequilibrium**' with a causative gene (see Chapter 66).

Recognition that the genome is organized into conserved haplotypes of 10 000–20 000 bp allowed application of **genome-wide association studies** (**GWAS**), which have revealed hundreds of new SNP–disease associations. Such studies offer the possibility of estimating the odds of disease in an individual (see Table 31.1 and calculation of the 'odds ratio'). However, given the multifactorial nature of disease these tests are not strictly diagnostic.

Table 31.1 Genetic association study.

	Affected	Unaffected controls	Total
Allele present	750	575	1325
Allele not present	250	425	675
Total	1000	1000	2000

$$\text{Odds of allele carrier having disorder} = \frac{750/1325}{575/1325} = \frac{750}{575} = 1.42$$

$$\text{Odds of non-carrier having disorder} = \frac{250/675}{425/675} = \frac{250}{425} = 0.59$$

$$\text{Odds ratio} = \frac{1.42}{0.59} = 2.41$$

32 Physical gene mapping

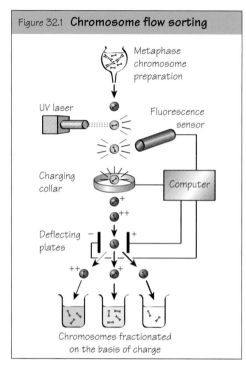

Figure 32.1 Chromosome flow sorting

Metaphase chromosome preparation

UV laser

Fluorescence sensor

Charging collar

Computer

Deflecting plates

Chromosomes fractionated on the basis of charge

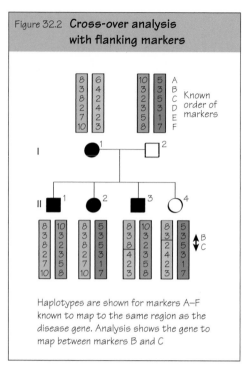

Figure 32.2 Cross-over analysis with flanking markers

A
B
C
D
E
F

Known order of markers

I

II

B
C

Haplotypes are shown for markers A–F known to map to the same region as the disease gene. Analysis shows the gene to map between markers B and C

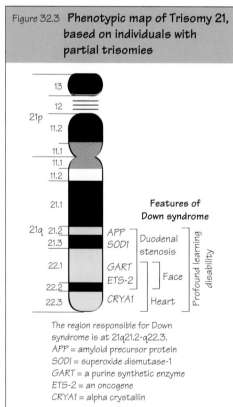

Figure 32.3 Phenotypic map of Trisomy 21, based on individuals with partial trisomies

21p

13
12
11.2
11.1
11.1
11.2

21q

21.1
21.2 — APP ⎫ Duodenal
21.3 — SOD1 ⎭ stenosis
22.1 — GART ⎫
22.2 — ETS-2 ⎭ Face
22.3 — CRYA1 — Heart

Features of Down syndrome

Profound learning disability

The region responsible for Down syndrome is at 21q21.2-q22.3.
APP = amyloid precursor protein
SODI = superoxide dismutase-1
GART = a purine synthetic enzyme
ETS-2 = an oncogene
CRYA1 = alpha crystallin

Table 32.1 Approaches for physical gene mapping

An average gene occupies about 1000 bp (1 kb) (1 cM is about 10^6 bp [1 Mb]). An average chromosome is about 150 cM or 150 Mb

Basis of method	Goal	Resolution (base pairs)
Somatic cell hybrids Flow cytometry	Chromosome assignment	$50–250 \times 10^6$
Chromosome rearrangements Gene dosage analysis Cross-over analysis	Regional mapping	$5–20 \times 10^6$
In situ hybridization Linkage analysis Restriction mapping Chromosome walking	Fine-scale mapping	$10^5–10^6$
Cloning in YACs Cloning in BACs DNA sequencing	Large-scale cloning Gene cloning Nucleotide sequence	$10^5–10^6$ $10^{3-5} \times 10^4$ $10^{3-5} \times 10^4$

BACs, bacterial artificial chromosomes
YACs, yeast artificial chromosomes

Overview

Physical mapping aims to identify the physical locations of genes on chromosomes and generally progresses sequentially at four levels:

1 chromosome assignment;
2 regional mapping;
3 high resolution mapping;
4 DNA sequencing (see Chapter 68).

These approaches are rapidly becoming only of historical interest so far as the practice of medicine is concerned, as genomic sequencing is concentrated on the discovery of genes associated with human phenotypes (Chapter 33).

Chromosome assignment
Patterns of transmission

Four locations are indicated by unique patterns of transmission. These are the X and Y chromosomes, the pseudoautosomal region and the mitochondria (see Chapters 10–12).

Chromosome flow-sorting, flow cytometry

A culture of dividing cells is arrested at metaphase (see Chapter 16) and the chromosomes released and stained with a fluorescent DNA stain. The preparation is then squirted through a fine jet, vertically downwards through an ultraviolet (UV) laser beam. As each chromosome fluoresces it acquires an electrical charge and is deflected by an electrical potential across its path. Deflection is proportional to intensity of fluorescence and this allows preparations of individual chromosomes to be amassed.

Such chromosome preparations can be used for making chromosome paints (see Chapter 35) or chromosome-specific 'dot-blots' on nitrocellulose membranes. Sequences can then be assigned to chromosomes merely by testing their capacity to hybridize with the dot-blots (see Chapter 67).

Somatic cell hybrids

A **somatic cell hybrid** is produced by fusing together two somatic cells or by incorporating a foreign genome into a cell. By careful selection, cloning and long-term maintenance it is possible to create cultures of mouse–human cells containing a single human chromosome along with most of the mouse genome. Chromosome assignment of the genes for human proteins synthesized in such cultures is then a matter of recognizing the human chromosome present.

Regional mapping
Family linkage studies

The frequency of cross-over between loci relates inversely to the physical distance between them, by a mathematical expression called **the mapping function**.

Autosomal traits have been assigned on the basis of co-transmission with cytogenetic features such as translocation breakpoints, or linkage to already assigned markers, an early objective being the identification of DNA markers at 10-cM intervals throughout the genome (see Chapter 31). The **positional cloning approach** involves mapping the disease gene by conventional linkage analysis with respect to the nearest reliable marker.

An alternative is the **candidate gene approach**. In this, one identifies genes known to map to the indicated region, or to have a role in relevant physiology. Patients are then screened for variants of these candidate genes.

Restriction mapping

DNA is digested with a restriction enzyme and subjected to electrophoresis, etc., as described for Southern blotting (see Chapter 67). By use of several enzymes that cleave DNA at different sites, it is possible to order the fragments by recognizing regions of overlap.

Cross-over analysis

This approach aims to map a gene by defining its haplotype with respect to adjacent markers before and after cross-over (see Figure 32.2).

Gene dosage

Normally every individual has two copies of every autosomal gene. Exceptions include heterozygotes for a deletion, and trisomics. Among these, the amount of primary gene product varies threefold. The location of a gene can sometimes be determined by relating quantity of enzyme to the chromosomal breakpoints (see Figure 32.3).

In situ hybridization

The technique of FISH provides a direct approach to gene mapping (see Chapter 35). If a probe recognizes a specific gene sequence, both chromosomal and regional assignment is straightforward.

High-resolution mapping
Cloning

A range of advanced techniques, such as **chromosome microdissection**, **jumping** and **walking**, involve mass production of DNA fragments of a variety of lengths. Before PCR was developed (see Chapter 69) the only way to amplify a chosen gene sequence was by cloning in a microorganism. The basic idea is to insert the gene into a bacterial **plasmid** or **bacteriophage** and allow this to proliferate in a bacterial culture (see Chapters 33 and 67). Larger DNA fragments are cloned in artificial bacterial vectors called **cosmids** and **bacterial artificial chromosomes** (**BAC**s), very large ones (50–1000 kb) in **yeast artificial chromosomes** (**YAC**s).

Fibre-FISH

Chromosomes are extended at interphase and this can be exploited to map genes by an adaptation of FISH called **fibre-FISH** or **DIRVISH** (**dir**ect **vis**ualization **h**ybridization). A liquid preparation of interphase DNA is applied to a microscope slide, which is tilted, causing the liquid to run down the slide and the chromosomes to become stretched along its length. Fluorescent probes directed against genes known to map to the same region are added to the slide and allowed to hybridize, when the order of the fluorescent spots indicates that of the genes along the chromosome.

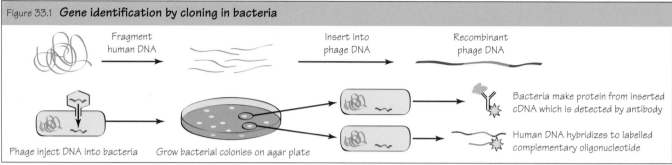

Figure 33.1 **Gene identification by cloning in bacteria**

Fragment human DNA → Insert into phage DNA → Recombinant phage DNA

Phage inject DNA into bacteria

Grow bacterial colonies on agar plate

Bacteria make protein from inserted cDNA which is detected by antibody

Human DNA hybridizes to labelled complementary oligonucleotide

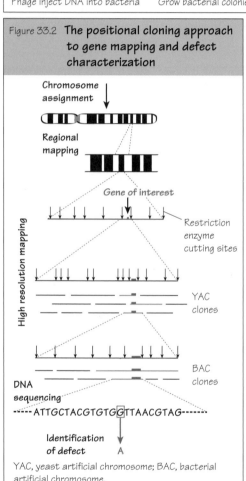

Figure 33.2 **The positional cloning approach to gene mapping and defect characterization**

Chromosome assignment

Regional mapping

Gene of interest

High resolution mapping

Restriction enzyme cutting sites

YAC clones

BAC clones

DNA sequencing

----ATTGCTACGTGTGGTTAACGTAG------

Identification of defect   A

YAC, yeast artificial chromosome; BAC, bacterial artificial chromosome.

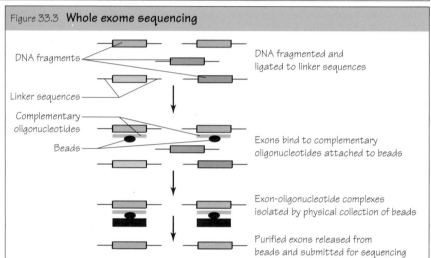

Figure 33.3 **Whole exome sequencing**

DNA fragments

Linker sequences

Complementary oligonucleotides

Beads

DNA fragmented and ligated to linker sequences

Exons bind to complementary oligonucleotides attached to beads

Exon-oligonucleotide complexes isolated by physical collection of beads

Purified exons released from beads and submitted for sequencing

Table 33.1 **Gene identification by exome sequencing**

	Patient 1		Patient 2	
	Dominant	Recessive	Dominant	Recessive
Mutations	4574	2874	4769	2865
Not in benign database	464	34	485	29
Predicted to be damaging	218	4	243	5
Common between two	5	1	5	1

Two unrelated patients have exome sequencing for a recessive disorder. Only one gene is found to have a mutation in both alleles (recessive) that is not in a database of benign variants, is also predicted to be damaging and is in the same gene in the two patients.

Overview

Identification of a gene associated with a human phenotype opens the door to molecular diagnosis and may provide insights into pathophysiology that can lead to new therapies. There has been an exponential increase in the number of genes connected with medically important phenotypes since the introduction of recombinant DNA technologies in the 1970s. With the completion of the human genome sequence and the development of high-throughput DNA sequencing technologies, the pace of gene discovery has accelerated markedly.

Identification of genes with known gene products

The earliest successes in human gene identification involved the discovery of genes that encode known gene products. The first such example was the recognition that an amino acid substitution in β-globin is the cause of sickle cell anaemia; the base substitution was inferred from the genetic code long before DNA sequencing was possible (see Chapters 25 and 68).

The advent of recombinant DNA technologies made it possible to introduce segments of human DNA into bacterial cells. 'Libraries' of

Medical Genetics at a Glance, Third Edition. Dorian J. Pritchard and Bruce R. Korf.

bacterial colonies could be made either from genomic DNA or from DNA copies of mRNA (cDNA) and colonies identified that had taken up a genomic or cDNA segment corresponding to a gene of interest. Relatively large segments of human DNA could be introduced into bacterial cells using modified bacteriophage vectors (see Figure 33.1). Colonies that had randomly taken up DNA corresponding to a gene of interest could be identified using hybridization probes that included a partial nucleotide sequence of the structural gene. This was inferred either from the amino acid sequence of its encoded protein, or by expression of the human cDNA in the bacteria. Antibody specific for the gene product was then used to identify that colony, which could then be grown in large quantities. This permitted detailed study of the human DNA, including sequencing of the relevant gene (Chapter 68). Variations on this approach led to identification of dozens of structural genes, including most of those involved in human inborn errors of metabolism (see Section 11).

Positional cloning

The early gene cloning approach was successful when the product was known in advance, but could not be employed in cases when it was unknown. Positional cloning, introduced in the mid 1980s, offered a new way to identify such genes. The principle was first to use linkage analysis to localize the site of the gene on the chromosome (Chapter 31). DNA in that region was then isolated through recombinant DNA methodologies, resulting in a large segment of purified DNA corresponding to the chromosomal region of interest.

Identification of the gene involved finding a chromosomal segment with the following properties: (i) it encodes an expressed sequence and one expressed in the tissue known to be involved in the phenotype (e.g. the DMD gene should be expressed in muscle); and (ii) the gene is mutated or deleted in individuals who express the disease phenotype, but not in the unaffected. In some cases, it was possible to look for regions displaying species' conservation or including sequence motifs (such as 'CpG islands') that indicate regions likely to encode genes (Chapter 21).

Some of the first successes were chronic granulomatous disease (Chapter 65), DMD (Chapter 11), hereditary retinoblastoma (Chapter 56), CF (Chapter 8), and neurofibromatosis (Chapters 9 and 56). In many, if not most cases, the genes identified were not previously recognized, or their products not suspected as having a role in the disorder.

Mapping studies by positional cloning accelerated greatly following completion of the human genome sequence, as once linkage had been established, candidate genes could be selected using annotated 'genome browsers'. Some corresponded to proteins of known function while others were inferred to be coding sequences from their structure (see Chapter 21). The most likely candidates could then be directly sequenced for mutations in affected individuals. If something was already known about their function it was sometimes possible to make an educated guess as to the gene most likely to be causative of that phenotype.

Positional cloning required a gene to be mapped. In rare cases this could be done by finding a chromosomal abnormality in affected individuals that, in effect, 'broke' the gene, and in so doing marked its location. However, in most cases genetic linkage data was needed and this required access to many families so that segregation of features of interest could be related to markers of known chromosomal location. Many genetic disorders, however, are exceedingly rare, seen only in a small number of individuals, often just one family member. This is particularly true for rare recessives or dominants due to new lethal mutations. In these the positional cloning approach has been less successful.

Gene identification by whole exome/whole genome sequencing

Recently an alternative approach has been developed, based on sequencing of the entire genome (**whole genome sequencing**, **WGS**) or, in **whole exome sequencing** (**WES**), just the protein-encoding portion, or **exome**. This is done by **massively parallel sequencing** (or 'next generation sequencing'), in which small segments of DNA from across the genome are simultaneously sequenced and the whole conceptually pieced together by computer (see Chapter 68).

WGS begins by isolation of DNA from one or more affected individuals and sometimes also from parents and/or unaffected siblings. The DNA is fragmented and those fragments that correspond to exons are 'captured' by hybridization to a set of synthetic oligonucleotides corresponding to almost all known exons in the human genome. This capture can be done in solution, with the oligonucleotides attached to beads, or to oligonucleotides immobilized (e.g. on glass) in a microarray. Either way, the captured fragments are washed free of the oligonucleotides, then subjected to massively parallel sequencing and analyzed computationally. Any individual will have thousands of DNA variants in an exome (and millions in a whole genome) when compared to a standardized human DNA sequence; finding the one that is relevant to the phenotype of interest is a massive bioinformatic puzzle. 'Benign' variants that have already been catalogued as occurring in the general population are filtered out of consideration, as are those that can be predicted by computer modelling to have little or no effect on gene function. One then looks for a variant expected to be deleterious either as a single allele (if a dominant is suspected), or for variants on two alleles of the same gene (if the trait is believed to be recessive). If (i) the same gene (although not necessarily the same variant) is affected in multiple, unrelated individuals that share a phenotype, or (ii) if the variant segregates with the disease phenotype in an affected family, or (iii) if the variant occurs as a *de novo* mutation in all affected individuals, it is likely that gene is the one responsible for the disease.

The exome comprises less than 5% of the genome (Chapter 19) yet most known pathogenic mutations reside within protein-coding segments. Focusing on the exome therefore offers a cheaper and faster approach to gene identification than WGS, though there is the risk that some exons may not be efficiently captured, and some genes of interest may not encode protein.

Although relatively new, this approach has already unlocked the genetic basis of a large number of Mendelian conditions. A concerted effort is now under way to find all the genes involved in Mendelian traits.

Figure 34.1 Linkage analysis in an autosomal dominant disorder

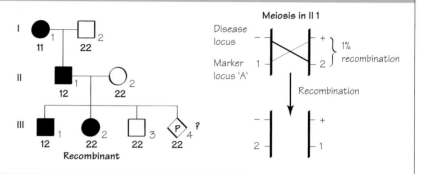

The two alleles at the disease locus are labelled '+' for wildtype and '−' for disease; alleles at marker locus 'A' are labelled '1' and '2'. At the right, the map of the region is shown, as well as the consequence of recombination. Unborn child III-4 has probably (99%) not inherited the '−' allele, but there remains a 1% chance that recombination occurred during formation of its paternal pronucleus.

Figure 34.2 Linkage analysis in an autosomal recessive disorder

Both parents are heterozygous, having alleles '1' and '2' at a polymorphic marker closely linked to the disease allele. The affected child has inherited allele '1' from both parents so, assuming no recombination, this is the allele in coupling with the disease allele in both parents. The second child can be offered testing; if she has genotype '11' she is likely to be affected, '22' unaffected and '12' heterozygous.

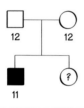

Figure 34.3 Comparative risk of disease

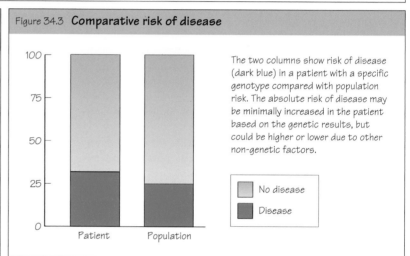

The two columns show risk of disease (dark blue) in a patient with a specific genotype compared with population risk. The absolute risk of disease may be minimally increased in the patient based on the genetic results, but could be higher or lower due to other non-genetic factors.

Overview

An approach to the management of genetic disease that is increasingly finding practical application is the direct detection of specific mutations. However, such strategies are not always possible. For example, in many Mendelian disorders the causative genes are unknown, or allelic or locus heterogeneity raise problems. The human gene map (Chapters 31 and 32) offers a powerful supplementary approach, based on tracking disease alleles through **closely linked polymorphic markers**. By their nature, multifactorial disorders also cannot be diagnosed directly by detecting any specific mutation, although **association studies** do permit estimation of the 'odds' of disease (Chapter 31). Both approaches provide statistical estimates of disease risk, but both are imprecise and subject to misinterpretation. Nevertheless they can still be useful in clinical practice. This chapter explores the application of the indirect strategies of chromosomal linkage analysis and genetic association to clinical diagnosis.

Linkage analysis
Principle

Linkage analysis depends on the concept that genes are organized in the same linear order in (virtually) every person. If a polymorphic locus is revealed to be closely linked to a disease locus, that linkage is true for (almost) all individuals. If a carrier of genetic disease is heterozygous for the polymorphism and the coupling phase of marker and disease alleles can be determined (see Chapter 31), then alleles at the polymorphic locus can be used as markers for the disease. Intragenic neutral polymorphisms can also be used in an adaptation of this approach and in such cases we assume zero recombination.

The polymorphisms most valuable as genetic markers are single nucleotide polymorphisms, microsatellites and VNTRs (see Chapters 19, 29 and 70). When linkage phase has been established in a family the marker locus can be assayed in the at-risk individual, in order to determine whether he or she has inherited the chromosome segment containing the disease allele, or alternatively its homologue carrying the normal allele. Since this requires no direct examination, or indeed knowledge, of the disease-causing mutation or its product, it can be considered a form of **indirect diagnosis**.

Disadvantages of the linkage approach are that the marker gene may not show sufficient heterozygosity in that family and that recombination can occur between disease and marker genes within the family. These problems can often be overcome in practice by means of several markers located either side of the disease locus. Linkage analysis is increasingly being replaced by direct analysis, but there are still situations where it is useful.

Autosomal dominant traits

In the dominant pedigree (see Figure 34.1), the affected individual, II-1, is heterozygous for both the disease gene and for alleles '*1*' and

Medical Genetics at a Glance, Third Edition. Dorian J. Pritchard and Bruce R. Korf.

'2' at locus 'A'. The 'A' locus is known from studies in other families to be closely linked to the disease gene, with a 1% rate of recombination between them. Individual II-1 has inherited both the disease allele and marker allele '1' from his diseased mother, so in this individual marker allele '1' is located on the same chromosome as the disease allele. His partner (II-2) is homozygous for the '2' allele at the marker locus. We can trace the inheritance of the disease allele in their children by determining whether marker allele '1' or '2' was inherited from the father. Child III-1 has inherited allele '1' and is affected, while III-3 has inherited '2' and is unaffected. Child III-2 is an exception as she inherited the '2' allele from her father, yet is affected. This is due to recombination, the probability of which is known from other studies to be 1%. If the unborn child, III-4, is a '22' homozygote, the probability he or she will be affected is only 1%, despite the existence of a recombinant sib. If necessary, additional polymorphic flanking markers can be used to confirm such deductions and increase the accuracy of analysis.

Autosomal recessive traits

Linkage-based diagnosis can also be performed with recessive traits to follow transmission of alleles from each parent to affected or unaffected children (see Figure 34.2). In such cases one must use the situation in an affected child to infer coupling phases in the parents.

X-linked traits

The same analysis can be done for X-linked traits, tracking the inheritance of the two X chromosomes from a heterozygous female. If the grandparental generation is not available for study, one can infer coupling phase from affected children, with the caveat that one or more might be recombinants. This caveat introduces some uncertainty, and thus decreases analytical power, but it is still better than the Mendelian estimate of 50% based on the equal probability of inheriting one or the other chromosome homologue.

Pitfalls in interpretation of linkage

• Clinical diagnosis must be firmly established, since linkage testing alone will not confirm or refute the original diagnosis.
• Different genetic loci are sometimes responsible for clinically indistinguishable disorders; such genetic heterogeneity can invalidate linkage data.
• There must be closely linked polymorphic markers that are heterozygous in the individual heterozygous for the disease allele from whom transmission is being tracked. Each family must be studied individually, although if there is linkage disequilibrium one particular linked allele can be non-randomly associated with disease (see Chapters 31 and 66).

• Multiple family members must be available and willing to participate. The proband may be deceased and his or her DNA not available.
• Finally, the outcome of a linkage analysis remains only a statistical probability; genetic recombination may always occur and can potentially lead to misdiagnosis.

Association analysis

Genetic association studies have revealed polymorphisms associated particularly with common multifactorial disorders such as asthma or type 2 DM (Chapters 52 and 59). These are for the most part SNPs in which a specific allele is found more frequently in affected individuals than controls. The association may indicate direct involvement of the polymorphic gene in pathogenesis, or only linkage disequilibrium with a nearby disease gene, but in either case, determination of the genotype of an individual can be used to assess the odds of disease (see Chapter 31). If its population prevalence is known this can be used to estimate the absolute risk of disease. Such calculations can be done on a gene-by-gene basis, or an individual can be genotyped simultaneously for hundreds of thousands of polymorphisms, yielding a risk profile for a large number of distinct multifactorial conditions.

Pitfalls in interpretation of association

As with linkage-based tests, interpretation of risk of a common disease based on association is subject to many caveats (see Figure 34.3).
• Genetic factors contribute only a part of the risk of any common disorder, with other factors, such as environmental, contributing the balance.
• Analysis of SNPs known to be associated with a condition may not account for all the genetic risk factors, which may include copy number changes, or unique constellations of rare variants, etc.
• Genetic risk factors for a given disease may differ between populations.
• Individuals need to distinguish between risk of disease and diagnosis. Those deduced to be at low risk can still develop the condition, while those at high risk may not. There is particular concern that low-risk individuals may make decisions that have long-term health implications irrespective of genotype, such as to abandon recommended exercise or dieting programmes.
• There may be little value in elucidating the risk of common disease if there are no established interventions that can help prevent eventual disease development. Nevertheless some commercial organizations have marketed genomic profiling of SNPs on a direct-to-consumer basis. This is controversial since such testing may bypass medical professional input to the consumer and important health inferences can be overlooked.

Figure 35.1 G-banding and labelling of chromosomes

Chromosome 7 is shown at resolutions of 450, 550 and 850 bands per haploid set. The indicated band is designated 7q31.32

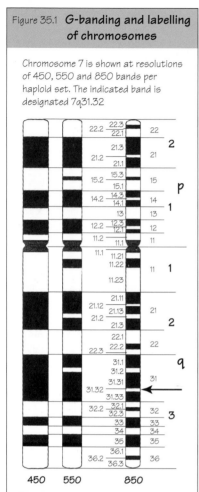

450   550   850

Figure 35.2 Three chromosome forms
(alternative representation, at metaphase)

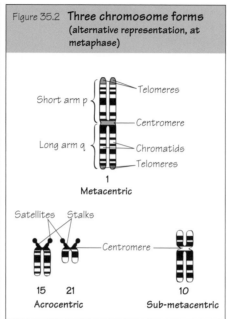

Short arm p
Telomeres
Centromere
Long arm q
Chromatids
Telomeres

1
Metacentric

Satellites   Stalks

Centromere

15   21
Acrocentric

10
Sub-metacentric

Conventional abbreviations used in cytogenetics

A-G	Chromosome groups	M	Monosomy
1-22	Autosome number	p	Short arm
del	Deletion	q	Long arm
der	Derivative chromosome	r	Ring chromosome
dup	Duplication	t	Translocation
i	Isochromosome	T	Trisomy
ins	Insertion	ter	Terminal
inv	Inversion		

See also Chapter 34

Figure 35.3 Use of FISH probes

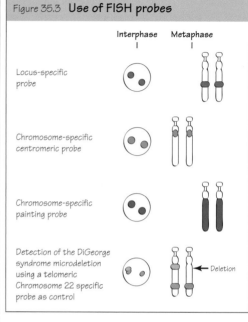

Interphase   Metaphase

Locus-specific probe

Chromosome-specific centromeric probe

Chromosome-specific painting probe

Detection of the DiGeorge syndrome microdeletion using a telomeric Chromosome 22 specific probe as control

Deletion

Overview

The study of number and structure of chromosomes is called **cytogenetics**. Traditionally it is performed on compacted chromosomes at a magnification of about 1000×, providing resolution to around 3 million base pairs, or one narrow chromosome band (see Chapter 15). By incorporation of molecular techniques this can be reduced to 2 kb (2000 bp).

Conventional cytogenetics uses mitotic chromosomes. The chorion (**syncytiotrophoblast**) and bone marrow normally contain sufficient dividing cells for examination, but most tissues require culturing *in vitro*, with an overall time schedule of about 10 days. **Molecular cytogenetics**, utilizing DNA probes, can be applied directly to interphase nuclei.

Preparation of a karyotype

A visual karyotype is prepared by arresting dividing cells at metaphase with a spindle inhibitor such as *colchicine* (see Chapter 16), spreading the cells on a glass slide and staining with Giemsa stain. Traditionally a photographic positive is then made and the chromosomes cut out and assembled on a card, in pairs in order of size, sometimes in conventional groups A–E (Figure 35.4). In modern practice, this step is replaced by digital imaging. Chromosomes 1, 3, 16, 19 and 20, with the centromere in the middle, are known as **metacentric**; 13, 14, 15, 21, 22 and Y, with the centromere near one end, are **acrocentric**. The rest are **sub-metacentric**. The short arm is symbolized 'p' (for petite) and the long arm 'q'.

Karyotype formulae are described in Chapter 36. Positions of genes along chromosome arms are defined by **region** number (from the centromere outwards), **band**, **sub-band** and **sub-sub-band** numbers, for example 12q24.32 refers to Chromosome 12, long arm, region 2, band 4, sub-band 3, sub-sub-band 2. **High-resolution banding** involves fixation before the chromosomes are fully compacted.

C-banding stains heterochromatin, **NOR staining** reveals the **N**ucleolar **O**rganizer **R**egions on the satellite stalks of the acrocentrics.

Fluorescent *in situ* hybridization (FISH)

FISH enables the specific localization of genes and the direct visualization of abnormalities at the molecular level. With chromosome-specific probes it allows rapid diagnosis or exclusion of a diagnosis of trisomy in amniotic fluid cells.

In a typical application, a labelled probe is denatured by heating, added to a metaphase chromosome spread on a microscope slide and incubated overnight to permit sequence-specific hybridization. Surplus probe is then washed off and the bound probe located by overlaying

Table 35.1 Single-gene disorders with cytogenetic effects.

Disorder	Inheritance	Cytogenetic effect
Ataxia telangiectasia	AR	Chromatid damage due to defective DNA repair; 7, 14 rearrangements
Bloom syndrome	AR	High frequency of sister chromatid exchange
Fanconi anaemia	AR	Chromosome breakage and translocation
Fragile X syndrome	XR	Chromosome breakage at Xq27.3
Roberts syndrome	AR	Premature separation of centromeres at metaphase
Xeroderma pigmentosum	AR	Defective repair of ultraviolet damage, sister chromatid exchange

the spread with a solution of fluorescent '**reporter molecule**'. Unbound reporter is washed off and a counterstain applied to reveal the chromosomes. Bound reporter, and hence the site of the gene of interest, is then located by its fluorescence under ultraviolet light.

Use of unique sequence probes
Microdeletions
Submicroscopic deletions can be detected with fluorescent probes directed against one or more unique sequences within the interval suspected to be deleted. **Microdeletion probes** are used in diagnosis of **DiGeorge/VCFS** at 22q11; **Wolf–Hirschhorn** at 4p16.3, **Prader–Willi** and **Angelman**, **Williams** and **Smith–Magenis syndrome**, etc. (see Chapter 39).

Translocations
FISH probes directed at the *BCR* and *abl* sequences can be used to reveal the Philadelphia chromosome (see Chapter 38) as two fluorescent signals on the derivative Chromosome 22; in normal cells the signals are on separate chromosomes. FISH probes to regions near the telomeres can be useful in identifying subtelomeric rearrangements that result in unbalanced karyotypes which may lead to mental retardation.

Sex chromosome rearrangements
In some phenotypic males lacking a Y chromosome, an SRY probe reveals the site to which the male-determining *SRY* locus (see Chapters 10 and 43) has been translocated from its normal site at Yp11, often to the X.

Chromosome painting
Chromosome painting has now largely been replaced by microarray methods (see Section 13), but may still be useful in some circumstances. When unique-sequence probes for one chromosome are pooled and labelled with the same fluorochrome this creates a '**chromosome paint**' that identifies that specific chromosome or its fragments after translocation.

In **reverse painting**, a battery of probes is made from an *abnormal* chromosome and hybridized to normal metaphase spreads, so allowing the derivation of the abnormal chromosome to be deduced. Such probes are created by assembling many copies of the abnormal chromosome using a **fluorescence activated chromosome sorter** (see Chapter 32).

Primed *in situ* hybridization
The primed *in situ* hybridization (PRINZ) technique involves setting up a polymerase chain reaction (PCR) *in situ* on a chromosome spread. Primers are added that define a specific genetic locus, resulting in a layer of target DNA at the site of interest. If a fluorescent base analogue is incorporated during the PCR reaction the sequence is rendered visible in one step. This method is rarely used now.

Comparative genome hybridization (CGH)
CGH can be used to detect partial monosomies or trisomies, chromosome deletions and amplifications. It is based on making test DNA and control DNA compete at hybridizing to the same target. The target can be either a metaphase spread, or an array of tiny samples of oligonucleotides on a glass slide. It is especially valuable in evaluation of individuals with intellectual disability and/or congenital anomalies and is beginning to be used in clinical evaluation of genetic rearrangements in cancer.

In **standard CGH**, test DNA is labelled with red fluorescent dye and control DNA with green. The two samples are mixed, hybridized competitively to metaphase chromosomes and photographed using a fluorescence microscope. Regions duplicated in the test cells hybridize with excess red-labelled DNA; regions deleted in the test cells light up as green, while unchanged regions appear yellow. The ratio of red to green FISH signal is automatically plotted along the length of each chromosome emphasizing regions where it deviates significantly from the 1 : 1 expectation. This is especially useful for inferring the state of progression of a cancer.

In **array CGH** DNA sequences rather than chromosomal band locations are identified, utilizing microarrays of DNA spotted onto glass slides (see Chapter 67). Each spot consists of oligonucleotides corresponding with the DNA sequence from a defined chromosomal region. It is possible to create arrays that cover the entire human genome and carry out rapid robotic scans for microdeletions and microduplications.

Multiplex PCR screening for aneuploidy
See Chapter 69.

Indications for chromosome analysis
The following are situations in which cytogenetic investigation is advised:
1 suspected chromosome abnormality;
2 multiple congenital anomalies and/or developmental retardation;
3 disorders of sexual function;
4 undiagnosed intellectual disability;
5 certain malignancies;
6 infertility or multiple miscarriage;
7 stillbirth and neonatal death.

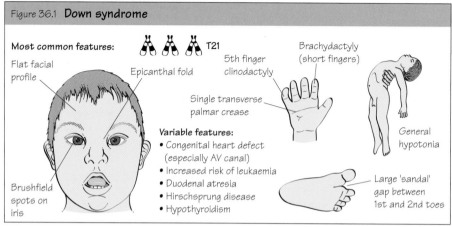

Figure 36.1 Down syndrome

Most common features:
- Flat facial profile
- Epicanthal fold
- 5th finger clinodactyly
- Single transverse palmar crease
- Brachydactyly (short fingers)
- Brushfield spots on iris
- General hypotonia

Variable features:
- Congenital heart defect (especially AV canal)
- Increased risk of leukaemia
- Duodenal atresia
- Hirschsprung disease
- Hypothyroidism
- Large 'sandal' gap between 1st and 2nd toes

T21

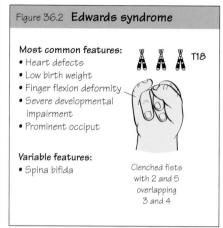

Figure 36.2 Edwards syndrome

Most common features:
- Heart defects
- Low birth weight
- Finger flexion deformity
- Severe developmental impairment
- Prominent occiput

Variable features:
- Spina bifida

Clenched fists with 2 and 5 overlapping 3 and 4

T18

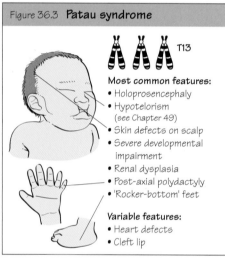

Figure 36.3 Patau syndrome

T13

Most common features:
- Holoprosencephaly
- Hypotelorism (see Chapter 49)
- Skin defects on scalp
- Severe developmental impairment
- Renal dysplasia
- Post-axial polydactyly
- 'Rocker-bottom' feet

Variable features:
- Heart defects
- Cleft lip

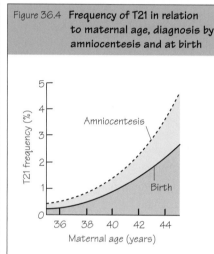

Figure 36.4 Frequency of T21 in relation to maternal age, diagnosis by amniocentesis and at birth

Amniocentesis

Birth

T21 frequency (%) vs Maternal age (years)

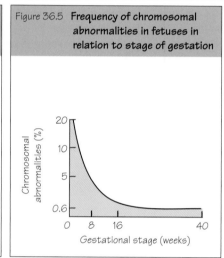

Figure 36.5 Frequency of chromosomal abnormalities in fetuses in relation to stage of gestation

Chromosomal abnormalities (%) vs Gestational stage (weeks)

Overview

Chromosomal disorders involve both abnormal numbers of chromosomes and aberrations in their structure (see Chapter 38). **Euploidy** means that the chromosome number per body cell is an integral multiple of the haploid number, N = 23, **aneuploidy** that it is other than an integral multiple. Aneuploidy is usually ascribed to failure of chromosome pairs to conjugate, or **non-disjunction** (non-separation) of chromosomes in Meiosis I; or non-disjunction, **premature disjunction,** or **anaphase lag** (delayed separation) in Meiosis II.

Diploidy describes the normal situation, a typical body cell in humans having 2N = 46 chromosomes. Women have 23 similar pairs, including a pair of X chromosomes, their **karyotype** formula being **46,XX**. In normal men there is an X and a Y chromosome, their karyotype being **46,XY**. The non-sex chromosomes are called **autosomes**. **Polyploidy** refers to multiples of the haploid number (e.g. **triploidy**, 3N = 69).

Trisomy (2N + 1) is presence of three copies of one chromosome. Possession of only a single copy of an autosome (2N−1) is called **monosomy**. Autosomal monosomies are nearly always incompatible with survival.

Chromosomal abnormalities are present in at least 10% of spermatozoa and 25% of oocytes. Approximately 50% of spontaneous first trimester miscarriages have a chromosome abnormality, including a high proportion of Trisomy 13 (T13) and T18 fetuses. The most common is T16, not seen in livebirths.

Aetiology

Trisomy 21, causing **Down syndrome (DS)**, T18, causing **Edwards syndrome (ES)** and T13, causing **Patau syndrome (PS)**, are the only autosomal trisomies compatible with survival to birth and all three syndromes can also be caused by translocations (see Chapter 38) or as somatic mosaics.

The majority (95% of DS and ES, 80% of PS) have complete trisomy and a severe clinical phenotype. The birth frequency of this class increases with maternal age, especially after 35 years of age. Nevertheless 75% of DS babies are born to women under 35, since most babies are born to younger mothers.

Around 4% of DS and ES and close to 20% of PS have major translocations involving the relevant chromosomes. Translocation DS almost always involves another acrocentric chromosome, that is 13, 14, 15, or 22; t14,21 is the most common. Translocations that lead to partial trisomy are associated with milder manifestation and longer survival.

Medical Genetics at a Glance, Third Edition. Dorian J. Pritchard and Bruce R. Korf.

92 © 2013 John Wiley & Sons, Ltd. Published 2013 by John Wiley & Sons, Ltd.

Table 36.1 Newborn and diagnostic features of the autosomal trisomies.

	Down syndrome	Edwards syndrome	Patau syndrome
Trisomic karyotype	47,XX,+21 or 47,XY,+21	47,XX,+18 or 47,XY,+18	47,XX,+13 or 47,XY,+13
Frequency	Overall corrected incidence ~1/700	1/3000–1/6000 live births	1/5000–1/8000 live births
Head and face	Small, flattened head, short neck with excess nuchal skin. Face broad. Tongue without a central fissure. Low nasal root, ears small	Microcephaly, fine features, elongated skull with prominent occiput, small, low-set ears with unravelled helices and large lobes, small mouth, micrognathia	Microcephaly with sloping forehead; facial features coarse; cleft lip and palate; micrognathia
Eyes	Eyes slanting upwards, with marked epicanthic folds; cataracts, squint and nystagmus (involuntary eye movements). Most have white speckles on the iris		Microphthalmia, anophthalmia, cyclopia or hypotelorism (closely spaced eyes)
Hands and feet	Half have a single palmar flexion crease. Limbs and fingers short, little finger in-turned, with single crease. Large 'sandal gap'. Webbing of toes 2 and 3	'Rocker bottom' feet with prominent heels; a distinctive way of clenching the fists with index and little fingers overlapping the middle ones; often a single palmar crease	'Rocker-bottom' feet; frequently a single palmar crease, postaxial polydactyly (6th finger present)
Muscle tone	Babies are always 'floppy' (hypotonic) and tend to be sleepy		
General	See text	Prenatal growth deficiency; abnormal muscle tone; major malformations of the renal and CN systems. Severe learning difficulty; most require complete care and can never walk or feed themselves	Midline malformations include failure of separation of the cerebral ventricles, and cardiac abnormalities. Frequently malformations of the CN and renal systems. Seizures common. Skills limited to those of a child of 2 years. All boys have undescended testes
Life expectancy	50–60 years	50% die in the first few weeks, 95% in the first year	50% die within the first month, 95% by 3 years
Problems requiring immediate attention	Congenital heart disease; oesophageal, anal or duodenal **atresia** (closure)	Pneumonia, **apnoea**, diaphragmatic hernia; **omphalocoele**, infection, heart defects, **spina bifida**	Special care with feeding; repair of oral/facial clefts; investigation of heart and renal systems; learning disability

Around 1–4% of patients with each syndrome show mosaic expression.

Recurrence risk for T21 is 0.5–1.0%, depending on maternal age; for translocation cases: 1–3% for male carriers; 10–15% for female.

Maternal serum screening in the second trimester detects 75–80% of DS pregnancies. This is based on 'triple' or 'quadruple testing' (see Chapter 72), followed by chromosomal analysis or FISH (see Chapter 35).

Down syndrome (DS)
Problems in infancy and childhood
Hearing deficit is a problem in 60–80% and epilepsy in 5–10%. About 20% have either an overactive or underactive thyroid gland. There is risk of obesity, sleep apnoea and skeletal problems, including dislocation of cervical vertebrae.

Acute lymphocytic leukaemia accounts for 5% of deaths in childhood. Upper respiratory tract infections are common.

Congenital heart disease affects around 40% of DS babies. The most common anomalies are failure of fusion of the interatrial and interventricular septa (AV canal) and/or retention of the (i.e. 'patent') **ductus arteriosus**. 'Failure to thrive' is among the first signs.

There is usually significant intellectual delay, with specific deficits in speech and auditory short-term memory.

Problems in adolescence and adulthood
More than 80% of DS patients survive beyond 10 years. Average adult height is ~150 cm, average IQ of young adults 40–45. Males are nearly always sterile and about 40% of females fail to ovulate.

Life expectancy is reduced and there are Alzheimer-like features in half those over 40 years of age.

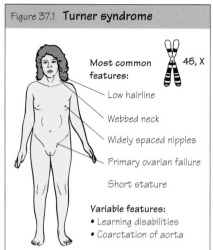

Figure 37.1 **Turner syndrome**

45, X

Most common features:
- Low hairline
- Webbed neck
- Widely spaced nipples
- Primary ovarian failure
- Short stature

Variable features:
- Learning disabilities
- Coarctation of aorta

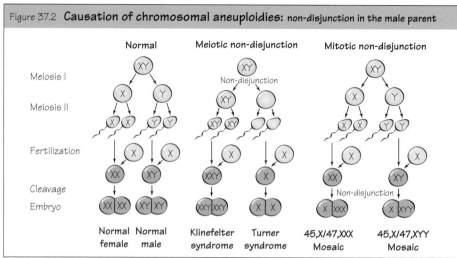

Figure 37.2 **Causation of chromosomal aneuploidies:** non-disjunction in the male parent

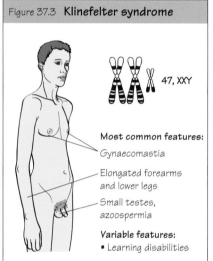

Figure 37.3 **Klinefelter syndrome**

47, XXY

Most common features:
- Gynaecomastia
- Elongated forearms and lower legs
- Small testes, azoospermia

Variable features:
- Learning disabilities

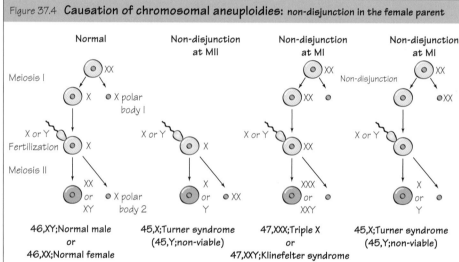

Figure 37.4 **Causation of chromosomal aneuploidies:** non-disjunction in the female parent

Overview

Monosomy of the X chromosome is the only whole body monosomy compatible with postnatal life, but the associated Turner syndrome demonstrates the requirement in both sexes for two active copies of the pseudoautosomal region, as well as several other X-linked genes. Monosomy X probably occurs in 1–2% of conceptions, but almost all are lost prenatally.

Karyotype formulae indicate the *total* number of chromosomes, together with the sex chromosome constitution.

Klinefelter syndrome

Genotype Karyotype **47,XXY**; or **48,XXXY**; **49,XXXXY**, etc.; abnormal presence of Barr bodies, one less than the number of X chromosomes (see Chapter 43).
Frequency 1/500–1/1000 male births.
Life expectancy Normal, but 50% die before birth.
Body form Phenotype is basically male, tall with elongated lower legs and forearms, but with a feminine body shape and low muscle mass.

There is **gynaecomastia** in one-third and risk of **osteoporosis** and breast cancer.
Fertility Small, soft testes (<10 mL, 2 cm); most are sterile or produce few sperm, as a result of atrophy of the seminiferous tubules. Testicles and penis remain small; there is low libido and impotence. Blood tests show high gonadotrophin and low testosterone levels. Pubic, axillary and chest hair are sparse and daily facial shaving is rarely necessary.
IQ 10–15 points reduced, representing around 1% of men in institutions for the learning disabled.
Other features There may be **scoliosis**, **emphysema**, varicose veins and leg ulcers, diabetes mellitus in 8% and thyroid problems are common.
Aetiology Around 15% show 46,XY/47,XXY mosaicism. Mental deficiency and physical abnormality increase with the number of supernumerary X chromosomes.
Management Klinefelter syndrome presents in childhood with clumsiness, learning difficulties and poor verbal skills.

Medical Genetics at a Glance, Third Edition. Dorian J. Pritchard and Bruce R. Korf.

Testosterone therapy by long-term implants should be initiated at the beginning of puberty. Fertility has been achieved using testicular sperm aspiration and **intracytoplasmic sperm injection (ICSI)** (Chapter 71).

Turner syndrome, X chromosome monosomy

Genetics Karyotype **45,X**; body cells abnormal for females in containing no Barr bodies. They can show X-linked recessive disease as in males.

Frequency 1/2000–1/3000 female births

Body form Phenotype basically female, but patients fail to mature; short stature from age of 3 years, no adolescent growth spurt. Mature height averages 145 cm (4 ft 9 in; 20 cm below average); shield-shaped chest with widely spaced nipples.

Head and face Heart-shaped face with micrognathia and low posterior hairline; excess skin forms a web between neck and shoulders; high arched palate with overcrowding of teeth.

Eyes High incidence of long or short sight, **strabismus**, **epicanthic folds**, **ptosis** of eyelids.

Ears Ears are low-set and posteriorly rotated, **otitis media** is frequent and can lead to conductive deafness.

Hands and feet Short fingers and toes, especially 4th metacarpals (in 50%), frail nails; increased carrying angle at elbow (**cubitus valgus**). There is often **lymphoedema** in the hands and feet of newborns.

Fertility Breasts, pubic hair and menstruation are usually absent. Ovaries may appear normal at birth, but atrophy progressively; some have borne children.

Heart Twenty per cent have heart defects, most commonly obstructive lesions of the left side (50% have a bicuspid aortic valve, 15–30% **coarctation**, that is narrowing, of the aorta) leading to hypertension in 30% and peripheral vascular problems. Life expectancy is reduced.

Cognition Patients may have difficulty with specific visual–spatial coordination tasks and mathematics.

Thyroid Hypothyroidism due to lymphocytic thyroiditis.

Other features Half have structural kidney defects; there is occult aneurysm of cerebral arteries, many **naevi** (moles).

Aetiology Sixty to 80% are caused by loss of the paternal-derived sex chromosome during paternal meiosis or early cell division in the embryo.

In 45,X fetuses the lymphatic system sometimes becomes obstructed, the common thoracic duct fails to empty and the posterior cervical area develops as a large, fluid-filled sack (**cystic hygroma**). Coarctation of the aorta may result from compression and the fluid imbalance may result in **hydrops** (heart failure and widespread swelling), culminating in collapse of the circulation, the primary cause of fetal death. Alternatively the cystic hygroma can recede, leaving a short neck with redundant skin, low posterior hairline and low-set ears.

Management Adolescents usually present with decreased growth or **primary amenorrhoea**.

Ultrasound scanning in the second trimester can reveal generalized oedema (**hydrops fetalis**), or swelling localized to the neck.

• *Sexual development.* Oestrogen administration at 12–13 years can ensure breast development, growth of pubic hair and maturation of the uterus and vaginal epithelium. Cyclic treatment with oestrogen and progesterone maintains female phenotype and prevents osteoporosis. Pregnancy can be achieved by *in vitro* fertilization with donor eggs.

• *Short stature.* Height can be increased by growth hormone administration.

• *Aorta.* Coarctation is indicated by a diminished femoral pulse, when surgical correction is recommended.

• *Eyes.* Optical checks and provision of spectacles, correction of strabismus.

• *Ears.* Regular hearing checks after otitis media bouts; treatment of 'glue ear'.

• *Hypothyroidism.* Thyroxine administration if necessary.

• *Hand–eye coordination.* Physical therapy.

Table 37.1 Chromosomal errors in Turner patients.

Proportion of Turner patients (%)	Chromosomal error
50	Monosomy: 45,X
30–40	Mosaicism: mostly 45,X/46,XX; a few 45X/45,XY
10–20	Isochromosomes, ring chromosomes, deletions, etc.

▶ **Problems requiring immediate attention**

• Possible heart surgery; treatment of hypothyroidism.

47,XYY syndrome

Genotype Karyotype 47,XYY

Frequency 1/1000 male births; 2–3% of males institutionalized because of learning problems or antisocial criminal behaviour.

Features Very tall stature, large teeth. Fertility is normal.

IQ Ten to twenty points below controls. Minor behavioural disorders such as attention deficit, hyperactivity, learning disabilities, sometimes problems in motor coordination. They can show aggression in childhood, emotional immaturity and impulsive behaviour. A slightly higher than normal proportion become involved in criminal activity.

Triple-X syndrome

Genotype Karyotype, **47,XXX** (and **48,XXXX**, **49,XXXXX**, etc.); each body cell contains one fewer Barr bodies than the number of X chromosomes.

Frequency 1/1000–1/1500 female births.

Features Generally tall with slender body shape. They have a mild reduction in intellectual skills and sometimes 'oppositional behaviour' and difficulty in interpersonal relationships. Abnormalities are in proportion to the number of X chromosomes they possess. The additional X is of maternal origin in 95% of cases.

Twenty five per cent are infertile, sometimes ascribed to 45,X oocytes in 45,X/47,XXX mosaics.

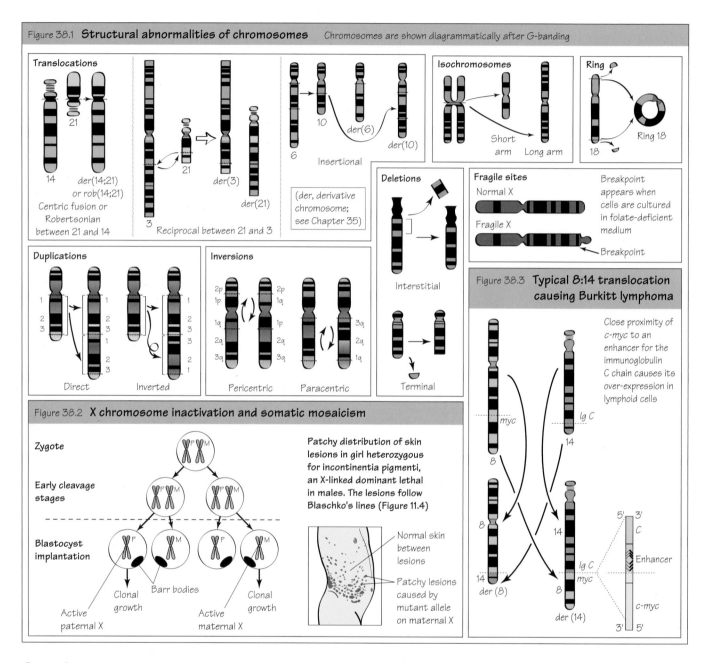

Figure 38.1 **Structural abnormalities of chromosomes** *Chromosomes are shown diagrammatically after G-banding*

Figure 38.3 **Typical 8:14 translocation causing Burkitt lymphoma**

Figure 38.2 **X chromosome inactivation and somatic mosaicism**

Overview

Chromosome abnormalities are a principal cause of pregnancy loss, an estimated 10–15% of conceptions having a chromosome abnormality of which 95% are lost before term. Close to 90% of the abnormalities are aneuploidies, the remainder being chromosome structural abnormalities. Around two-thirds of the structural abnormalities arise in oocytes, one-third in sperm, the latter increasing with paternal age.

Structural aberrations include **translocations, deletions, ring chromosomes, duplications, inversions, isochromosomes, centric fragments** and **fragile sites**. Most of these result from unequal exchange between homologous repeated sequences on the same or different chromosomes, or when two chromosome breaks occur close together and enzymic repair mechanisms link the wrong ends.

Somatic mosaicism

Mosaicism refers to the existence in the body of more than one genetically distinct cell line following a single fertilization event (c.f. **chimaerism**, in which different cell lines result from multiple fertilizations). Both yield incidence patterns that depart from general rules.

If an abnormal birth occurs in a family with no previous history of that disorder, it could be caused by a new mutation in a single germ cell, in which case the risk of recurrence would be negligible. If the mutation occurs throughout a mosaic patch of tissue that includes germ cells, the recurrence rate is usually estimated as around 1% or up to 6% for highly mutable genes such as **osteogenesis imperfecta** and **Duchenne muscular dystrophy** (see Chapter 11).

Medical Genetics at a Glance, Third Edition. Dorian J. Pritchard and Bruce R. Korf.

X chromosome inactivation (see Chapter 43) creates a mosaic for expression of the two X chromosomes in normal women, which in heterozygotes can allow pathological expression of X-linked recessive alleles. For example, a woman heterozygous for recessive colour blindness is colour blind if the normal X is inactivated in all her photoreceptor cones (see Chapter 10). Her genetic status as a heterozygote would be revealed, however, if she produced both normal and colour-blind sons.

Translocations

A translocation involves transposition of chromosome material usually between chromosomes. Three types are recognized: **centric fusion** or 'Robertsonian', **reciprocal** and **insertional**.

Centric fusion or 'Robertsonian translocations' (code: 'rob')

Centric fusion arises from breaks at or near the centromeres of two chromosomes, followed by their fusion. The long arms of Chromosomes 13, 14, 15, 21 and 22 only are involved, especially 13 with 14 (rob13;14), and 14 with 21 (rob 14;21). These are all **acro-centric** chromosomes with very small short arms (see Chapter 35), the latter carrying multiple copies of the ribosomal RNA genes (see Chapter 23). Their tendency to undergo centric fusion possibly relates to their joint contribution to the function of the nucleolus (see Chapter 14).

Although centric fusion involves loss of rRNA genes, sufficient intact copies remain on other chromosomes for no serious consequence to result. The carrier of a pair of centrically fused chromosomes may therefore have only 45 chromosomes, but be quite healthy as the overall loss is insignificant. This is a **balanced translocation**. However, such balanced translocation carriers run into problems at meiosis, with the result that a woman could have many miscarriages and individuals of either sex can have offspring with effective T21 and Down syndrome (see Chapter 39).

Reciprocal translocations (code: 't')

Reciprocal translocation involves interchromosomal exchange. Either arm of any chromosome can be involved and carriers are usually healthy. The medical significance is therefore usually for *future* generations, as carriers can produce chromosomally unbalanced fetuses.

X-linked recessive disease can arise in heterozygous females as a consequence of X–autosome translocation. For example, the reciprocal translocation between chromosomes X and 1, formulated as 46,X,t(X;1)(p21;q31) (see Chapter 35) interferes with X inactivation, as the translocation breakpoint occurs between that gene and the inactivation centre.

Reciprocal translocations can also activate genes in cancers, as in Burkitt lymphoma (see Figure 38.3 and Chapters 39 and 56).

Insertional translocations (code: 'ins')

Insertional translocation involves insertion of a deleted segment interstitially at another location. It is extremely rare and balanced carriers are usually healthy, but may produce chromosomally unbalanced offspring with either a duplication or a deletion.

Deletions (code: 'del')

Deletion of part of a chromosome can be **interstitial** or **terminal**. Interstitial deletions can arise from two breaks, followed by faulty repair, from unequal crossing-over in a previous meiosis, or as a consequence of a translocation in a parent. The error is described using the code 'del' followed by a description of the missing region in a separate set of brackets. For example, DiGeorge syndrome, caused by a deletion at 22q11.22, is formulated: del(22)(q11.22). A terminal deletion of the long arm of Chromosome 1 from band 21 would be formulated: 46,XX,del(1)(q21;qter) (see Chapter 35).

The smallest deletions detectable by **high-resolution banding** (see Chapter 35) are of about 3 megabases (i.e. 3 million base pairs). Since a gene may be as short as 1 kb (1000 bases), visible deletions tend to indicate loss of many genes. They are generally characterized by mental handicap and multiple congenital malformations (see Chapter 45). Several syndromes are ascribed to microscopically invisible **microdeletions** and when several genes are deleted together the term **contiguous gene syndrome** is applied to the corresponding phenotype (see Chapter 40).

Ring chromosomes (code: 'r')

If two breaks occur in the same chromosome the broken ends can fuse as a ring. Acentric rings are lost, but if the ring contains a centromere it can survive subsequent cell division. Clinically a ring represents two deletions. They can double by sister chromatid exchange, leading to effective trisomy, or be lost, resulting in monosomy. They are sometimes associated with growth failure and mental handicap.

Duplications (code: 'dup')

Duplication is the presence of two adjacent copies of a chromosomal segment and can be either 'direct' (or 'tandem'), or 'inverted'. Duplications may originate by unequal crossing-over in a previous meiosis, or as a consequence of translocation, inversion, or presence of an isochromosome (see below) in a parent. Duplications are more common, but generally less harmful than deletions. An example is **cat eye syndrome** involving **iris coloboma** formulated: dup(22)(p13;q11).

Inversions (code: 'inv')

Inversions arise from two chromosomal breaks with end-to-end switching of the intervening segment. If this includes the centromere it is **pericentric**, if not, the inversion is **paracentric**. They can lead to chromosomally unbalanced gametes following crossing-over.

Isochromes (code: 'iso')

An isochromosome has one chromosome arm deleted and the other duplicated. In live births the commonest involves the long arm of the X, resulting in Turner syndrome due to short arm monosomy. Most cause spontaneous abortion.

Fragile sites (code: 'fra')

A fragile site is an apparent gap in a chromosome. Some are common (or 'universal'), others are rare and sensitive to folate levels in the medium in which the cells under examination are cultured. These are inherited in a Mendelian fashion, a well known example being the defect associated with fragile X syndrome (see Chapter 11).

Figure 39.1 **Meiosis in a 14/21 translocation carrier produces familial Down syndrome**

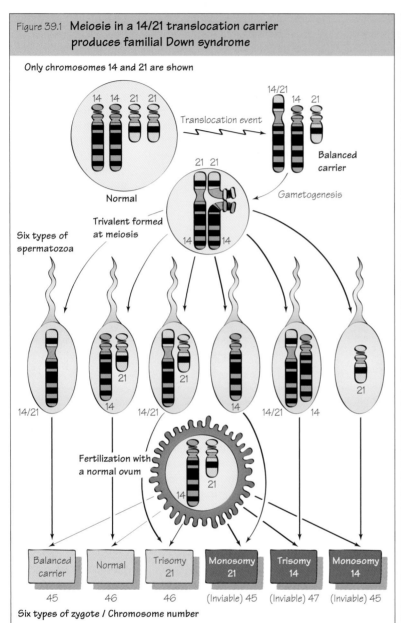

Only chromosomes 14 and 21 are shown

Figure 39.2 **Derivation of the Philadelphia chromosome by reciprocal exchange between chromosomes 9 and 22**

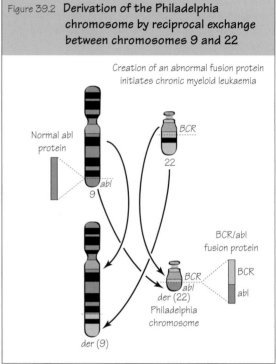

Creation of an abnormal fusion protein initiates chronic myeloid leukaemia

Figure 39.3 **Girl with karyotype 46,XX,del(5)(p15.2) showing Cri-du-chat syndrome**

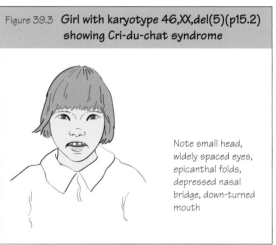

Note small head, widely spaced eyes, epicanthal folds, depressed nasal bridge, down-turned mouth

Figure 39.5 **Girl with karyotype 46,XX,del(7(q11.23) showing Williams-Beuren syndrome**

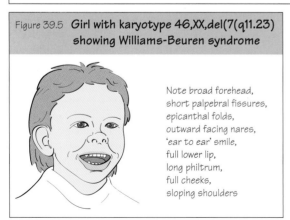

Note broad forehead, short palpebral fissures, epicanthal folds, outward facing nares, 'ear to ear' smile, full lower lip, long philtrum, full cheeks, sloping shoulders

Figure 39.4 **Girl with karyotype 46,XX,del(4p) showing Wolf-Hirschhorn syndrome**

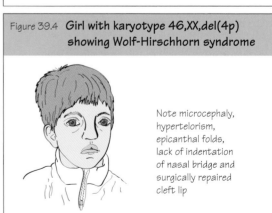

Note microcephaly, hypertelorism, epicanthal folds, lack of indentation of nasal bridge and surgically repaired cleft lip

Overview

Very rarely a patient suffers simultaneously from what appear to be several quite different genetic disorders. This is usually due to disruption of an extended section of a chromosome, among the most obvious of which are interchromosomal translocations. Translocations can be balanced in the individuals in which they arose, but cause errors in subsequent generations due to unequal segregation of genetic material at meiosis. A well known example is translocation Down syndrome. Faults can also occur due to rearrangement of structural genes with respect to control elements. The latter is rare as a cause of inherited disease, but common in tumorigenesis, a well-known example being the Philadelphia chromosome (see Chapters 39 and 57). Damage also occurs to genes at the chromosomal breakpoints, but even when gene function is disrupted there may be no phenotypic consequence if the other, unaffected allele can perform sufficient of the function alone. If a 50% decrease in product does cause an adverse effect, the normal allele is said to be 'haploinsufficient', as in some cases of Sotos syndrome. Due to X-chromosome inactivation in females, a special category of abnormality arises from translocation between the X and an autosome.

Congenital abnormalities are increasingly being ascribed to small deletions. Large deletions and medium-scale deletions known as segmental aneuploidies may be rendered visible by fluorescence in situ hybridization (FISH) to banded chromosomes (see Chapter 35). Smaller microdeletions and microduplications are addressed in the next chapter.

Segmental aneuploidies are small-to-medium scale deletions associated with well-recognized syndromes that occur repeatedly. At the DNA level they are characterized by series of repeats of 1 kb or more in length, flanking the sequence of genes that become deleted or duplicated. Those repeats are thought to be normally responsible for helping homologous chromosomes to align in register, side by side during zygotene of Meiosis I (Chapter 18), misalignments causing Non-Alleleic Homologous Recombination (NAHR), with loss of chromosomal material by one homologue and gain by its partner. Examples include Cri-du-chat, Wolf–Hirschhorn, Williams–Beuren, DiGeorge/velocardiofacial, Smith–Magenis, and Prader–Willi syndromes (see Chapter 27).

Although chromosomal syndromes are typically quite variable, several generalizations are nevertheless possible:
• Most chromosomal abnormalities are associated with developmental delay in childhood and intellectual handicap in teenagers and adults.
• Most produce characteristic facial appearances.
• Most are associated with retarded growth.
• Many include congenital malformation of the heart.
   (See Chapter 49 for explanation of dysmorphic terms.)

It is important that every child with multiple congenital abnormalities should be examined for chromosome damage at an early stage. If a condition is suspected, antenatal diagnosis is generally possible by chorionic villus sampling at 10–12 weeks, or amniocentesis at 16 weeks (see Chapter 72).

Deletions and segmental aneuploidies
Cri-du-chat; Lejeune syndrome

Frequency 1/20 000–1/50 000; possibly 1% of profoundly learning disabled.

Genetics 46,XX,del(5)(p15.2)

Features The newborn baby has a low birthweight and makes a distinctive cry similar to that of a kitten due to under-development of the larynx (French: 'cri du chat': 'cry of the cat'). Typically there are microcephaly, hypertelorism, epicanthic folds, divergent strabismus, low-set ears, hypotonia, severe breathing problems and often failure to thrive. Patent ductus arteriosus is present in 30%. The face is round in children, elongated in adults; severe intellectual handicap (IQ ~35).

Management A structured exercise regime is recommended, plus verbal stimulation and correction of squints.

Lifespan Survival into adulthood sometimes occurs.

▶ Problems requiring immediate attention

Surgical correction of congenital heart disease; severe respiratory and feeding difficulties.

Wolf–Hirschhorn syndrome

Frequency 1/50 000; male:female ratio 3:4.

Genetics e.g. 46,XY,del(4)(p16.1); balanced translocation in 10%.

Features Microcephaly, hypertelorism, epicanthic folds; lack of indentation of the nasal bridge is described as resembling the protective nosepiece of an ancient Greek helmet. Hypotonic at birth and muscle tone remains poor; cleft lip with or without cleft palate (CL ± P); low-set ears, short upper lip, heart defects, convulsions, hypospadias and undescended testes, severe learning difficulties. There is failure to thrive, but lifespan can be into the teens.

Management Developmental checks are necessary.

▶ Problems requiring immediate attention

Nasogastric feeding; heart surgery; correction of facial clefts and hypospadias; selection of appropriate anticonvulsant.

Williams–Beuren syndrome; infantile hypercalcaemia
Frequency 1/10 000

Genetics 1.5-Mb microdeletion: del(7)(q11.23); possibly inherited as AD.

Features Broad forehead, short palpebral fissures, starry pattern of irides, tip-tilted nose with low bridge and outward facing nostrils, long philtrum, full cheeks, large mouth with full lips; excessive vomiting; sleeplessness; slow growth rate. Children have a 'cocktail party manner', with outgoing attitude, hyperactivity and advanced facility in language, but become withdrawn as adults and sensitive especially to loud noise. There are also mental retardation, supravalvular aortic stenosis (SVAS), multiple peripheral pulmonary arterial stenoses, dental malformations, short stature with sloping shoulders and visual–spatial cognitive deficiency.

Aetiology Deletion of a segment of 7q carrying about 20 contiguous genes including the elastin structural locus. Elastin is expressed in the

Chromosome structural abnormalities, clinical examples – continued

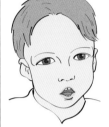

Note characteristic square face with micrognathia

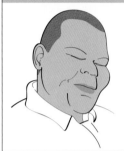

Note small crown, small nose, low-set ears and excessive body bulk

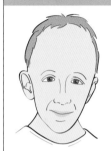

Note prominent forehead, triangular face, hypertelorism, down-slanting palpebral fissures

aortic wall, its deficiency causing SVAS (see Chapters 47 and 48). LIMK1 can also be lost, this is a kinase expressed in the brain and likely to be involved in visual spatial cognition.

Management Dietetic advice, energetic play. Intellectual disability prevents independency.

▶ Problems requiring immediate attention

Special care is needed with feeding; regulation of serum calcium; possible need for cardiac surgery.

DiGeorge anomaly, velocardiofacial syndrome (VCFS)

Frequency 1/4000 live births; one of the commonest microdeletion syndromes.

Genetics Deletion of 3 Mb (3 million base pairs): del(22)(q11.2), sometimes related to unbalanced translocation of 22q; can be inherited as AD.

Features Recognizable facial appearance with micrognathia and congenital short or cleft palate; thymic hypoplasia causing T-cell deficiency and parathyroid hypoplasia depressing serum calcium levels; heart malformations particularly of the cardiac outflow tract (see Chapter 48). About half have partial growth hormone deficiency and 40% of adults have schizophrenia-like episodes.

Aetiology Deletion of multiple contiguous genes with primary effect on migration of neural crest cells to the cervical region (see Chapters 42).

Lifespan Many die in their first year.

Management Investigation for cardiac abnormality, calcium and parathyroid status and renal anomalies, prevention of infection.

▶ Problems requiring immediate attention

Surgery for cardiac abnormality and cleft palate; serum calcium and growth hormone regulation.

Smith–Magenis syndrome

Frequency >1/25 000 live births.

Genetics del(17)(p11.2); mutations in *RAI1* gene.

Features Small head, midface hypoplasia, small nose; ears low-set and of unusual shape. Initially delayed growth, but excessive weight gain in older children, despite unexceptional appetite (c.f. P-WS; see Chapter 27). Seizures, learning difficulties and speech delay. Most often recognized by aggressive or hyperactive, self-harming behaviour, persistent disturbed sleep and characteristic 'self-hugging'. Congenital heart disease in a third, scoliosis develops in late childhood in more than half, middle ear infections and hearing impairment in two-thirds.

Aetiology Haploinsufficiency of the **RAI1 (retinoic acid induced 1) gene** responsible for synthesis of a protein necessary for brain cell development.

Management Speech and hearing therapy; dietetic advice.

▶ Problems requiring immediate attention

Cardiac surgery; treatment of ear infection; use of melatonin to control sleep pattern.

Autosomal translocations
Translocation Down syndrome

About 4% of Down syndrome cases involve a Robertsonian translocation between the long arm of Chromosome 21 and another acrocentric, usually 14 (see Chapters 36 and 38).

Consider an individual defined as 45,XX,der(14;21)(q10;q10). This woman lacks one normal 14 and one normal 21 and instead has a chromosome derived by reciprocal translocation between the entire long arms of 14 and 21. Since there is little genetic information in either short arm her phenotype is essentially normal. However, during meiosis the abnormal derivative chromosome may segregate in either of several ways to yield an ovum which, if fertilized by a normal sperm, could create a fetus with either translocation Down syndrome, with effective T21, or monosomy 21 (M21); effective T14, or M14. Embryos with the latter three karyotypes fail to survive to term, and additional prenatal losses reduce the frequency of liveborn Down syndrome babies to 10–15%. The equivalent figure for fathers with the balanced 14;21 translocation is 1–2%.

By comparison, the recurrence risk for a Down syndrome pregnancy with a karyotypically normal woman under 30 years is around 1%.

Sotos syndrome, cerebral gigantism
Frequency Rare

Genetics 5;8 translocation with breakpoint at 5q35; mutations in *NSD1* gene at 5q35.

Features Large head with prominent forehead, hypertelorism with outwardly down-slanting palpebral fissures, characteristic nose in childhood and prominent chin. Usually high birthweight, hypotonia, feeding difficulties, often motor delay and ataxia. Cerebral ventricles may appear dilated on MRI or CT scan. Children are tall with long arms, large hands and feet, and advanced bone age.

Aetiology Haploinsufficiency of the *NSD1* (**nuclear SET domain 1**) **gene**, a transcription factor and regulator.

Management Psychological problems related to stature. Scoliosis can develop in adolescence.

The Philadelphia chromosome
The 'Philadelphia chromosome' is a derivative of Chromosomes 22 and 9, created by reciprocal translocation. The modified 22 carries the coding for an abnormal 'fusion protein' with increased enzymic activity that initiates chronic myeloid leukaemia (see Chapters 39 and 57).

X-autosome translocations
Female Duchenne muscular dystrophy (DMD)
In female somatic cells one X-chromosome is inactivated at an early stage, creating mosaic representation of heterozygous X-linked genes (see Chapters 11, 38 and 43). This generally is sufficient to protect female heterozygotes from X-linked disorders that affect males (Chapter 38). However, X-inactivation in the female carrier of an X-autosome translocation can sometimes create lethal genetic imbalance in half her body cells, causing those cells to die. The result is that the same X-chromosome is expressed in every cell and if that chromosome carries a disease allele the individual can express the X-linked disease like a male. This is the explanation for some female cases of Duchenne muscular dystrophy.

40 Contiguous-gene and single-gene syndromes

Figure 40.1 (a) Woman with karyotype 46,XX,del(11)(p13) showing WAGR syndrome

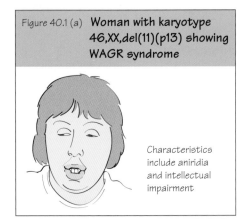

Characteristics include aniridia and intellectual impairment

Figure 40.1 (b) Chromosome 11 showing region deleted in WAGR

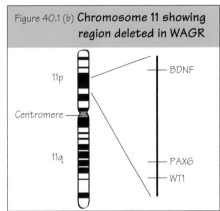

11p

Centromere

11q

BDNF

PAX6

WT1

Figure 40.2 Girl with karyotype 46,XX,del(8)(q24.11;q24.13) showing Langer-Giedion syndrome

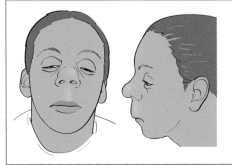

Note ptosis of eyelids, bulbous nose, elongated philtrum, sparse hair

Figure 40.3 Girl with karyotype 46,XX, del(1)(p36;pter) showing '1p36 syndrome'

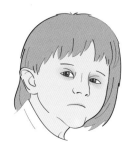

Note short, wide head, pointed chin, sunken eyes, mid-face hypoplasia, straight eyebrows

Figure 40.4 MRI scan and face of child with karyotype 46,XY,del(17)(p13.3) showing Miller-Dieker syndrome

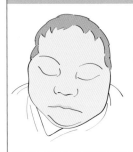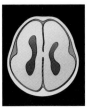

Note typical 'Figure 8' appearance of brain section and smooth cortical surface. Note also narrow forehead, small nose with antiverted nostrils, up-slanting palpebral fissures, protruding upper lip and micrognathia.

Medical Genetics at a Glance, Third Edition. Dorian J. Pritchard and Bruce R. Korf.

Overview

'Microdeletions' and microduplications are detectable by comparative genome hybridization (CGH) at levels below those of conventional microscopic resolution, that is less than 5 Mb (see Chapter 35). This approach can be applied to whole, extended chromosomes, as in FISH, or in **array CGH**, to spots of cloned DNA oligonucleotides distributed in arrays on glass slides. Three categories of disorder are thereby distinguished, in order of diminishing size:

- segmental aneuploidies (see Chapter 39)
- contiguous-gene syndromes
- single-gene syndromes.

Contiguous-gene syndromes (CGSs) are seen primarily in males with X-chromosome deletions. The classic case is an unfortunate boy with Duchenne MD (see Chapter 11), who also had **chronic granulomatous disease**, retinitis pigmentosa, **McLeod phenotype** (a red blood cell disorder) and intellectual handicap. The combination was caused by the combined loss of a short series of structural genes adjacent to that for DMD at Xp21.

Such microdeletions are relatively common at Xp21 and proximal Xq, but rarely seen in some parts of the X, possibly because deletion of most sections is lethal. CGSs are much less common on the autosomes because of the usual presence of the normal homologue. Exceptions are the relatively rare haploinsufficient, or dosage-sensitive, genes, for example those causing **WAGR, Langer–Giedion** and **Miller–Dieker lissencephaly syndromes**.

Typically any gene generally affects only a single step in a biochemical pathway, or one organ, system or cell type. The existence of multiple clinical features due to a single defective allele is called **pleiotropy**, usually ascribable to expression in more than one location or situation, as in **Rubinstein–Taybi syndrome**, or to cascade effects as in **Alagille syndrome**. In the cytogenetic context, 'single-gene syndrome' generally refers to deletion or duplication of a small chromosomal segment containing essentially just one gene. Rubinstein–Taybi and Alagille syndrome are examples, as are some cases of Angelman syndrome (see Chapter 27). A small percentage of unexplained cases of intellectual handicap are due to terminal deletions, including **1p36 syndrome**.

It is interesting to compare the consequences of monosomy of a region due to deletion, with trisomy due to duplication; for example Miller–Dieker and **17p13.3 duplication syndrome** (see below).

Contiguous gene deletion syndromes

WAGR syndrome
Frequency 1/10 000

Genetics CGS: del(11)(p13) (Figure 40.1b).

Features Wilms (embryonal renal) tumour, **A**niridia, **G**enitourinary abnormalities (including gonadal tumours), **R**etardation of growth and development (hence **WAGR**).

Aetiology Loss of gene *PAX6* confers aniridia; loss of *WT1* (**Wilms tumour suppressor 1**) causes Wilms tumour (see Chapter 56); loss of *BDNF* (**brain-derived neurotropin factor**) relates to retardation (see Figure 40.1a).

Management A *WT1* DNA probe can be used for antenatal diagnosis.

Langer–Giedion syndrome, trichorhinophalangeal syndrome Type II
Frequency Rare.

Genetics CGS: del(8)(q24.11-q24.13); AD

Features Large, laterally protruding ears, bulbous nose, elongated upper lip; sparse scalp hair, short fingers and toes, winged scapulae, multiple **exostoses** (tumorous bony overgrowths), redundant skin, intellectual handicap.

Aetiology Combines the clinical features of trichorhinopharyngeal syndrome Type I and multiple exostoses Type I due to mutations in *TRPS1* and *EXT1* (at 8q24.12), respectively. Protein EXT1 (**exostosin 1**) normally forms a complex with EXT2 that catalyses polymerization of heparan sulphate. The complex is an essential factor in a signal transduction cascade that regulates chondrocyte differentiation, ossification and apoptosis.

Management Analgesia for joint pain. Monitoring of growth and development. May require hip replacement in 5th or 6th decade.

1p36 deletion syndrome
Frequency 1/ 5000 livebirths; the most common terminal deletion syndrome.

Genetics CGS: del(1)(p36;pter)

Features Small head unusually short and wide, straight eyebrows, sunken eyes, midface hypoplasia with flat nasal bridge, asymmetric ears, pointed chin, hypotonia, developmental delay, severe learning difficulties, epilepsy, patent ductus arteriosus (see Chapter 47) and other cardiomyopathy, hearing impairment, hypermetropia.

Aetiology Defects due to haploinsufficiency of several genes near the 1p terminus.

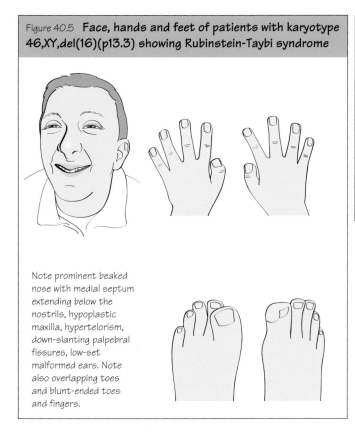

Figure 40.5 **Face, hands and feet of patients with karyotype 46,XY,del(16)(p13.3) showing Rubinstein-Taybi syndrome**

Note prominent beaked nose with medial septum extending below the nostrils, hypoplastic maxilla, hypertelorism, down-slanting palpebral fissures, low-set malformed ears. Note also overlapping toes and blunt-ended toes and fingers.

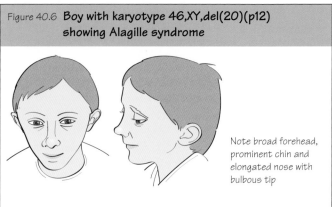

Figure 40.6 **Boy with karyotype 46,XY,del(20)(p12) showing Alagille syndrome**

Note broad forehead, prominent chin and elongated nose with bulbous tip

▶ Problems requiring immediate attention

Treatment of heart defects and seizures.

Azoospermia

Frequency This deletion may be responsible for 10–20% of cases of idiopathic (i.e. occurring without apparent extrinsic cause) **azoospermia** and severe **oligospermia** (i.e. complete lack or severe deficiency of sperm).

Genetics Microdeletion del(Y)(11.2).

Features Male infertility.

Aetiology Deletions cause loss of genes within the **AZF** (**azoospermic factor**) region, including three subregions responsible for different phases of spermatogenesis.

Miller–Dieker lissencephaly syndrome

Frequency Rare

Genetics Visible or submicroscopic contiguous gene deletion: del(17)(p13.3); AR; (c.f. 17p13.3 microduplication below).

Features Classic **lissencephaly** (smooth brain), subtle brain defects include **microcephaly**. Prominent occiput, narrow forehead, upslant-ing palpebral fissures (see Chapter 49), small nose and chin, cardiac malformations, hypoplastic male genitalia, macrosomia, mild developmental delay. Severe intellectual handicap, seizures, EEG abnormalities, attention deficit hyperactivity disorder, psychomotor retardation. Death usually in early childhood.

Aetiology Haploinsufficiency of one or more genes at 17p13.3.
Management Sometimes correction of **omphalocele** (umbilical hernia), attention to feeding problems.

▶ Problems requiring immediate attention

Correction of feeding problems by fitting of gastrostomy tube; management of seizures.

Contiguous gene duplication syndrome

17p13.3 Microduplication

Genetics CGS: dup(17)(p13.3); (c.f. Miller–Dieker syndrome above).

Features This defect is due to duplication of the region deleted in the Miller–Dieker syndrome. Prominent forehead and a pointed chin. Class I: autistic features, speech and motor delay, subtle dysmorphic facial features and hand or foot malformations (not illustrated), a tendency to postnatal overgrowth. Class II: moderate to mild developmental and psychomotor delay, hypotonia, microcephaly, severe growth retardation, no dysmorphism.

Aetiology Class II involves duplication of gene *PAFAH1B1* and sometimes of *CRK* and *YWHAE*. Class I involves duplication of *YWHAE* but not *PAFAH1B1*.

Single-gene syndromes

Rubinstein–Taybi or broad thumb–great toe syndrome

Frequency 1/125 000, but 1/500 in institutions for severe mental handicap.

Genetics del(16)(p13.3); AD.

Features Broad thumbs and great toes flattened at ends and sometimes bifid or overlapping; widely separate from other toes. Wide-set eyes, blue sclerae, long down-slanting palpebral fissures (see Chapter 49), ptosis, long eyelashes, strabismus and refractive errors. Large convex nose, small mouth with high palate, teeth crowded. Excess body hair, flame-shaped **naevi** (moles). Vertebral and sternal abnormalities, heart defects, absent or extra kidney, pulmonary stenosis, undescended testes. Microcephaly, mental retardation, developmental delay, final height only at 50th centile (see Chapter 49). Brain tumours in later life. Patients nevertheless are generally happy, sociable and friendly.

Aetiology **CREB binding protein** (**CREBBP**) is a histone acetyltransferase that functions as a transcription factor for Gli proteins concerned with patterning of skeletal elements. The deletion creates a haploinsufficiency that leads to this syndrome.

Management Correction of eye defects and undescended testes, surgery on feet, attention to obesity and dental issues. Speech therapy and instruction in self-help skills.

▶ **Problems requiring immediate attention**

Treatment of constipation, convulsions, ear and urinary infections.

Alagille syndrome, type I

Frequency 1/100 000 live births.

Genetics Seven per cent of patients have deletion of **jagged-1** (*JAG1*): del(20)(p12); AD.

Features Prolonged neonatal jaundice or cardiac murmurs in 70%. Hypoplasia of hepatic ducts, hepatosplenomegaly, hypercholesterolaemia, renal disease and hypertension. Characteristic facies in older children, with broad forehead, pointed chin and elongated nose with a bulbous tip. Growth retardation and rickets. Significant intracardiac lesions with increased mortality: atrial and ventricular septal defects, tetralogy of Fallot, patent ductus arteriosus (see Chapter 48). 'Butterfly hemivertebrae' and abnormalities of ribs and hands.

Aetiology *JAG1* encodes a ligand critical to the **notch** gene signalling cascade important in the developmental regulation of bile duct formation. Deficiency of the jagged-1 protein leads to a paucity of bile ducts and cholestatic liver disease underlying cardiac disease, CNS vasculopathy, renal disease, etc.

▶ **Problems requiring immediate attention**

Cardiac surgery, treatment for jaundice, renal disease and hypertension.

Figure 41.1 Fertilization and implantation (uterus not to scale)

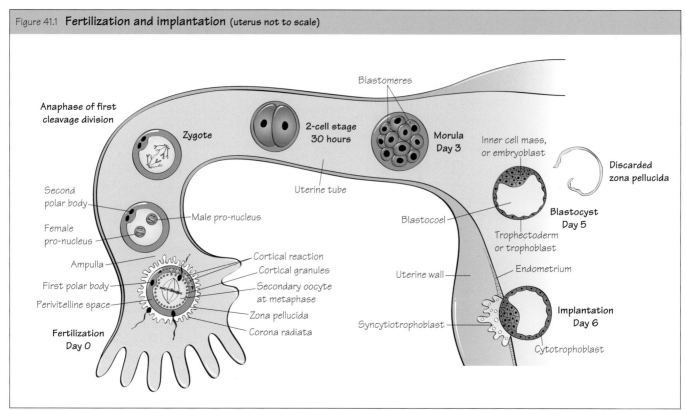

- Blastomeres
- Anaphase of first cleavage division
- Zygote
- 2-cell stage 30 hours
- Morula Day 3
- Inner cell mass, or embryoblast
- Discarded zona pellucida
- Uterine tube
- Second polar body
- Male pro-nucleus
- Blastocoel
- Trophectoderm or trophoblast
- Blastocyst Day 5
- Female pro-nucleus
- Ampulla
- Cortical reaction
- Cortical granules
- Secondary oocyte at metaphase
- Uterine wall
- Endometrium
- First polar body
- Perivitelline space
- Zona pellucida
- Corona radiata
- Syncytiotrophoblast
- Implantation Day 6
- Fertilization Day 0
- Cytotrophoblast

Figure 41.2 Formation of the embryonic disc

Figure 41.3 Embryonic disc

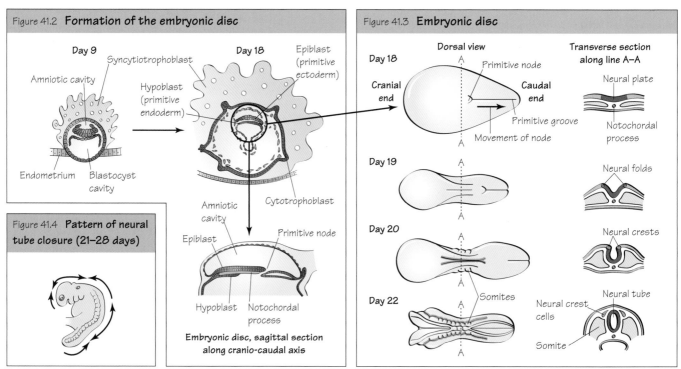

Figure 41.2 labels:
- Day 9
- Syncytiotrophoblast
- Epiblast (primitive ectoderm)
- Day 18
- Amniotic cavity
- Hypoblast (primitive endoderm)
- Endometrium
- Blastocyst cavity
- Cytotrophoblast
- Amniotic cavity
- Epiblast
- Primitive node
- Hypoblast
- Notochordal process
- Embryonic disc, sagittal section along cranio-caudal axis

Figure 41.4 Pattern of neural tube closure (21–28 days)

Figure 41.3 labels:
- Dorsal view
- Transverse section along line A–A
- Day 18
- Primitive node
- Neural plate
- Cranial end
- Caudal end
- Primitive groove
- Notochordal process
- Movement of node
- Day 19
- Neural folds
- Day 20
- Neural crests
- Day 22
- Somites
- Neural crest cells
- Neural tube
- Somite

Medical Genetics at a Glance, Third Edition. Dorian J. Pritchard and Bruce R. Korf.

106 © 2013 John Wiley & Sons, Ltd. Published 2013 by John Wiley & Sons, Ltd.

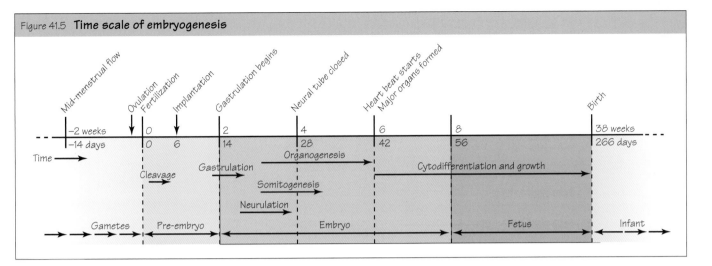

Figure 41.5 **Time scale of embryogenesis**

Overview

Fertilization by a sperm initiates **embryogenesis**. Mitosis ensues and the **pre-embryo** implants in the uterus. The **embryo** proper develops from a few internal cells, through creation of three **embryonic germ layers**. **Organogenesis** involves interactions between these and is completed by 6–8 weeks. During the subsequent period of **growth** and **cytodifferentiation** the individual is called a **fetus**.

The pre-embryo (weeks 0–2)

The secondary oocyte is shed into the peritoneal cavity and directed into the adjacent **uterine** (Fallopian) **tube**, where fertilization must take place within 24 hours. The sperm performs four functions: (i) *stimulation of metaphase II in the secondary oocyte*; (ii) *restoration of the diploid number of chromosomes*; (iii) *initiation of cleavage*; and (iv) *determination of sex*.

The sperm passes through the **corona cells** on the oocyte surface and adheres to the **zona pellucida**. The **acrosome** in the sperm head then releases enzymes that digest a tunnel through the zona pellucida, allowing the sperm to pass into the **perivitelline space** and fuse with the oocyte membrane. The sperm head is then engulfed by the oocyte and entry of more sperm prevented by a rapid **cortical reaction**. The oocyte nucleus completes metaphase II, expels the second polar body and maternal and paternal **pro-nuclei** fuse to form the **zygote**.

Mitosis of the pre-embryo is called **cleavage** and the resultant **blastomeres** are smaller after each division. The 16-cell **morula** passes down the uterine tube aided by peristalsis and ciliary movement. A space called the **blastocoel** forms off-centre in the morula to create the **blastocyst**, which swells and bursts from the zona pellucida. Two different cell types are now recognizable, the flattened **trophectoderm** cells of the outer **trophoblast** and an eccentrically placed **inner cell mass** or **embryoblast**.

On day 6 the blastocyst implants in the endometrium lining the uterus. Some trophoblast cells fuse to form the invasive **syncytiotrophoblast**, the remainder constituting the **cytotrophoblast**. The blastocyst now takes nourishment from the mother and grows rapidly as it sinks further into the endometrium.

The inner cell mass exposed ventrally to the blastocoel flattens to form the **primitive endoderm**, or **hypoblast**, while the remainder forms the **primitive ectoderm**, or **epiblast**, within which develops the **amniotic cavity**. The double-layered disc called the **embryonic disc** forms from the epiblast and hypoblast at 7–12 days, *from which the embryo proper develops*.

The embryo (weeks 2–8)

Gastrulation is the process that creates the **embryonic mesoderm** and initiates activity of the embryo's own genes. The **primitive streak** first appears in the epiblast at the caudal (tail) end of the embryonic disc, extends towards its centre and then develops the **primitive groove** in its amniotic (i.e. dorsal) surface. At the cranial (head) end of this develops the **primitive** (or **Hensen's**) **node**.

Epiblast cells migrate across the disc, through the primitive groove and into the space above the hypoblast. These become the embryonic mesoderm, creating the three **germ layers**: **ectoderm** from the epiblast, **mesoderm**, and **endoderm** from the hypoblast together with some epiblast cells that merge with it. Mesoderm cells that migrate anteriorly and accumulate in the midline form the **notochordal process**, which later extends caudally.

The epiblast thickens to form the **neural plate** and a **neural fold** arises on either side of the central axis. These curve over, contact and from 22 days fuse in five separate movements to create the **neural tube**, which later becomes the spinal cord. Along the dorsal edges of the neural folds are the **neural crest cells** that migrate out to give rise to several cell types: nerve, bone, supporting structures of the heart, adrenalin-secreting and pigment cells, etc.

As the primitive node moves caudally down the midline, blocks of mesoderm on either side rotate to create 42–44 pairs of segmental **somites**, the most caudal five to seven of which subsequently disappear (see Chapter 42).

The fetus (weeks 8–38)

The ectoderm is the origin of the outer epithelium and CNS and, with mesoderm, peripheral structures such as the limbs; mesoderm forms muscles, circulatory system, kidneys, sex organs and together with endoderm, the internal organs; endoderm gives rise to the gut and digestive glands. The rudiments of all the major organs are formed through 'inductive' tissue interactions by about 6 weeks, when the heart starts beating. Thereafter development mainly involves increase in the number and types of cells.

Expected date of delivery (EDD)

Birth is generally considered to occur at 38 weeks from conception, or 40 weeks (280 days) from the first day of the woman's last normal menstrual period (LMP). There are variations among women in cycle length and times of ovulation, the modal EDD being around 283 days from the LMP. This has important implications with respect to birth induction; modern practice favours final dating by ultrasound.

Figure 42.1 Structure of the four paralogous HOX clusters

Order of expression is from the right (3') to left (5')

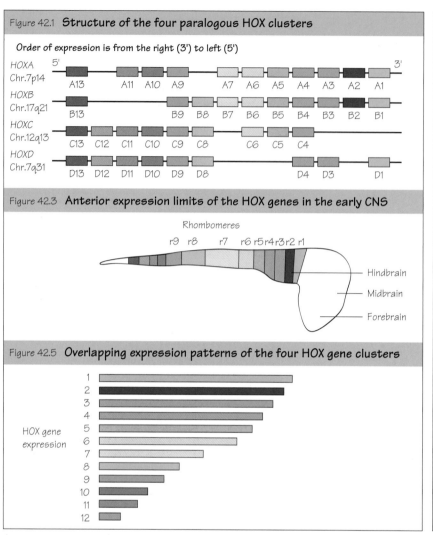

HOXA Chr.7p14
HOXB Chr.17q21
HOXC Chr.12q13
HOXD Chr.7q31

Figure 42.3 Anterior expression limits of the HOX genes in the early CNS

Rhombomeres

r9 r8 r7 r6 r5r4r3r2 r1

Hindbrain
Midbrain
Forebrain

Figure 42.5 Overlapping expression patterns of the four HOX gene clusters

HOX gene expression

1
2
3
4
5
6
7
8
9
10
11
12

Figure 42.2 Pattern of migration of neural crest cells into the branchial arches

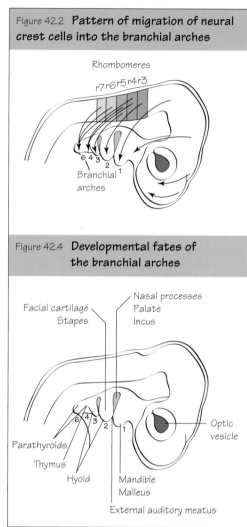

Rhombomeres

r7 r6 r5 r4 r3

Branchial arches

Figure 42.4 Developmental fates of the branchial arches

Facial cartilage
Stapes

Nasal processes
Palate
Incus

Parathyroids
Thymus
Hyoid

Mandible
Malleus

External auditory meatus

Optic vesicle

Figure 42.6 P–D, D–V axis definition in the limb bud

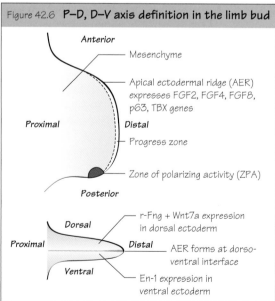

Anterior
Mesenchyme
Apical ectodermal ridge (AER) expresses FGF2, FGF4, FGF8, p63, TBX genes
Distal
Progress zone
Zone of polarizing activity (ZPA)
Proximal
Posterior

Dorsal
r-Fng + Wnt7a expression in dorsal ectoderm
Proximal
Distal
AER forms at dorso-ventral interface
Ventral
En-1 expression in ventral ectoderm

Figure 42.7 A–P axis definition in the limb bud

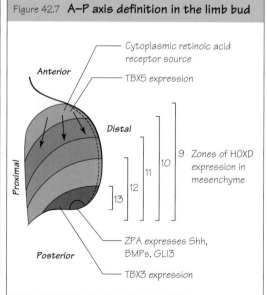

Cytoplasmic retinoic acid receptor source
Anterior
TBX5 expression
Distal
Proximal
9 Zones of HOXD expression in mesenchyme
10
11
12
13
ZPA expresses Shh, BMPs, GLI3
Posterior
TBX3 expression

Figure 42.8

Mesenchymal condensates in the forelimb

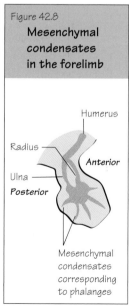

Humerus
Radius
Anterior
Ulna
Posterior
Mesenchymal condensates corresponding to phalanges

Medical Genetics at a Glance, Third Edition. Dorian J. Pritchard and Bruce R. Korf.

Overview

The human body shows regular features of anatomical organization that constitute what is known as 'body patterning'. Many of the important genes involved code for RNA transcription factors that bind to DNA, or protein morphogens that bind to cell surface receptors on target tissues.

Some of the gene names seem bizarre, as they are derived from research on other species.

Genes identified in non-human species are conventionally written in lower case, with an upper case capital if dominant (e.g. *Shh*), the equivalent human genes being written in upper case (e.g. *SHH*).

The main body
Differentiation along the antero-posterior axis

The antero-posterior axis is defined by the primitive streak, initiation and maintenance of which relates to the caudal movement of the primitive node and the sequential expression of members of four gene clusters, *HOXA*, *B*, *C* and *D*. Each cluster contains a very similar series of up to 13 genes encoding transcription factors, each containing the **homeobox** DNA binding domain.

HOX genes located at the 3′ (number 1) end are expressed earlier than those located 5′ and there is direct linear correlation between the position of each *HOX* gene in its cluster and its temporal and spatial expression. This derives from the graded sensitivity of gene expression controlling sequences to a common control molecule.

Primitive node function requires expression of the *Nodal* gene and its associated morphogen is believed to be **retinoic acid**, which it secretes increasingly abundantly as it moves in the caudal direction. More posterior target cells are thus exposed to larger concentrations of retinoic acid, with progressive activation of more *HOX* genes.

The fate of the neural crest (NC) cells is defined by the specific *HOX* genes that are active at their origin. NC cells from the fore- and midbrain migrate and differentiate into the mesenchyme of the first pharyngeal pouch, those of the anterior hindbrain to the mesenchyme of the second pharyngeal pouch. Cervical NC cells move into the third, fourth and sixth pharyngeal arches.

The first embryonic pharyngeal arch forms the mandible and malleus, the first cleft the external auditory meatus and the mesenchyme of the first pharyngeal pouch, the nasal processes, palate and incus. The second arch forms part of the hyoid apparatus, the stapes and facial cartilage. The third arch also contributes to the hyoid cartilage. The third and fourth pouches become the thymus and parathyroids. The fourth and sixth arches form the laryngeal cartilages, the fifth arch degenerates.

The blood vessels within the arches form the aortic and pulmonary systems.

There is evidence that the gene *TBX1* may be important specifically for the arteries of the fourth arch, and **DiGeorge syndrome**, with partial absence of the thymus and facial malformation, etc. (see Chapter 39) is due to a Chromosome 22 microdeletion involving *TBX1*.

Differentiation of left from right

In the normal condition, **situs solitus**, the right (R) lung is trilobed, the left (L) bilobed, the apex of the heart points to the left, the spleen and stomach are on the left, the liver is on the right and the small bowel loops in a counter-clockwise direction. In **situs inversus** there is complete mirror-imaging, but usually no disease symptoms. **Situs ambiguous** involves randomization of the arrangement of heart, lung, liver, spleen and stomach about the midline and is often associated with congenital heart defects. Mirror image bilateral symmetry of the whole body is called **isomerism**, that of individual organs **heterotaxia**, and both are associated with a variety of pathologies.

The first observable sign of L/R asymmetry is looping of the heart tube to the right and the first relevant molecular signal detectable is of **sonic hedgehog** (**Shh**) protein from the notochord. Cilia at the primitive node, powered by the motor protein **dynein**, then cause asymmetrical flow of perinodal fluid, which activates the genes for **Nodal** protein and **Lefty-2** (*LEFTB*), specifically on the left side of the embryo. Both are members of the **transforming growth factor-β** (**TGF-β**) family of signalling proteins and Nodal is responsible for the rightward looping of the heart tube. These initiate signalling pathways that activate left-hand-specific transcription factors, including **Pitx2** and **eHAND**, which promotes differentiation of the left ventricle, while **dHAND** promotes differentiation of the right ventricle. **Lefty-1** (*LEFTA*) prevents leakage of signals across the midline.

Situs inversus, isomerism and heterotaxia are produced by mutations in *LEFTA*, *LEFTB* and *NODAL*, while **Kartagener syndrome** involves random situs and other problems due to immotile cilia. Mutations in the zinc finger proteins, **ZIC3** and **GLI3** (see Chapter 22), cause rare abnormalities of asymmetry including **Greig cephalopolysyndactyly** and **Pallister–Hall syndrome**.

Discrepancies in L/R asymmetry in MZ and conjoined twins indicate normal diffusion of lateralizing influence from the left, the twin arising on the R most commonly showing randomization.

Dorso-ventral differentiation

Bone morphogenetic protein-4 (**BMP-4**) is emitted by the primitive node and induces ventral characteristics, but on its dorsal side proteins **noggin** and **chordin** are also expressed and these bind directly to BMP-4 and prevent it activating its receptor dorsally. **Sonic hedgehog** (**Shh**) protein expressed in the notochord is responsible for dorso-ventral patterning of the neural tube. Mutations and duplications of *SHH* can cause **holoprosencephaly** (non-division of the forebrain) and **cyclopia** (a single, central eye).

The limbs
The proximo-distal axis

The limb bud grows by proliferation of mesenchyme cells in the '**progress zone**' less than a millimetre below the **apical ectodermal ridge** (**AER**) at its tip. At this stage the mesenchyme cells receive progressively changing instructions mediated by **fibroblast growth factors**, FGF2, **4** and **8**, that define the extent of their proliferation, depending on which bony elements they are to form.

Limb abnormalities are a feature of **Apert syndrome**, in which there are mutations in the FGF2 receptor (*FGFR2*). Expression of *p63* is crucial for sustaining the AER, and *p63* mutations cause split hands and feet, called **ectrodactyly**.

The antero-posterior axis

At the posterior margin of the limb bud is the **ZPA**, or **zone of proliferating activity**, the source of morphogens that define the form, number and location of the digits. These diffuse anteriorly and generate a nested, overlapping pattern of *HoxD* and *HoxA* expression.

Mutations of *HOXD13* cause **synpolydactyly** (fusion of the middle digits). Defects in the anterior and posterior elements of the upper limbs occur in **Holt–Oram** and **ulnar–mammary syndromes**, caused by mutations in *TBX5* and *TBX3* specifying thumb and little finger respectively.

43 Sexual differentiation

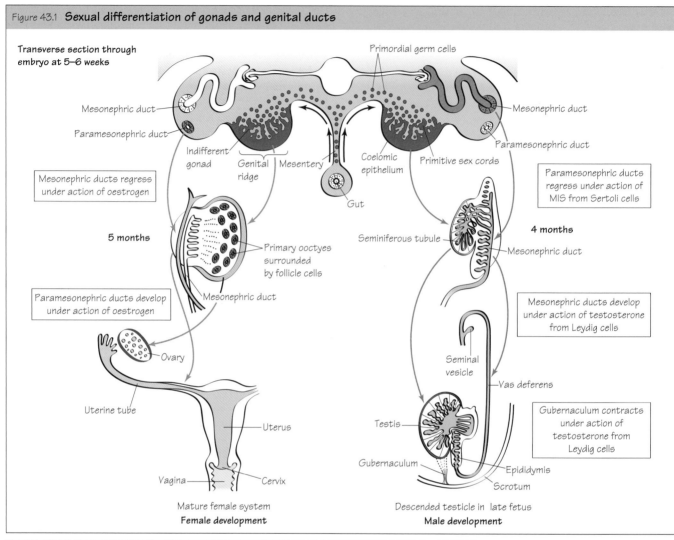

Figure 43.1 **Sexual differentiation of gonads and genital ducts**

Transverse section through embryo at 5–6 weeks

Primordial germ cells

Mesonephric duct

Paramesonephric duct

Indifferent gonad

Genital ridge

Mesentery

Coelomic epithelium

Gut

Primitive sex cords

Mesonephric duct

Paramesonephric duct

Mesonephric ducts regress under action of oestrogen

Paramesonephric ducts regress under action of MIS from Sertoli cells

5 months

4 months

Seminiferous tubule

Mesonephric duct

Primary ooctyes surrounded by follicle cells

Paramesonephric ducts develop under action of oestrogen

Mesonephric duct

Mesonephric ducts develop under action of testosterone from Leydig cells

Ovary

Seminal vesicle

Vas deferens

Uterine tube

Uterus

Testis

Gubernaculum

Gubernaculum contracts under action of testosterone from Leydig cells

Vagina

Cervix

Epididymis

Scrotum

Mature female system
Female development

Descended testicle in late fetus
Male development

Figure 43.2 **Sexual differentiation of external genitalia**

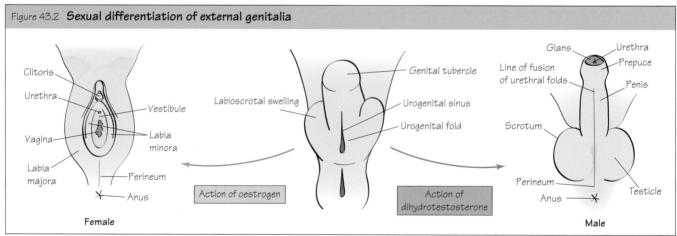

Clitoris

Urethra

Vestibule

Vagina

Labia minora

Labia majora

Perineum

Anus

Labioscrotal swelling

Genital tubercle

Urogenital sinus

Urogenital fold

Glans

Urethra

Line of fusion of urethral folds

Prepuce

Penis

Scrotum

Perineum

Testicle

Anus

Action of oestrogen

Action of dihydrotestosterone

Female

Male

Medical Genetics at a Glance, Third Edition. Dorian J. Pritchard and Bruce R. Korf.

Overview

Sexual differentiation is initiated at fertilization, depending on whether the sperm carries an X or a Y chromosome. At the blastocyst stage in XX embryos, one X chromosome in every cell is permanently inactivated, otherwise development of the sexes is similar until the *SRY gene* on the Y chromosome is activated and certain structures, including the brain, become progressively masculinized.

X chromosome inactivation

At the late blastocyst stage cells inactivate all but one of their X chromosomes. The nuclei of normal XX female cells therefore come to contain one inactive X, which can be seen at interphase as a **Barr body** in addition to their active X. Presence or absence of a Barr body is the basis of the original Olympic sex test (now long since supplanted; see Chapter 11). The choice of whether it is the paternal or maternal X which becomes inactive is random in each somatic cell, but in descendent cells it remains the same. Every woman therefore develops as a mosaic with respect to expression of her two X chromosomes. In the extraembryonic trophoblast cells the paternal X is preferentially inactivated. In oogonia the inactive chromosome is reactivated.

Genes in the pairing (**pseudo-autosomal**) region and several other sites on the X are not subject to inactivation, accounting for the variety of abnormalities of XXY and XO individuals (see Chapter 37).

Early development

At the beginning of week 5, up to 2000 **primordial germ cells** migrate from the endoderm cells of the yolk sac and infiltrate the **primitive sex cords** within the mesodermal **genital ridges**, which are developments of the coelomic epithelium. The paired **indifferent gonad** is identical in males and females.

The ovary

In the early ovary the primitive sex cords break down, but the surface epithelium proliferates and gives rise to the **cortical cords**, which split into clusters, each surrounding one or more germ cells. The latter, now called **oogonia**, proliferate then enter meiosis as **primary oocytes**.

The testis

The *SRY* gene carried only on the Y chromosome is expressed in week 7 in the cells of the primitive sex cords. Its product is a zinc finger transcription factor that binds to DNA in those same cells, leading to a masculine gene expression pattern. These cells proliferate into the **testis cords**.

Leydig cells derived from the original mesenchyme of the gonadal ridge move in around the 8th week and until weeks 17–18 synthesize male sex hormones, or **androgens**, including **testosterone**, which initiate sexual differentiation of the genital ducts and external genitalia. By the 4th month the male gonads also contain **Sertoli cells** derived from the surface epithelium of the gonad (see Chapter 44).

Genital ducts

Initially both sexes have two pairs of genital ducts: **mesonephric** (or **Wolffian**) and **paramesonephric** (or **Mullerian**). In females the mesonephric ducts regress under the action of **oestrogens** produced by the maternal system, placenta and fetal ovaries, but the paramesonephric ducts remain and become the **uterine tubes** and **uterus** (see Chapter 44).

In males the Sertoli cells produce **Mullerian inhibiting substance** (**MIS**), which causes the paramesonephric ducts to degenerate.

Testosterone binds to an intracellular receptor protein and the hormone–receptor complex then binds to specific control sites in the DNA and regulates transcription of tissue-specific genes. In male embryos testosterone converts the mesonephric ducts into the **vas deferens**, **seminal vesicle** and **epididymis**.

External genitalia

The external genitalia are derived from a complex of mesodermal tissue located around the **urogenital sinus**. At the end of the 6th week in both sexes this consists of the **genital tubercle** anteriorly, the paired **urogenital folds** on either side and lateral to these the **labioscrotal swellings**.

In females oestrogen stimulates slight elongation of the genital tubercle to form the **clitoris**, while the urogenital folds remain separate as the **labia minora**. The urogenital sinus remains open as the **vestibule** and the labioscrotal swellings become the **labia majora**.

The tissues around the **urogenital sinus** synthesize **5-α-reductase**, which in males converts **testosterone** secreted by the Leydig cells to **dihydrotestosterone**. Under the action of this hormone the genital tubercle elongates into the **penis**, pulling the urethral folds forward to form the lateral walls of the **urethral groove**. At the end of the 3rd month the tops of the walls fuse to create the **penile urethra**, while the urogenital sinus becomes the **prostate** (see Chapter 44).

Descent of the testis

Usually in the 7th month the testes descend from the peritoneal cavity between the peritoneal epithelium and pubic bones and into the **scrotum**. This is mediated finally by the **gubernaculum** contracting under the influence of testosterone, but descent may not be completed until birth.

Puberty

Puberty is triggered by hormones secreted by the **pituitary gland** acting on ovaries, testes and adrenal glands. In girls, usually between ages 10 and 14 years, the ovaries respond by secreting oestrogen that stimulates breast growth. About a year later **menstruation** commences, accompanied by maturation of the uterus and vagina and broadening of the pelvis. Testosterone synthesis is stimulated in the adrenal glands and is responsible for growth of pubic and axillary hair in girls. Menstruation ceases at **menopause**, at around 50 years.

In boys, starting at about 11–12 years, the testes enlarge and synthesis of androgens is reactivated. The testis cords acquire a lumen, so forming the **seminiferous tubules**, which link up with the urethra. The androgens enhance growth of the penis and larynx and initiate spermatogenesis.

Medical issues

Disorders of sexual differentiation are dealt with in Chapter 44. Failure of testicular descent is called **cryptorchidism**. Tumours arising from primordial germ cells are known as **teratomas**; they can contain several well-differentiated tissues (e.g. hair, bone, sebaceous gland, thyroid tissue) and are usually benign (see Chapter 55).

44 Abnormalities of sex determination

Figure 44.1 Summary of main events in sex determination

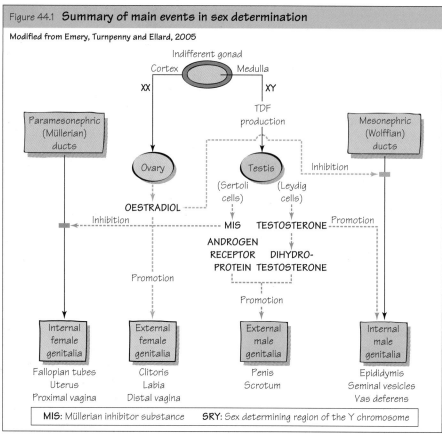

Figure 44.2 Genetic errors of steroidogenesis in the adrenal cortex

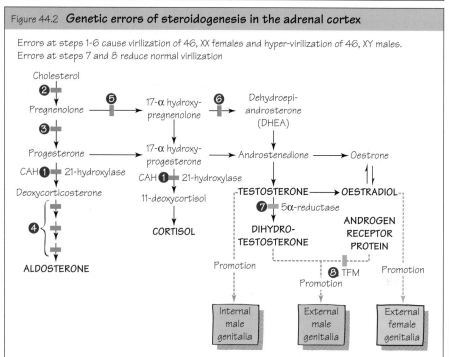

Figure 44.3 Appearance of infants with campomelic dysplasia

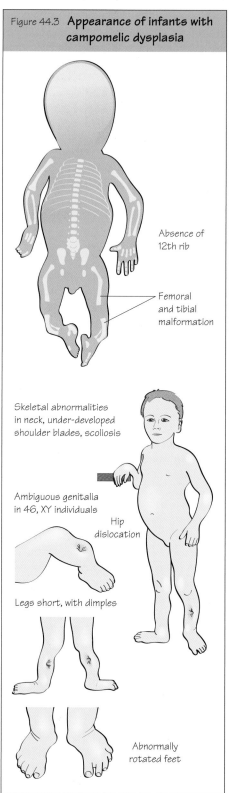

Medical Genetics at a Glance, Third Edition. Dorian J. Pritchard and Bruce R. Korf.

112 © 2013 John Wiley & Sons, Ltd. Published 2013 by John Wiley & Sons, Ltd.

Overview

Sexual differentiation begins in the early 'indifferent' gonads with secretion of oestrogen or androgen, depending on whether the Y-chromosome is absent or present. Male conversion is mediated by the **testis determining factor (TDF)**, a DNA-binding protein that is the product of the **sex determining region (SRY)** on the Y chromosome. Subsequently steroidogenesis is triggered in the adrenal cortex and this becomes responsible for much of later sexual differentiation and maturation. The roles and interactions of the hormones in normal sexual development are summarized in Figure 44.1. Figure 44.2 illustrates the steps in the relevant biochemical pathways at which pathogenic disruption most frequently occurs.

Disorders of sexual differentiation have been divided into five categories:

1 *congenital development of ambiguous genitalia* – e.g. virilization of a 46,XX individual by exposure to androgens, due to **congenital adrenal hyperplasia**;

2 *congenital disjunction of internal and external sexual anatomy* – e.g. female external anatomy in a 46,XY individual with testes, due to **androgen insensitivity**;

3 *incomplete development of sexual anatomy* – e.g. failure of gonadal development;

4 *sex chromosome anomalies* – e.g. **Turner** or **Klinefelter syndrome** (see Chapter 37);

5 *disorders of gonadal development* – e.g. individuals with an ovary on one side and a testis on the other, or a mixture of ovarian and testicular tissue.

Problems in genetic females

Virilization arising from defects at six or more steps in the biosynthesis of **aldosterone** and/or **cortisol** (**hydrocortisone**) creates ambiguous genitalia. All are inherited as autosomal recessives. By far the most significant is **congenital adrenal hyperplasia (CAH, causing adrenogenital syndrome)**; due to **21-hydroxylase deficiency** (21-OHD; Step 1 in Figure 44.2). This so-called '**classic OHD**' causes deficiency of **aldosterone** and **cortisol** and build-up of adrenocortical steroids proximal to the block, many of which have androgenic properties. About 25% suffer excessive salt excretion and circulatory collapse at 2–3 weeks. Reduced cortisol production stimulates **adrenocorticotrophic hormone (ACTH)** secretion and overgrowth of the adrenal glands.

An estimated 1% of the inhabitants of New York, of Jewish, Hispanic, Slavic and Italian origin, have '**non-classic OHD**', with defects in one of five or so enzymes of related function (Figure 44.2 Steps 2–6).

Other causes of ambiguous sexuality in females are maternal androgen ingestion and androgen-secreting tumours. There can also be abnormal representation of the *SRY* gene on the X in an XX individual, due to illegitimate crossover between the X and Y in the father.

Problems in genetic males

Swyer syndrome individuals have a 46,XY karyotype, but a normal female phenotype due to the inheritance of a Y chromosome that lacks the *SRY* region, this being replaced with the corresponding sequence from the end of the X chromosome. **Androgen insensitivity syndrome (testicular feminization, or TFM)** allows development of female external genitalia in XY individuals due to lack of the receptor for **dihydrotestosterone** (Figure 44.2 Step 8). Classically they present with a convincing external female phenotype, but lack of onset of menstrual periods, or inguinal hernia containing a testis, which can develop malignant cancer (**gonadoblastoma**).

Males with deficiency in **5α-reductase**, responsible for converting **testosterone** into **dihydrotestosterone**, may initially be classified as girls, but require reclassification at puberty when the deficiency is corrected by a surge of androgen from late-developing testes (Figure 44.2 Step 7).

Other causes of ambiguous sexuality are **Klinefelter syndrome** (e.g. 47,XXY; see Chapter 37) and 45,X/46,XY mosaicism due to loss of the Y from a progenitor cell during embryogenesis. There can also be absence of the *SRY* gene from the Y chromosome due to previous illegitimate crossover between the X and Y.

One target of TDF is the *SOX9* gene at 17q24, defects in this causing **campomelic dysplasia,** with bowing of the long bones, especially the tibia and femur, anomalies of ribs and vertebrae and frequently sex reversal from male to female phenotype ('campomelic' is derived from the Greek for 'bent limb'). There are characteristic skin dimples over the bent bones, especially in the lower leg (Figure 44.3). The *SOX9* gene codes for a transcription-regulating protein that recognizes the DNA sequence CCTTGAG. It normally controls transcription of Type II collagen and proteoglycan during chondrocyte differentiation and with steroidogenic factor I regulates transcription of Muellerian inhibiting substance (Chapter 43). Its deficiency therefore leads to both skeletal malformations and defects in male sexual development. Weakening of the cartilage of the upper respiratory tract can cause the larynx to collapse.

> ▶ **Problems requiring immediate attention**
>
> Difficulty with breathing.

Production of cholesterol is deficient in **Smith–Lemli–Opitz syndrome** and involves hypovirilization of boys (see Chapter 60) due to androgen deficiency, as cholesterol is a precursor of androgens. Males with 'non-classic OHD' may have hypervirilization, with increased penis size.

45 Congenital abnormalities, pre-embryonic, embryonic and of intrinsic causation

Figure 45.1 Frequency of all birth defects

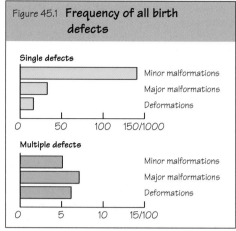

Single defects
- Minor malformations
- Major malformations
- Deformations

0   50   100   150/1000

Multiple defects
- Minor malformations
- Major malformations
- Deformations

0   5   10   15/100

Figure 45.2 Frequency of major congenital malformations in relation to development

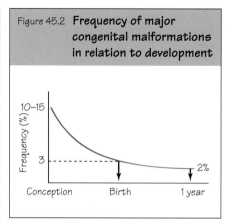

Frequency (%)

10–15

3

2%

Conception   Birth   1 year

Figure 45.3 Relative frequency of birth defects in girls and boys

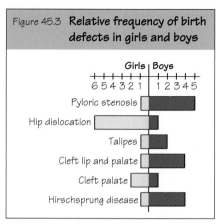

Girls | Boys

6 5 4 3 2 1 | 1 2 3 4 5

- Pyloric stenosis
- Hip dislocation
- Talipes
- Cleft lip and palate
- Cleft palate
- Hirschsprung disease

Figure 45.4 Cause of major congenital malformations

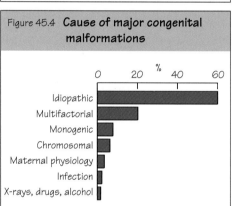

%
0   20   40   60

- Idiopathic
- Multifactorial
- Monogenic
- Chromosomal
- Maternal physiology
- Infection
- X-rays, drugs, alcohol

Figure 45.5 Organ-specific critical periods (see Chapter 41)

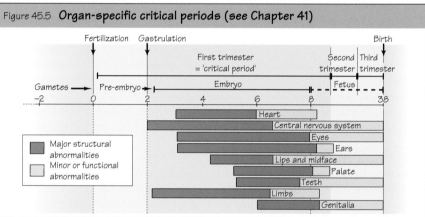

Fertilization   Gastrulation   Birth

First trimester = 'critical period'   Second trimester   Third trimester

Gametes → Pre-embryo → Embryo   Fetus

-2   0   2   4   6   8   38

Major structural abnormalities
Minor or functional abnormalities

- Heart
- Central nervous system
- Eyes
- Ears
- Lips and midface
- Palate
- Teeth
- Limbs
- Genitalia

Figure 45.6 The Potter sequence

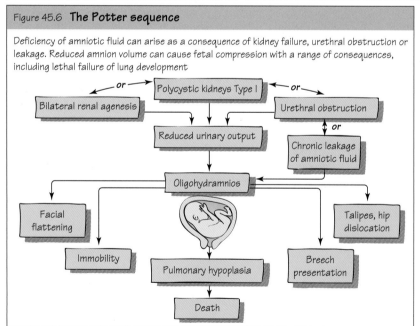

Deficiency of amniotic fluid can arise as a consequence of kidney failure, urethral obstruction or leakage. Reduced amnion volume can cause fetal compression with a range of consequences, including lethal failure of lung development

- Bilateral renal agenesis or Polycystic kidneys Type I or Urethral obstruction
- Reduced urinary output
- Chronic leakage of amniotic fluid or
- Oligohydramnios
- Facial flattening
- Immobility
- Pulmonary hypoplasia
- Talipes, hip dislocation
- Breech presentation
- Death

Figure 45.7 Causation of neural tube defects

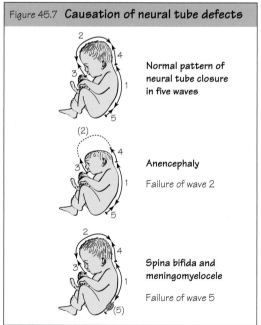

Normal pattern of neural tube closure in five waves

Anencephaly
Failure of wave 2

Spina bifida and meningomyelocele
Failure of wave 5

Medical Genetics at a Glance, Third Edition. Dorian J. Pritchard and Bruce R. Korf.
© 2013 John Wiley & Sons, Ltd. Published 2013 by John Wiley & Sons, Ltd.

Overview

The word '**congenital**' means 'existing at birth' and includes all 'birth defects' regardless of causation. Congenital abnormalities are apparent in 1/40 newborn babies and account for 20–25% of infant deaths. At birth 0.7% of babies have *multiple major* abnormalities, 2–3% a *single major* defect and 14% a *single minor* defect (Table 71.1). Probably 15–25% of congenital abnormalities have a recognized genetic, 10% an environmental and 20–25% a multifactorial basis. Twinning accounts for 0.5–1.0% (see Chapter 53) and 40–60% are **idiopathic**, that is of unknown causation.

For medico-legal purposes malformations are regarded as 'congenital' only if recognized within the first 2 weeks after birth.

Classification of defects
Single abnormalities

1 **Malformations** are due to errors occurring in the initial formation of structures, for example cleft lip with or without palate (CL ± P), polydactyly; most are multifactorial (see Chapters 50 and 51).
2 **Disruptions** are due to disturbances after an organ has been formed, for example **phocomelia** resulting from a vascular problem.
3 **Deformations** are mechanical distortions, for example clubfoot (**talipes**). They frequently resolve completely soon after birth.
4 **Dysplasias** are abnormalities in tissue organization, for example in the differentiation of blood cells from vessels; most are monogenic.

Multiple abnormalities

1 **Sequences** are cascades of effects, for example **Pierre–Robin sequence**, in which a primary defect in mandibular development produces secondary **glossoptosis** (drooping tongue) and cleft palate.
2 **Syndromes** are groups of anomalies that consistently occur together due to a single underlying cause, for example Down syndrome due to trisomy 21.
3 **Associations** are where traits coincide more often than expected by chance.

The overall frequency of **multiple malformations** is 7/1000, apart from Down syndrome, the most frequently diagnosed being Beckwith–Wiedeman (see Chapter 27), DiGeorge and Williams–Beuren syndromes (Chapter 39), **CHARGE** syndrome (Chapter 40), Noonan syndrome and **VATER** association.

Noonan syndrome
Frequency 1/2000 births.

Genetics Defect in tyrosine phosphatase, non-receptor-type 11 (*PTPN11*) at 12q22 in most patients, other genes involved in the Ras signalling pathway (Chapter 54) mutated in others.

Features Similar to Turner syndrome (Chapter 37), but affecting both sexes: short stature, neck webbing, increased carrying angle at the elbow, also learning difficulties, hypertelorism, down-slanting palpebral fissures, low-set ears and congenital heart disease. Pulmonary stenosis is the most common heart lesion, but there are also aventricular (ASD) and ventricular septal defect (VSD) and hypertrophic cardiomyopathy (see below). Some have bleeding problems and a quarter have chest deformity.

CHARGE syndrome
CHARGE involves the co-occurrence of **C**oloboma, **H**eart defects, cho**A**nal atresia, **R**etarded growth, **G**enital abnormalities and abnormal **E**ars. Mutation occur in either *CHD7* or *SEMA3E* genes.

VATER/VACTERL association
VATER involves **V**ertebral defects, **A**nal atresia, **T**racheo-o**E**sophageal fistula (i.e. abnormal fusion) and **R**enal defects. **VACTERL** also includes **C**ardiac and **L**imb defects.

Timing and aetiology
Pre-embryo
Damage to the pre-embryo generally results in spontaneous abortion or regulative repair, so few errors in newborns are ascribable to pre-implantation damage. The following are exceptions:
1 **monozygotic twinning** (see Chapter 53);
2 **germ layer defects**, e.g. **ectodermal dysplasia** affecting skin, nails, hair, teeth and stature.

Embryo
The **first trimester**, especially between weeks 2 and 8, is the **critical period**. The palate and lips, eyes, ears, brain, neural tube and heart are all particularly susceptible at this stage and the CNS, eyes, lips and midface, teeth and genitalia remain especially vulnerable throughout gestation.

The following errors are most important during the first trimester:
1 **failure of cell migration**, e.g. **neural crest cells**, **DiGeorge syndrome**;
2 **failure of embryonic induction**, e.g. **anophthalmia**;
3 **failure of tube closure**, e.g. the **neural tube defects** (see Chapter 51);
4 **developmental arrest**, e.g. **cleft lip** (see Chapter 50);
5 **failure of tissue fusion**, e.g. **cleft palate** (see Chapter 51);
6 **defective morphogenetic fields**, e.g. **sirenomelia**;

The foundations of **consequent disturbances** are laid at this stage, for example the **Potter sequence**.

The Potter/oligohydramnios sequence
Babies are sometimes born with the combination of squashed facial features, severe talipes, dislocated hips, growth deficiency and lethal pulmonary hypoplasia. Such babies typically adopted breech presentation. The features arise from the 'Potter sequence', involving prolonged deficiency of amniotic fluid, called **oligohydramnios**.

Oligohydramnios develops due to defective urinary output by the baby, or chronic leakage. This leads to fetal compression and immobility, with the consequences described. The primary causes of reduced urinary output are bilateral **renal agenesis** (1/3000 births), **polycystic kidney disease Type 1** and obstruction of the urethra. The recurrence risk for subsequent pregnancies is 1/33.

Renal agenesis classes as a *malformation*, which through oligohydramnios causes secondary *deformations*, the combination constituting a *syndrome* and the series of events, a *sequence*.

Defects of the CNS
Neural tube defects (NTDs)
NTDs arise from failure of closure of the neural tube at the end of week 3 (see Chapter 41). An anterior defect results in either **anencephaly** or **encephalocele** (absence or protrusion of the brain). A posterior defect can lead to lumbosacral **myelocele** or **meningomyelocele** (protruding spinal cord exposed, or covered by meninges), **spina bifida** and leg deformity (see Chapter 51).

Holoprosencephaly
Holoprosencephaly is failure of cleavage of the embryonic forebrain, resulting in severe mental impairment and abnormal facies, in

severe cases cyclopia. Survival is usually less than 1 month in severe cases.

It can be associated with Triploidy 13 (see Chapter 36) and Smith–Lemli–Opitz syndromes (see Chapter 60), maternal diabetes mellitus (see Chapter 46) and several deletions and mutations in various genes.

Isolated hydrocephalus

This is enlargement of the brain ventricles without NTD. It can arise from intracranial haemorrhage, infection or genetic defect, or be idiopathic.

Management involves insertion of a cerebrospinal fluid (CSF) drain, usually to the peritoneum.

Prenatal diagnosis is by serial ultrasound in the second trimester.

Lissencephaly (smooth brain)

This is caused by defective neuronal migration at 3–5 months. It can be associated with epilepsy and mental retardation and is a feature of Miller–Dieker syndrome and other disorders (see Chapter 40). As an isolated condition it has an empiric recurrence risk of 10% (see Chapter 13).

Macrocephaly and microcephaly

These terms apply to head circumferences greater than the 97th and less than the 3rd centile (see Chapter 49). **Microcephaly vera** (i.e. without other abnormalities) is usually AR, but there is a variety of causes of each.

Congenital heart defects

Heart development occurs at 3–8 weeks and developmental defects occur in 7/1000 live births. Congenital heart defects can result in inadequate oxygenation of blood and/or poor perfusion of tissues (see also Chapters 48 and 51).

Gastro-intestinal (GI) tract defects

Oesophageal atresia

This arises from an error in the formation of the oesophagus and can lead to **polyhydramnios** (excessive amniotic fluid because of failure to swallow). There may be associated tracheo-oesophageal fistulae. It occurs in 1/2500 live births, is multifactorial, associated with tetralogy of Fallot, ano-rectal agenesis and NTD and requires urgent surgical correction.

Pyloric stenosis

See Chapters 46 and 50.

Duodenal atresia

At week 7 the midgut is solid; **duodenal atresia** occurs when the lumen fails to open. The frequency is 1/330, 35% of cases being associated with T21.

Surgical correction is required urgently.

Hirschsprung disease (HSCR); congenital intestinal aganglionosis

This is a defect in peristaltic activity of the hindgut, due to failure of migration of neural crest cells (see Chapter 42). Typically there is no passage of meconium in the first 48 hours. The frequency is 1/5000 live births, (3 ♂ : 1 ♀). Inheritance is due to mutation in single genes or may be multifactorial. The recurrence risk is 3–4% in the absence of monogenic causation. Management requires surgical removal of affected tissue.

Imperforate anus

This has a frequency of 1/5000. It is multifactorially inherited and corrective surgery is urgent.

Figure 46.1 **Major birth defects (total 30–40/1000 births)**

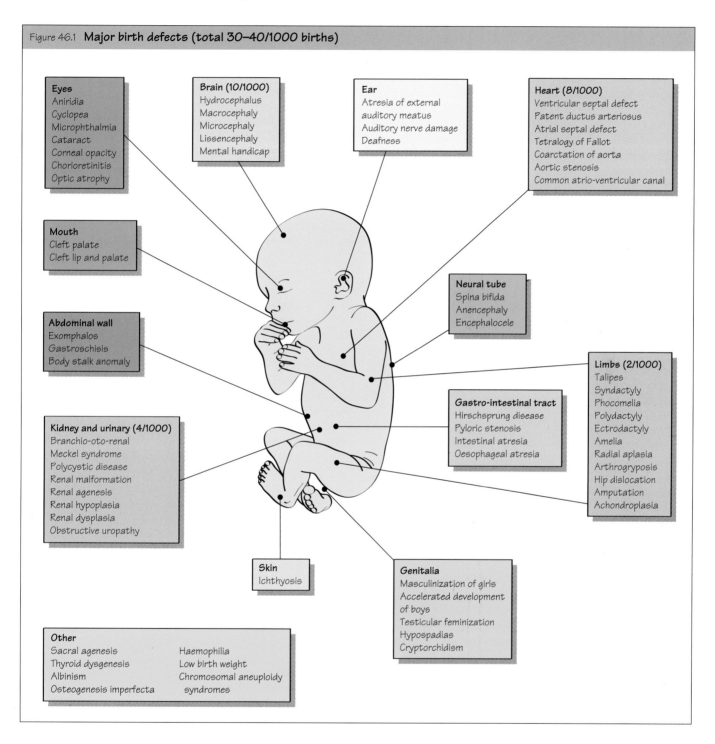

Eyes
Aniridia
Cyclopea
Microphthalmia
Cataract
Corneal opacity
Chorioretinitis
Optic atrophy

Brain (10/1000)
Hydrocephalus
Macrocephaly
Microcephaly
Lissencephaly
Mental handicap

Ear
Atresia of external
auditory meatus
Auditory nerve damage
Deafness

Heart (8/1000)
Ventricular septal defect
Patent ductus arteriosus
Atrial septal defect
Tetralogy of Fallot
Coarctation of aorta
Aortic stenosis
Common atrio-ventricular canal

Mouth
Cleft palate
Cleft lip and palate

Neural tube
Spina bifida
Anencephaly
Encephalocele

Abdominal wall
Exomphalos
Gastroschisis
Body stalk anomaly

Limbs (2/1000)
Talipes
Syndactyly
Phocomelia
Polydactyly
Ectrodactyly
Amelia
Radial aplasia
Arthrogryposis
Hip dislocation
Amputation
Achondroplasia

Kidney and urinary (4/1000)
Branchio-oto-renal
Meckel syndrome
Polycystic disease
Renal malformation
Renal agenesis
Renal hypoplasia
Renal dysplasia
Obstructive uropathy

Gastro-intestinal tract
Hirschsprung disease
Pyloric stenosis
Intestinal atresia
Oesophageal atresia

Skin
Ichthyosis

Genitalia
Masculinization of girls
Accelerated development
of boys
Testicular feminization
Hypospadias
Cryptorchidism

Other
Sacral agenesis
Thyroid dysgenesis
Albinism
Osteogenesis imperfecta
Haemophilia
Low birth weight
Chromosomal aneuploidy
syndromes

Medical Genetics at a Glance, Third Edition. Dorian J. Pritchard and Bruce R. Korf.
© 2013 John Wiley & Sons, Ltd. Published 2013 by John Wiley & Sons, Ltd.

Overview

The 'embryonic' period ends at about 9 weeks, when the rudiments of all the major organs have been formed. In the subsequent 'fetal' period the main processes are growth and morphogenesis and there is extensive **programmed cell death**, or **apoptosis**.

Partial chromosomal duplication or deficiency may cause postnatal **neurodevelopmental delay**, pre- or postnatal **growth delay**, **dysmorphism** or death. The aetiology of two-thirds of congenital defects is unknown or multifactorial, but a genetic component is suspected in about a third. Other pathogenic influences include abnormal maternal physiology and infection, exposure to medicines and non-prescription drugs, environmental chemicals and external physical influences. Extrinsic agents, especially chemicals, that cause birth defects are called **teratogens**.

The practical application of **dysmorphology** is outlined in Chapter 49. For genital defects, see Chapter 44.

Pathogenic mechanisms

1 **Absence of normal apoptosis**, e.g. **finger webbing**;
2 **disturbances in tissue resorption**, e.g. **anal atresia**;
3 **failure of organ movement**, e.g. **cryptorchidism**;
4 **destruction of formed structures**, e.g. **phocomelia** due to interference in blood supply;
5 **hypoplasia** (reduced proliferation), e.g. **achondroplasia** (see Chapter 4);
6 **hyperplasia** (enhanced proliferation), e.g. **macrosomia**;
7 **constriction by amniotic bands** (strands of broken amnion), e.g. limb amputation;
8 **restriction of movement**, e.g. talipes.

Maternal illness

Diabetes mellitus (see Chapter 52)

High maternal blood glucose levels in early pregnancy due to Type 1 diabetes mellitus is associated with a two- to three-fold increase in congenital abnormalities, including heart disease, neural tube defects, sacral agenesis, femoral hypoplasia, holoprosencephaly and **sirenomelia**. The causative influence is high maternal blood glucose levels in early pregnancy.

Phenylketonuria (see Chapter 8)

Uncorrected high maternal blood levels of phenylalanine can cause severe mental retardation, microcephaly and congenital heart disease.

Epilepsy

There is a two to four times increased incidence (to 5–10%) of birth defects in babies exposed prenatally to antiepileptic drugs, and the number increases if more than one drug is used. They include NTDs (in about 10%), oral clefting, genitourinary abnormalities, and heart and limb defects. Learning difficulties and behaviour problems are increased. Sodium valproate exposure is associated with the highest incidence, NTDs and characteristic facies. The recommended maternal medication is single drug treatment if possible, avoiding sodium valproate.

Other predisposing conditions are **systemic lupus erythematosus** and **Graves disease** (see Chapter 65).

Maternal infection

Microorganisms that cause multiple malformations are summarized by the acronym, **TORCH**, for *Toxoplasma*, **O**ther (e.g. syphilis, *Treponema pallidum*), *Rubella*, *Cytomegalovirus* and *Herpes simplex*. The most important are *Toxoplasma*, *Rubella* and *Cytomegalovirus*.

Toxoplasmosis

Maternal infection with the Protozoan, *Toxoplasma gondii*, confers a 20% risk to the fetus during the first trimester, rising to 75% in the second and third trimesters.

Rubella (German measles)

Rubella virus causes cardiovascular malformations in 15–20% of all babies infected in the first trimester.

Cytomegalovirus (CMV)

Risk is greatest if infection occurs during the first trimester. About 5% of infected pregnancies result in fetal damage.

Congenital deformations

Congenital dislocation of the hip

Incidence is 1/1000 (6♀ : 1♂). It is multifactorial, positively associated with breech birth and neuromuscular disorder and commonest in populations in which babies are swaddled.

Talipes equinovarus (club foot)

The feet are **plantar-flexed** and inverted (i.e. soles facing inwards). The incidence is 1/1000 live births; (3♂ : 1♀) (see Table 51.2).

Amputations

In 1/5000 live births there is limb amputation due to constriction by 'amniotic bands' formed by premature rupture of the amnion. It is frequently associated with oligohydramnios (see Chapter 45).

Congenital myotonic dystrophy

This can occur in association with hypotonia, respiratory insufficiency, mental retardation and can be lethal (see also Chapter 28).

Anterior abdominal wall defect

The overall incidence is 1/6000 live pregnancies.
• **Omphalocele** is a persistent midgut hernia into the umbilical cord; associated with T13 (30%) and congenital heart disease (10%).
• **Gastroschisis** is extrusion of the bowel through the abdominal wall.

Pyloric stenosis

Hypertrophy and hyperplasia of the pyloric sphincter muscles lead to projectile vomiting, constipation and dehydration in early infancy (see Chapter 50).

Limb malformations

Overall frequency 2/1000

Polydactyly is a feature of many syndromes, including T13, but can be inherited as AD or be of unknown aetiology.

Arthrogryposis is a heterogeneous group of malformations characterized by stiffness and contracture of the knee, elbow and/or wrist joints and often dislocation of the hips. They are classified as: myopathic; neuropathic; affecting connective tissue; restricting fetal movement.

The role of chemicals

Teratogenesis accords with the following principles.
1 Susceptibility may depend on the genotype of the zygote.

2 Maternal genotype affects drug metabolism, resistance to infection.
3 Susceptibility depends on developmental stage at time of exposure.
4 Severity of defect depends on dose and duration of exposure.
5 Individual teratogens have specific modes of action.
6 Abnormality is expressed as malformation, growth retardation, functional disorder or death.

Teratogenic medicines

These include:
• **abortifacients**, e.g. the folic acid antagonist *aminopterin*;
• **antiabortifacients**, e.g. *diethylstibestrol* causing malformations of reproductive systems;
• **androgens** can cause masculinization of female external genitalia;
• **anticonvulsants** used by epileptics; *valproate* (see above), *trimethadone, diphenylhydantoin, phenytoin, carbamazepine*;
• **sedatives and tranquilizers:** *thalidomide, lithium*;
• **anticancer drugs:** *methotrexate, aminopterin*;
• **antibiotics:** *streptomycin* can cause inner ear deafness; *tetracycline* inhibits skeletal calcification;
• **anticoagulants:** *warfarin, dicumarol*;
• **antihypertensive agents:** *ACE inhibitors*;
• **antithyroid drugs;**
• **vitamin A analogues**, e.g. *retinoids* used to treat acne.

Thalidomide

Thalidomide, prescribed as a sedative or antinausea agent, created severe abnormalities in 10 000 babies before medical recognition in 1961. The most common was **phocomelia**, with absence of long limb bones, ear defects, microphthalmia and CL ± P. Around 40% died of severe abnormalities of the heart, kidneys or GI tract. Thalidomide is currently used in the treatment of leprosy.

Non-prescription drugs

• **Fetal alcohol syndrome.** Children born to mothers who consumed excess alcohol during pregnancy can have midface hypoplasia, short palpebral fissures, a long smooth philtrum and mild developmental delay.
• **LSD** (lysergic acid diethylamide), '**angel dust**' or **PCP** (phenylcyclidine), **quinine** and birth control pills are all **teratogenic**.
• **Tobacco** smoking causes growth retardation and premature delivery.

Environmental chemicals

Lead, **methylmercury** and **hypoxia** are the most widely recognized hazards.

Physical agents

• **Prolonged hyperthermia** in early pregnancy can cause microcephaly, microphthalmia and neuronal migration defects.
• **Ionizing radiation and X-rays** in large doses can cause microcephaly and ocular defects, the most sensitive period being 2–5 weeks. Radiation also has mutagenic and carcinogenic effects (Chapter 26).

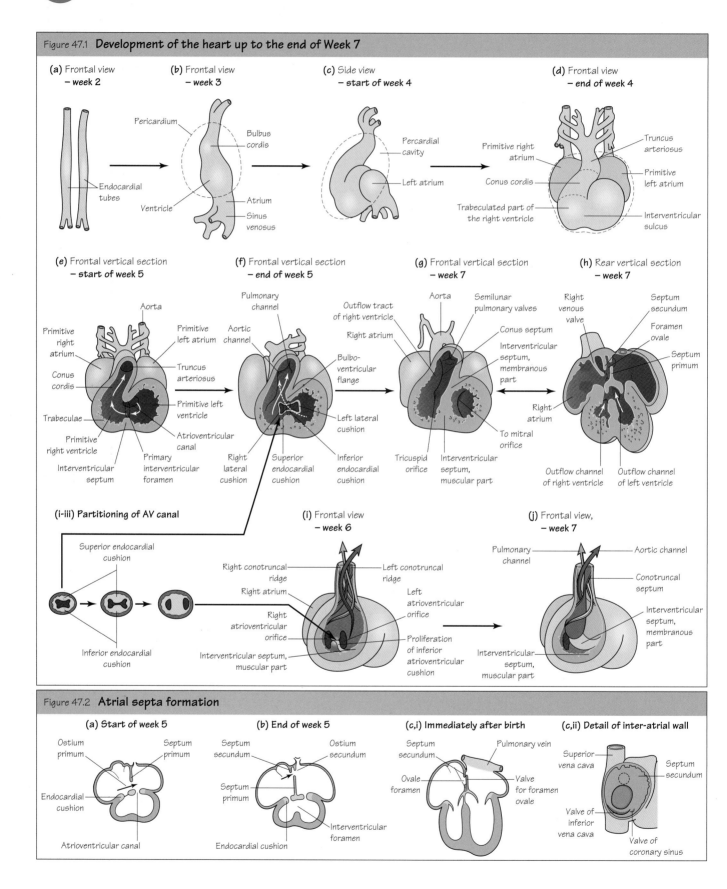

Figure 47.1 **Development of the heart up to the end of Week 7**

(a) Frontal view – week 2

Endocardial tubes

(b) Frontal view – week 3

Pericardium
Bulbus cordis
Ventricle
Atrium
Sinus venosus

(c) Side view – start of week 4

Percardial cavity
Left atrium

(d) Frontal view – end of week 4

Primitive right atrium
Conus cordis
Trabeculated part of the right ventricle
Truncus arteriosus
Primitive left atrium
Interventricular sulcus

(e) Frontal vertical section – start of week 5

Aorta
Primitive right atrium
Conus cordis
Trabeculae
Primitive right ventricle
Interventricular septum
Primitive left atrium
Aortic channel
Truncus arteriosus
Primitive left ventricle
Atrioventricular canal
Primary interventricular foramen

(f) Frontal vertical section – end of week 5

Pulmonary channel
Bulbo-ventricular flange
Right lateral cushion
Superior endocardial cushion
Left lateral cushion
Inferior endocardial cushion

(g) Frontal vertical section – week 7

Aorta
Outflow tract of right ventricle
Right atrium
Tricuspid orifice
Semilunar pulmonary valves
Conus septum
Interventricular septum, membranous part
To mitral orifice
Interventricular septum, muscular part

(h) Rear vertical section – week 7

Right venous valve
Right atrium
Outflow channel of right ventricle
Septum secundum
Foramen ovale
Septum primum
Outflow channel of left ventricle

(i-iii) Partitioning of AV canal

Superior endocardial cushion
Inferior endocardial cushion

(i) Frontal view – week 6

Right conotruncal ridge
Right atrium
Right atrioventricular orifice
Interventricular septum, muscular part
Left conotruncal ridge
Left atrioventricular orifice
Proliferation of inferior atrioventricular cushion

(j) Frontal view, – week 7

Pulmonary channel
Interventricular septum, muscular part
Aortic channel
Conotruncal septum
Interventricular septum, membranous part

Figure 47.2 **Atrial septa formation**

(a) Start of week 5

Ostium primum
Endocardial cushion
Septum primum
Atrioventricular canal

(b) End of week 5

Septum secundum
Septum primum
Ostium secundum
Endocardial cushion
Interventricular foramen

(c,i) Immediately after birth

Septum secundum
Ovale foramen
Pulmonary vein
Valve for foramen ovale

(c,ii) Detail of inter-atrial wall

Superior vena cava
Septum secundum
Valve of inferior vena cava
Valve of coronary sinus

Overview

The heart comes into existence very early in development and, of course, plays a vitally important survival role throughout development and later life. This means that its own development at any particular time is intrinsically related to performance of its function at that time. The fluid dynamic forces that exist within the heart due to the blood flow it continuously maintains are exploited in the further moulding of its form. Much of the anatomy of the heart is therefore not coded specifically in the genome, but is 'epigenetic', arising as the physical consequence of previous structure.

A major reconstruction occurs within the heart and adjacent vessels at birth, as the source of oxygenated blood switches from the placenta to the lungs. This must, of necessity, occur correctly within a very small number of minutes.

Initial development

During the 2nd week of development the heart consists of a pair of thin-walled, muscular tubes beneath the floor of the pharynx. By the 3rd, they have fused into a single chamber, which is pumping, this action being an intrinsic response of cardiac myoblasts to low K+ ion concentration. Two large veins bring blood to the heart and a single large artery, the **truncus arteriosus** directs it forward into the general circulation. As the heart elongates it curves back on itself in an S-curve (see Figure 47.1a–c).

The atrial part of the heart tube is initially a pair of structures that merge to create a common **atrium** linked to the early embryonic **ventricle** by the **atrioventricular canal (AVC)**. The former anterior end of the heart tube (the **bulbus cordis**) later becomes the outflow tract of the ventricles and, with the **conus cordis** and **truncus arteriosus**, becomes the proximal portion of the aorta (Figure 47.1d,e).

The caudal, inflow end of the primitive heart is called the **sinus venosus**. This is initially bifurcated, but the right sinus horn and veins enlarge and become incorporated into the right atrium, while the left gets obliterated. Inflow of blood is assisted by development of right and left **venous valves**.

Formation of cardiac septa

The major septa are formed at 27–37 days by two different kinds of process. At some sites **endocardial cushions** develop and thicken, narrowing down the channels between them. Abnormal cushion morphogenesis is a primary cause of cardiac malformation. Septa are also formed by expansion of the lumen of the chamber on each side, usually in conjunction with proliferation of neighbouring tissues.

Septum formation in the atrium

The common atrium becomes divided into left and right chambers by development of vertical septa. At the end of the 4th week the **septum primum** forms as a sickle-shaped crest descending from its roof, continued communication between the subchambers being allowed by a passage called the **ostium primum** (Figure 47.2a). At its lower edge the septum primum makes contact with the endocardial cushion below, which through its upward extension closes the ostium primum (Figure 47.2b). Before complete closure a new aperture, the **ostium secundum**, forms dorsally by programmed cell death within the septum primum.

Finally a second interatrial septum forms, the **septum secundum**, extending down from the roof on the right side of the ostium secundum, leaving an oval window called the **foramen ovale**. Behind this the ventral portion of the septum primum forms a valvular flap that ensures one-way flow from the right atrium to the left (Figure 47.2c).

Septum formation in the ventricles

At the end of heart loop formation the initially smooth-walled interior develops fibrous **trabeculae** in two areas on either side of what will later become the **interventricular septum**, separating the **primitive right** and **primitive left ventricles** (Figure 47.1e).

The **muscular interventricular septum** (MIVS) forms by gradual fusion of the medial walls of the primitive ventricle, leaving just the **primary interventricular foramen** between right and left ventricles (Figure 47.1e). Its complete closure is later accomplished by outgrowth of the inferior endocardial cushion along the top of the MIVS, which fuses with the **conus septum** above, creating the **membranous part of the interventricular septum** (Figure 47.1g). Blood from the two ventricles is then separately channelled into the two compartments of the conus, kept separate by the **conotruncal septum** (Figure 47.1f,g; see below).

Between the 6th and 9th weeks triple sets of **semilunar valves** form at the entries to both the pulmonary artery and aorta (Figure 47.1g).

Septum formation in the atrioventricular canal

Up to the end of the 4th week inflowing blood from the sinus venosus passes through the large atrioventricular canal directly into the common ventricle. During the 5th week the AVC develops a central division that results in inflowing blood being directed separately into the primitive left and the primitive right ventricles. This occurs through growth and merger of the **superior and inferior atrioventricular endocardial cushions** (Figure 47.1f).

Following this fusion, each endocardial cushion becomes surrounded by proliferating mesenchymal tissue, which then hollows out, leaving tough sheets of connective tissue covered by endothelium, anchored to the ventricular wall by muscular cords. These take on the role of valves guarding the atrioventricular orifices: the two-part **bicuspid** or **mitral valve** around the left AVC and the three-part tricuspid around the right (Figure 47.1g).

Septum formation in the truncus arteriosus and conus cordis

During the 5th week elongated swellings appear on the inside walls of the truncus arteriosus and conus cordis that grow and fuse, eventually creating the spirally twisted **conotruncal septum** that divides the lumen into a **pulmonary channel** taking blood from the left ventricle (LV) toward the lungs and an **aortic channel**, which becomes the outflow tract of the right ventricle (RV) (Figure 47.1i,j).

Circulatory changes at birth See Chapter 48.

Figure 48.1 Changes in blood flow in the heart at birth

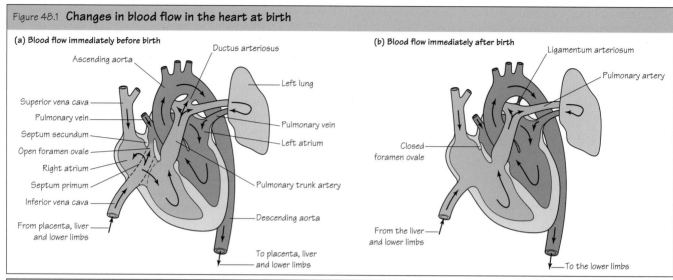

(a) Blood flow immediately before birth

Ascending aorta
Ductus arteriosus
Left lung
Superior vena cava
Pulmonary vein
Septum secundum
Open foramen ovale
Right atrium
Septum primum
Inferior vena cava
From placenta, liver and lower limbs
Pulmonary vein
Left atrium
Pulmonary trunk artery
Descending aorta
To placenta, liver and lower limbs

(b) Blood flow immediately after birth

Ligamentum arteriosum
Pulmonary artery
Closed foramen ovale
From the liver and lower limbs
To the lower limbs

Figure 48.2 Defects in septum formation

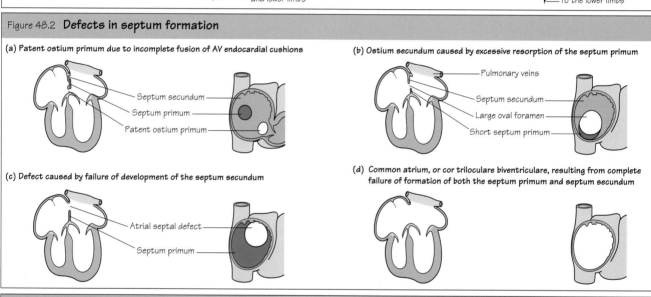

(a) Patent ostium primum due to incomplete fusion of AV endocardial cushions

Septum secundum
Septum primum
Patent ostium primum

(b) Ostium secundum caused by excessive resorption of the septum primum

Pulmonary veins
Septum secundum
Large oval foramen
Short septum primum

(c) Defect caused by failure of development of the septum secundum

Atrial septal defect
Septum primum

(d) Common atrium, or cor triloculare biventriculare, resulting from complete failure of formation of both the septum primum and septum secundum

Figure 48.3 Major heart defects

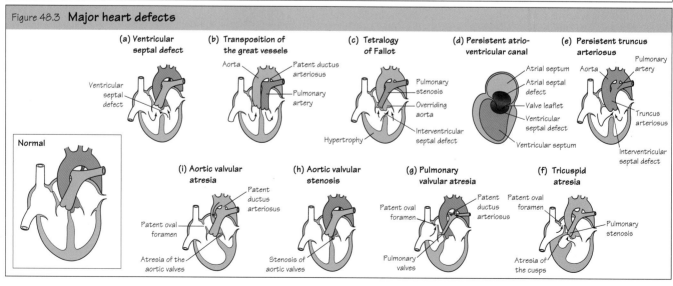

(a) Ventricular septal defect

Ventricular septal defect

(b) Transposition of the great vessels

Aorta
Patent ductus arteriosus
Pulmonary artery

(c) Tetralogy of Fallot

Pulmonary stenosis
Overriding aorta
Hypertrophy
Interventricular septal defect

(d) Persistent atrio-ventricular canal

Atrial septum
Atrial septal defect
Valve leaflet
Ventricular septal defect
Ventricular septum

(e) Persistent truncus arteriosus

Pulmonary artery
Aorta
Truncus arteriosus
Interventricular septal defect

Normal

(i) Aortic valvular atresia

Patent ductus arteriosus
Patent oval foramen
Atresia of the aortic valves

(h) Aortic valvular stenosis

Stenosis of aortic valves

(g) Pulmonary valvular atresia

Patent oval foramen
Patent ductus arteriosus
Pulmonary valves

(f) Tricuspid atresia

Patent oval foramen
Pulmonary stenosis
Atresia of the cusps

Medical Genetics at a Glance, Third Edition. Dorian J. Pritchard and Bruce R. Korf.

122 © 2013 John Wiley & Sons, Ltd. Published 2013 by John Wiley & Sons, Ltd.

Overview

Around 8% of cardiac malformations have genetic bases such as unbalanced chromosome constitutions, 2% are caused by environmental agents and 90% are multifactorial. Of all children with chromosomal abnormalities 33% have congenital heart defects. (See also Cardiomyopathy section, Chapter 52.)

Most heart defects arise as structural errors that become exacerbated as the continuously pumping embryonic heart is forced to compensate (see Chapter 47).

Circulatory changes at birth

Before birth there are two short-circuits in the circulatory system causing blood to bypass the lungs. These are the open foramen ovale linking the two atria and the short, muscular **ductus arteriosus (DA)** linking the pulmonary trunk artery to the aorta.

Before birth deoxygenated blood from the lower limbs, mixed with oxygenated blood from the placenta, enters the RA from the **inferior vena cava**, most of it passing through the foramen ovale and into the LA. A portion, however, blocked by the septum secundum, mixes with oxygen-desaturated blood returning from the head and arms via the **superior vena cava (SVC)** (see Figure 48.1a).

From the LA blood enters the LV and **ascending aorta** to the heart musculature and the brain. Desaturated blood from the SVC flows via the RV into the pulmonary trunk artery, although most then passes through the DA to mingle with that in the **descending aorta** en route to the placenta for reoxygenation.

Changes occurring at birth are caused by cessation of placental blood flow and the beginning of respiration, which triggers muscular contraction of the walls of the DA, with diversion of much blood to the lungs and increased pressure in the LA. Pressure in the RA simultaneously decreases, the septum primum presses against the septum secundum and the foramen ovale closes (Figure 48.1b). Complete fusion of the two septa normally occurs over the first year.

A relic of the DA remains in later life as the **ligamentum arteriosum**.

Clinically significant defects

In **dextrocardia** the heart develops on the dextral side of the thorax due to looping of the heart tube to the wrong side. It often accompanies transposition of the viscera, or **situs inversus**.

Abnormalities in endocardial cushion formation are responsible for **atrial** (Figure 48.2a–d) and **ventricular septal defects** (Figure 48.3a), **transposition of the great vessels** (Figure 48.3.b) and **tetralogy of Fallot**. The latter occurs in about 10/10000 births, due to unequal division of the conus, resulting from anterior displacement of the conotruncal septum. This creates a set of four characteristic abnormalities: (i) a narrow RV outflow tract, called **pulmonary infundibular stenosis**; (ii) IVS defect; (iii) an overriding aorta that arises directly above the defective IVS; and (iv) hypertrophy of the RV wall (Figure 48.3c).

The conotruncal endocardial cushions contain migratory neural crest cells. Abnormalities in neural crest development can cause defects here and associated defects in the head, face and neck, as in **Treacher–Collins syndrome (mandibulofacial dysostosis), Robin sequence, Goldenhaar syndrome (hemifacial microsomia) and DiGeorge syndrome** (Chapter 39).

Persistent AV canal (Figure 48.3.d) arises when the relevant cushions fail to fuse, and is combined with defects in both the A and V parts of the AV septum.

Atrial septal defects (ASDs) occur in 6.4/10000 births, twice as many girls as boys being affected. They include **patent ostium primum** (Figure 48.2a), **absence of the septum secundum** (Figure 48.2c), **absence of both septum primum and septum secundum** (Figure 48.d) and **excessive resorption of the septum primum** (Figure 48.2b). Ostium primum defect is usually combined with a cleft tricuspid valve.

Premature closure of the oval foramen causes massive RA hypertrophy with underdevelopment of the left side of the heart, death occurring usually soon after birth. By contrast, incomplete fusion of the septum primum and septum secundum occurs in about 20% of individuals and is virtually symptomless. This is known as **probe patency of the oval foramen**.

Ventricular septal defects (VSDs) involving the membranous part of the septum are the most common cardiac malformation, occurring in isolation (Figure 48.3a) in 12/10000 births and also with abnormalities in partitioning of the conotruncal region. **Persistent truncus arteriosus** (Figure 48.3e) (0.8/10000 births) results when the conotruncal ridges fail to develop correctly and is always accompanied by a defective IVS.

Transposition of the great vessels (4.8/10000 births) occurs when the conotruncal septum descends without spiralling, so that the aorta originates from the RV and the pulmonary artery from the LV (Figure 48.3b). It is usually accompanied by patency of the DA and often a defect in the IV septum.

Tricuspid atresia (Figure 48.3f) is characterized by absence of fusion of the tricuspid valves and involves obliteration of the right AV orifice. It is always associated with (i) patency of the oval foramen; (ii) VSD; (iii) under-development of the RV; and (iv) hypertrophy of the LV.

Valvular stenosis or **atresia** of the pulmonary artery (Figure 48.3g) or aorta (Figure 48.3h) (both 3–4/10000 births) occur when their semilunar valves are abnormally fused. When this occurs in the pulmonary artery, the DA always remains open. An extreme situation is **aortic valvular atresia** (Figure 48.3i), when the aorta becomes completely blocked and the aorta, LV and LA remain undeveloped, the DA also usually remaining open.

Patent ductus arteriosus is a feature of several conditions. This is due to failure of closure of the DA at birth and occurs in 8/10000 babies.

Figure 49.1 Facial development

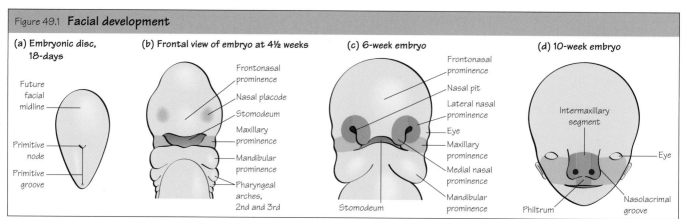

(a) Embryonic disc, 18-days

Future facial midline
Primitive node
Primitive groove

(b) Frontal view of embryo at 4½ weeks

Frontonasal prominence
Nasal placode
Stomodeum
Maxillary prominence
Mandibular prominence
Pharyngeal arches, 2nd and 3rd

(c) 6-week embryo

Frontonasal prominence
Nasal pit
Lateral nasal prominence
Eye
Maxillary prominence
Medial nasal prominence
Mandibular prominence
Stomodeum

(d) 10-week embryo

Intermaxillary segment
Eye
Nasolacrimal groove
Philtrum

Figure 49.2 Cleft lip malformations

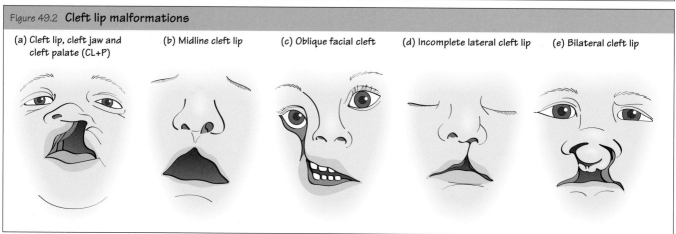

(a) Cleft lip, cleft jaw and cleft palate (CL+P)

(b) Midline cleft lip

(c) Oblique facial cleft

(d) Incomplete lateral cleft lip

(e) Bilateral cleft lip

Figure 49.3 Growth charts

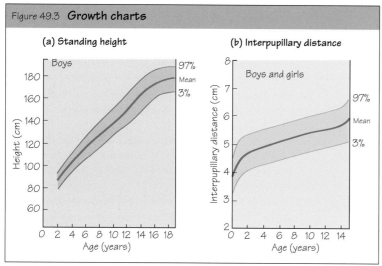

(a) Standing height

Boys
97%
Mean
3%
Height (cm)
180
160
140
120
100
80
60
0 2 4 6 8 10 12 14 16 18
Age (years)

(b) Interpupillary distance

Boys and girls
97%
Mean
3%
Interpupillary distance (cm)
8
7
6
5
4
3
2
0 2 4 6 8 10 12 14
Age (years)

Figure 49.4 Facial features utilized in dysmorphology

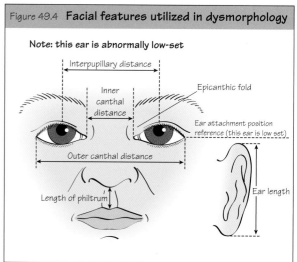

Note: this ear is abnormally low-set

Interpupillary distance
Inner canthal distance
Epicanthic fold
Ear attachment position reference (this ear is low set)
Outer canthal distance
Length of philtrum
Ear length

Medical Genetics at a Glance, Third Edition. Dorian J. Pritchard and Bruce R. Korf.

Overview

Anatomical features are considered **dysmorphic** if their measures or structures lie outside the normal range. **Dysmorphology** is the discipline concerned with their identification, delineation, diagnosis and management.

Quantitative characters vary with age and sex, but measures of different features in a normal subject should all lie within the same part of their respective ranges. An exceptional measure reflects abnormality. Since some dysmorphic features relate to age, re-examination at a later date can be helpful.

Two to four per cent of newborn babies have a physical anomaly and currently over 2000 dysmorphic diagnoses are listed. Multiple dysmorphic features enable identification of known syndromes and among the most distinctive and disturbing are those that affect the face.

Table 49.1 Some well-recognized malformation syndromes.

Apert syndrome (acrocephalosyndactyly)	Edwards syndrome
	Fragile X syndrome
Beckwith–Wiedemann syndrome	Noonan syndrome
	Patau syndrome
CHARGE syndrome	Rubinstein–Taybi syndrome
Cleidocranial dysostosis	Smith–Lemli–Opitz syndrome
Cri du chat syndrome	Treacher Collins syndrome
Crouzon disease (craniofacial dysostosis)	(mandibulofacial dysostosis)
	Turner syndrome
De Lange syndrome	VATER association
DiGeorge syndrome	Williams syndrome
Down syndrome	Wolf–Hirschhorn syndrome

Fetal alcohol syndrome

Fetal alcohol syndrome is indicated by the combination of growth deficiency, microcephaly, short palpebral fissures, a smooth philtrum, a thin upper lip and intellectual disability. Since teratogenic causation is initiated 4 weeks after the last menses, it frequently occurs before the mother is aware she is pregnant. **Midline cleft lip** is a rare, later consequence of **holoprosencephaly** (failure of division of the forebrain), due to incomplete merger of the medial nasal prominences (see below).

Development of the face

The face is derived mainly from **pharyngeal arches 1** and **2 (PA 1, PA 2)** (see Chapter 42). These have cores of originally paraxial mesenchyme, ectoderm externally and internally an epithelium of endoderm. The voluntary muscles of the face are derived from mesoderm and its bone largely from migratory neural crest (NC) cells. These originate in the neuroectoderm of the early brain and migrate around the forebrain and optic cup into the facial region (Chapter 42).

At 4.5 weeks, at the centre of the future face is the **stomodeum** surrounded by the first pair of PAs. Five mesenchymal 'prominences' can then be discerned: caudal to the stomodeum, the paired **mandibular prominences**, which will later form the lower jaw; the lateral **maxillary prominences** formed from the dorsal portion of PA 1, which will develop into the upper jaw; and the central **frontonasal prominence** between the **nasal placodes**. In the 5th week the latter invaginate, creating a ridge around each that constitute the **lateral** and **medial nasal prominences**.

During the following 2 weeks the maxillary prominences grow, compressing the medial nasal prominences toward the midline, where they merge to create the **intermaxillary segment**. This is composed of a **labial component** that forms the **philtrum** and upper lip, an **upper jaw component** carrying the four incisor teeth and a **palatal component** that forms the **primary palate** (see Chapter 51).

The bridge of the nose is formed from the frontal prominence, the merged medial nasal prominences provide its crest and tip and the lateral nasal prominences its sides and the outer walls of the nostrils. The maxillary prominences enlarge to form the cheeks and upper jaws. The mandibular prominences merge medially to become the lower lip and lower jaw.

Facial clefts

Oblique facial clefts can arise due to failure of a maxillary prominence to merge fully with its adjacent lateral nasal prominence.

The main part of the palate is formed by the pair of **palatine shelves** that grow inward from the maxillary processes in about the 6th week and fuse a week later, although fusion typically occurs 1 week earlier in females than males (see Chapter 51). The line of fusion between the triangular primary palate and the palatine shelves is called the **incisive foramen** and marks the boundary between the sites of 'anterior' and 'posterior' palatal clefts.

Anterior facial clefts are due to incomplete fusion of the maxillary prominence with the medial nasal prominence on one or both sides. These can vary from barely visible to a deep cleft through the nose, or a split in the maxilla between lateral incisor and canine tooth. They also include **lateral cleft lip (CL)**, **cleft upper jaw** and **cleft between primary and secondary palates**. Posterior clefts include 'cleft palate' **(CP)** and **cleft uvula**.

A third category, **cleft lip with or without cleft palate (CL ± P)** is due to clefting both anterior and posterior to the incisive foramen (see Chapter 51).

Anticonvulsant drugs such as **phenobarbital** and **diphenylhydantoin** early in pregnancy increase the risk of cleft palate (see Chapter 46).

Classification of abnormal developmental features

A variety of congenital anomalies have been delineated, the understanding of which is important in providing counselling to families (see Chapters 46 and 50). These are classified as follows:

- **malformations** – abnormal tissue formation, e.g. polydactyly;
- **deformations** – physical distortion of otherwise normally formed tissue, e.g. moulding of the fetal head due to uterine fibroids;
- **disruptions** – damage to previously normally formed tissue, e.g. amputation of a limb due to entrapment by an amniotic band;
- **dysplasias** – abnormal cellular development, e.g. neuronal **heterotopia** (i.e. presence of normal tissue at abnormal sites) in the brain.

Malformations may also be classified in terms of occurrence of features.

- **isolated malformation**, e.g. extra digit on one hand;
- **sequence** – primary malformation which leads to secondary effects on tissue formation, e.g. cleft palate in an infant with under-development of the jaw (**Pierre–Robin sequence**), in which upward displacement of the tongue in a very small mouth interferes with palatal closure (see Chapter 51);
- **association** – tendency of multiple malformations to occur together non-randomly, usually for unknown reasons, e.g. **VATER** and **VACTERL associations** (see Chapter 45);

- **syndrome** – a set of abnormal phenotypic features that frequently occur together due to a basic underlying cause, e.g. Down syndrome.

Assessment of development

Childhood development is monitored with regard to eight interconnected aspects:

1 hearing;
2 vision;
3 gross motor skills;
4 fine motor skills;
5 comprehension of language;
6 linguistic self expression;
7 behaviour and emotional development;
8 social skills.

Assessment involves checks on rate of development, qualitative scope of development in that aspect, and final level of achievement.

Clinically important growth parameters

Human growth charts show mean values and ranges plotted against age. Individuals who lie outside the third and 97th centiles are considered abnormal. Suboptimal growth and weight gain in infants and toddlers come within the term '**failure to thrive**' and their assessment requires careful physical examination, serial measurements and history taking.

The following measurements may be taken if there are specific concerns about disproportionate growth.

1 Standing height:
  (a) overall height;
  (b) lower segment: floor to upper border of pubis;
  (c) upper segment: overall height minus lower segment.
2 Sitting height.
3 Linear growth, i.e. change in body length over time.
4 Arm span.
5 Weight.
6 Head circumference: maximum occipitofrontal circumference is an indirect measure of brain size:
  (a) **microcephaly** can reflect poor brain growth or premature fusion of skull sutures;
  (b) **macrocephaly** may indicate high intracranial fluid pressure.
7 Eyes:
  (a) **hypertelorism** is a feature of nearly 400 syndromes, describing abnormally widely spaced orbits;
  (b) **hypotelorism** refers to abnormally closely spaced orbits, found in some 40 syndromes and often indicative of a brain malformation (holoprosencephaly);

  (c) **telecanthus** refers to an increase in the distance between the inner canthi with normal inter-orbital distance and is a feature of around 90 syndromes;
  (d) **blepharophimosis** is reduction in the length of the palpebral fissures and features in over 100 syndromes;
  (e) **epicanthic folds** are skin folds over the inner canthi;
  (f) **upwards slant** of the eyes means that the inner canthi are lower than the outer, as in Down syndrome (see Chapter 36);
  (g) **downwards slant** describes eyes with the inner canthi higher than the outer, as in Cri-du-chat syndrome (see Chapter 39).
8 Ears: maximum ear length and ear position are recorded. Ears are described as low-set if the upper border of their attachment is below a line through the outer canthi and the occipital protuberance at the back of the skull.
9 Head shape:
  (a) **brachycephaly** describes short anteroposterior skull length;
  (b) **dolichocephaly** refers to long anteroposterior skull length.
10 Testicular volume.
11 Limbs:
  (a) **syndactyly** indicates digital fusion, osseous (**synphalangism**), or cutaneous (**webbing**);
  (b) **polydactyly** describes extra digits on the **preaxial** (radial/tibial), or **postaxial** (ulnar/fibular) side;
  (c) **clinodactyly** describes an incurved digit, most often the fifth finger (see Down syndrome, Chapter 36).

Diagnosis in dysmorphology

Correct classification of congenital anomalies has implications for diagnosis and hence for management, prognosis and counselling. Tissue samples should be taken from malformed stillbirths and fetuses for laboratory investigation.

A systematic approach to diagnosis would involve the following:
- **Family pedigree construction** (see Chapter 2).
- **Pregnancy history**. Record drug exposure (e.g. treatment for maternal epilepsy), excess alcohol intake, maternal physiological disorders such as diabetes, and infection (see Chapter 46).
- **Physical examination.**
- **Laboratory investigations**, e.g. chromosome or microarray analysis, skeletal survey or brain imaging.
- **Differential diagnosis**. Illustrated texts and computerized databases can be used for reference (see Appendix).
- **Conclusion**. Currently in perhaps 50% of cases a secure diagnosis cannot be reached.

50 Principles of multifactorial disease

Figure 50.1 Polygenic basis of stature

In this theoretical model height is considered to be controlled by two genes, each with two codominant alleles, A/a and B/b. Alleles A and B make positive, and a and b negative contributions to height. The basis of a normal distribution is created, with individuals of medium height most frequent

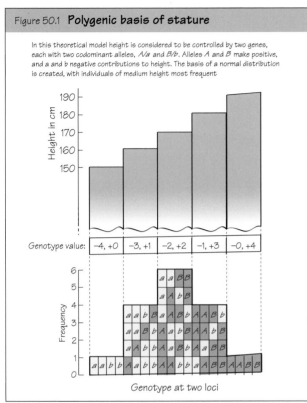

Figure 50.2 Normal distribution of stature in men

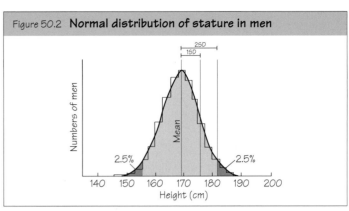

Figure 50.3 The multifactorial threshold model

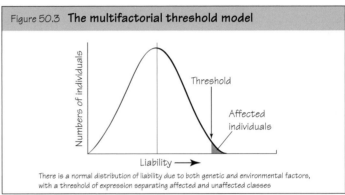

There is a normal distribution of liability due to both genetic and environmental factors, with a threshold of expression separating affected and unaffected classes

Figure 50.4 Recurrence risks in relatives

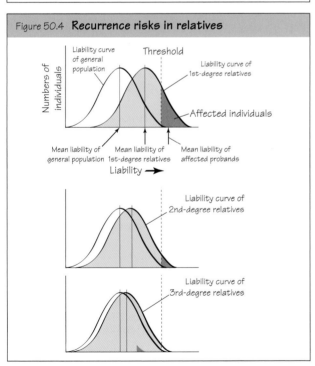

Figure 50.5 The effect of sex-related differential thresholds on recurrence risks (based on pyloric stenosis)

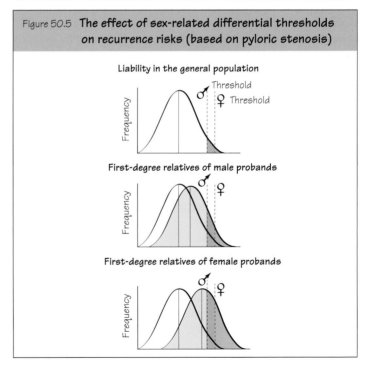

Medical Genetics at a Glance, Third Edition. Dorian J. Pritchard and Bruce R. Korf.
© 2013 John Wiley & Sons, Ltd. Published 2013 by John Wiley & Sons, Ltd.

Table 50.1 Some continuously variable traits.

Height
Weight
Intelligence
Finger ridge count
Blood pressure
Skin colour
Head circumference

Table 50.2 The greater responsibility of genotype in causation of Type 1 compared to that of Type 2 diabetes.

	Pop. incidence (%)	Freq. (empiric risk) in sibs (%)	λs (relative risk in sibs)
Type 1 diabetes (UK)	0.4	6.0	6.0/0.4 = 15.0
Type 2 diabetes (Europe)	10.0	35.0	35.0/10.0 = 3.5

Overview

Mendelian traits show **discontinuous variation** in that alternative phenotypes are distinctly different. With some characters variation is **continuous**, with no natural boundaries. This chapter explains how discontinuous and continuous variation can be seen as two aspects of the same genetic system.

Continuous variation

Quantitative characters such as height, skin colour and intelligence quotient (IQ) typically show continuous variation, their frequency distributions approximating a **normal curve** definable by its mean and **standard deviation** (**SD**). Such distributions are generated by the combined action of many genes, that is they are **polygenic** (see Figure 50.1), or together with environmental factors, **multifactorial**.

'Variance' is a measure of the variation in a character and equals the square of the SD.

In a normal distribution, 68% of the population is included within one SD of the mean, 95% within two and 99.7% within three SDs. The concept of a **normal range** is fundamental, especially in paediatrics, where height, weight, head circumference, etc. are measured routinely (see Chapter 49). Individuals that are outside two SDs from the mean (i.e. the 2.5% at either extreme) are regarded clinically as 'abnormal'.

Heritability (h^2)

Heritability refers to the proportion of variation in a character that can be ascribed to variation in genotype, as distinct from environment, and is expressed as a fraction of one (e.g. 0.8) or as a percentage (e.g. 80%).

The heritability of a continuous trait can be estimated from the **correlation coefficient** between the values in relatives. If the heritability is high, so is the correlation between first-degree relatives. For discontinuous multifactorial traits, heritability can be derived from a variety of data, including concordance rates of twins (see Chapter 53).

Estimation of risk

If there is no discernible pattern of inheritance on which to base predictions, **empiric risks**, calculated from observed incidence in relatives, are used in counselling. Data on different kinds of relatives of many probands are combined and average incidence figures derived. In contrast to the situation with single-gene disorders, recurrence risks are found to differ substantially between populations, because both allele frequencies and environmental factors vary between them.

The **relative risk** (λ, lambda) is the ratio of the risk for a class of family members to that for the general population. The relative risk for a sib is coded as λs. Despite the greater *empiric* risk for siblings of Type 2 diabetes patients, comparison of λs values reveals the greater responsibility of genotype in causation of Type 1 than Type 2 diabetes (Table 50.2).

Discontinuous variation, multifactorial threshold traits

Sometimes there are indications of genetic causation, but only a few family members are affected and the pattern of inheritance remains obscure. One explanation conceives an underlying normal distribution of **liability** to disease, due to an assemblage of harmful genetic and environmental factors, truncated by a threshold for disease manifestation. Disease liability for an individual depends on the combination of predisposing alleles and environmental conditions operating in that individual, and the proportion of the population beyond the threshold represents the population incidence. We all lie somewhere within the liability range for each condition, affected individuals beyond the threshold, and all those near the threshold having a greater than average probability of producing diseased offspring. Such conditions are known as **multifactorial threshold traits**.

Despite its intellectual appeal, the multifactorial threshold model should be viewed as an hypothesis rather than a fact and recent work suggests that very many fewer genes are often involved than was formerly imagined (see Chapter 51).

Rules for identification of a multifactorial threshold trait

1 *Disorders can be common (>1/5000 births; although they can also be rare!).* In comparison, seriously disabling *monogenic* conditions, if dominant and fully penetrant, are usually eliminated by disease, reduced fertility, early death, or failure to mate, and are therefore very rare.

2 *The disorder runs in families, but there is no distinctive pattern of inheritance.*

3 *The concordance rate in MZ twins is significantly greater than in DZ* (see Chapter 53).

4 *The frequency of disease in second-degree relatives is much lower than in first-degree, but declines less rapidly for more distant relatives.*

5 *Recurrence risk is proportional to the number of family members already affected.* This is because the occurrence of several affected family members indicates a particularly high concentration of harmful alleles.

6 *Recurrence risk is proportional to the severity of the condition in the proband.* This is because severity of expression and recurrence risk both depend on the concentration of adverse alleles.

7 *Recurrence risk is higher for relatives of the less-susceptible sex.* This is because disease expression in the less-susceptible sex requires the higher concentration of harmful alleles (see Pyloric stenosis, below).

Examples

Cleft lip with or without cleft palate (CL ± P)

(See also Chapter 49 and diagrams in Chapter 51.)

CL ± P is causally distinct from **cleft palate** alone (which occurs in 1/2000 malformed births). It is caused by failure of fusion of the lateral palatal shelf outgrowths of the maxillae with one another and/or with the anterior primary palate. It sometimes extends into the lip and includes chromosomal, teratogenic, monogenic and multifactorial forms.

A critical feature is the adhesive maturity of the cells on the surfaces of the lateral and medial processes in relation to their relative physical locations. Fusion of lateral and medial elements requires unimpeded movement of the palatal shelves past the tongue (see Figure, 51.1).

CL ± P affects about 1/1000 Europeans (0.1%), twice as many Japanese and half as many African-Americans. European recurrence risks in relatives are:

- first degree = 4%;
- second degree = 0.6%;
- third degree = 0.3% (Rule 4 above; also see Figure 50.4).

Severity of expression varies from unilateral cleft lip alone (UCL) to bilateral cleft lip with cleft palate (BCL + P). As Table 50.3 shows, the incidence of CL ± P (of all types) in first-degree relatives is directly related to severity of expression in the proband (Rule 6 above).

Sixty to eighty per cent of CL ± P patients are male and the incidence in sibs of male probands is 5.5%; 20–40% of patients are female and the incidence in their sibs is 7% (Rule 7 above).

Pyloric stenosis

Pyloric stenosis occurs in 5/1000 male but only 1/1000 female infants (see Chapter 46). Affected females are three times as likely as males to have affected offspring (Rule 7 above; see also Table 50.4). The sons of affected women have the highest risk, at about 20% (see Figure 50.5). The mean incidence in brothers of probands of both sexes combined is markedly higher than that in sisters. The mean incidence in the sibs (of both sexes) of female probands is markedly higher than when the proband is male. The highest risk category is male relatives of female probands.

Table 50.3 The incidence of cleft lip with or without cleft palate (CL ± P) (of all types) in first degree relatives in relation to severity of expression in the proband.

Phenotype of proband	Incidence in first degree relatives (=empiric risk for)
UCL	0.04 or 4%
UCL + P	0.05 or 5%
BCL	0.07 or 7%
BCL + P	0.08 or 8%

BCL, bilateral cleft lip alone; BCL + P, bilateral cleft lip with cleft palate; UCL, unilateral cleft lip alone; UCL + P, unilateral cleft lip with cleft palate.

Table 50.4 Recurrence risks (%) for pyloric stenosis in relation to gender of affected probands. (Source: Carter CO. (1976) Genetics of common single malformations. *Br Med Bull* **32**: 21–6.)

	Male probands		Female probands		Unweighted mean
	London	Belfast	London	Belfast	
Brothers	3.8	9.6	**9.2**	**12.5**	**8.8**
Sisters	2.7	3.0	3.8	3.8	3.3
Unweighted mean	4.8		7.3		

51 Multifactorial disease in children

Figure 51.1 Formation of the palate

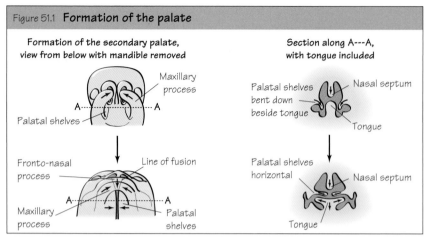

Formation of the secondary palate, view from below with mandible removed

- Maxillary process
- Palatal shelves
- Fronto-nasal process
- Line of fusion
- Maxillary process
- Palatal shelves

Section along A---A, with tongue included

- Palatal shelves bent down beside tongue
- Nasal septum
- Tongue
- Palatal shelves horizontal
- Nasal septum
- Tongue

Figure 51.2 The mature palate

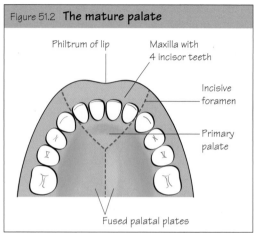

- Philtrum of lip
- Maxilla with 4 incisor teeth
- Incisive foramen
- Primary palate
- Fused palatal plates

Figure 51.3 The threshold model applied to creation of cleft palate

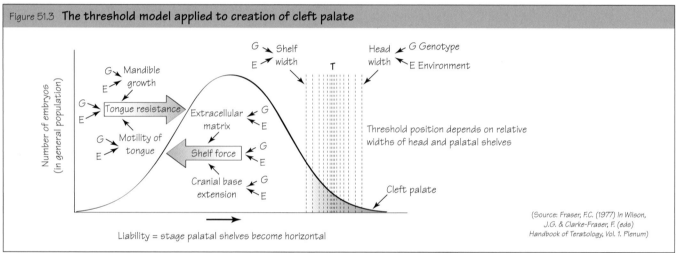

- G → Mandible growth ← E
- G → Tongue resistance ← E
- G → Motility of tongue ← E
- G → Shelf width ← E
- Extracellular matrix → G / E
- Shelf force → G / E
- Cranial base extension → G / E
- Head width
- G Genotype
- E Environment
- T
- Threshold position depends on relative widths of head and palatal shelves
- Cleft palate

Number of embryos (in general population)

Liability = stage palatal shelves become horizontal

(Source: Fraser, F.C. (1977) In Wilson, J.G. & Clarke-Fraser, F. (eds) Handbook of Teratology, Vol. 1. Plenum)

Overview

The diseases that collectively occupy the attention of most health-care practitioners show clustering within families, but are not inherited by Mendelian rules. They are common because the causative alleles are also carried and transmitted by healthy individuals.

The traditional explanation was polygenic causation, with many genes of minor effect acting together (see Chapter 50), but with advancing knowledge this explanation seems less convincing.

In summary:
- In many diseases there is just *one dominant allele, which is incompletely penetrant* (see Chapter 9).
- In *most* common diseases there are *probably no more than two AD disease alleles acting together* (see Chapter 53).
- A few common diseases are **oligogenic**, that is there is *more than one major disease allele acting with others of lesser effect*.
- Common inherited diseases are usually **genetically heterogeneous**, that is *genes at different loci are responsible for similar disease symptoms in different families*.

Methodology

Recognizing the relative importance of genotype and environment in causation of the common diseases can make the difference between health and disease for many people and their analysis demands a variety of approaches.

Twin studies

If a disease has a major genetic component, identical or **monozygotic (MZ)** twin pairs tend to have a high degree of **concordance** for disease (i.e. if one is affected the other usually is also), whereas in non-identical **dizygotic (DZ)** twins concordance is much lower. If MZ and DZ concordances are similar, genotype is deemed unimportant (see Chapter 53).

Family studies

If there is genetic causation the relative risk for a patient's relatives is higher than in the general population and increases with degree of relationship (see Table 51.1 and Chapter 50).

Adoption studies

Incidence of disease in children of affected parents adopted into unaffected families can show to what extent genetic predisposition is causative, as compared to a shared home environment.

Population studies

Study of migrant groups or different ethnic groups in the same environment can reveal genetic involvement.

Table 51.1 Empiric recurrence risks (%) for first, second and third-degree relatives of patients with some common childhood disorders. (Source: Jorde LB, Carey JC, Bamshad MJ & White RL. *Medical Genetics*, 3rd edition. Mosby, St Louis, Missouri 2003.)

Disorder	Population frequency (%)	First degree (%)	Second degree (%)	Third degree (%)
CL ± P	0.10	4.0	0.7	0.30
Talipes	0.10	2.5	0.5	0.20
Congenital dislocation of hip	0.20	5.0	0.6	0.40
Infantile autism	0.04	4.5	0.1	0.05

CL ± P, cleft lip with or without palate.

Polymorphism association analysis

This approach seeks association of disease with specific alleles of a **candidate gene** (see Chapter 32).

Linkage studies

Linkage studies look for co-transmission of disease with polymorphisms of possible linked **genetic markers** (see Chapter 32).

Biochemical studies

Biochemical studies investigate abnormal activity of enzymes involved in implicated biochemical pathways.

Animal models

Animal models can provide insight into the biochemistry and help with gene mapping, but are notoriously misleading.

Examples

Neural tube defects (NTDs)

Frequency 6/1000 livebirths among Northern Chinese; 5/1000 in England and Wales, reduced now to 1/1000 by folic acid supplementation, ultrasound scanning and termination.

Features NTDs arise from failure of closure of the neural tube at the end of week 3 (see Chapters 41, 45, 72, 73 and 74). An anterior defect can result in either **anencephaly** (partial or complete absence of the cranial vault, calvarium or cerebral hemispheres) or **encephalocele** (protrusion of the brain into an enclosed sack). Two-thirds of anencephalics are stillborn and term deliveries die within a few days; encephalocele is also rarely compatible with survival.

A posterior NTD can lead to lumbosacral **myelocele**, **meningomyelocele** (protruding spinal cord exposed, or covered by meninges) or **spina bifida** and about 75% of patients with posterior NTD have secondary hydrocephalus, which can lead to mental retardation.

Genetics NTD is associated with T13 and T18 (Chapter 36) and the AR **Meckel syndrome**. Isolated cases are mostly multifactorial. The empiric recurrence risk for siblings is 2–5%, reducible to 0.5% by medical intervention. For first-degree relatives in general the risk is 1/30, for second degree 1/70, for third degree 1/150. In Hungary where the population incidence is 1/300, sibling risk was found to increase from 3%, to 12%, to 25% after one, two and three affected offspring (see Table 51.2).

Table 51.2 Empiric recurrence risks (%) for some common multifactorial disorders of childhood in relation to health status of parents.

Disorder	Unaffected parents having a second affected child (%)	Affected parent having an affected child (%)	Affected parent having a second affected child (%)
Asthma	10	26	–
Cleft palate	2	7	15
CL ± P	4	4	10
Congenital heart defects	1–4	1–4	10
Cryptorchidism	10	–	–
Dislocation of hip	6	12	36
Epilepsy (idiopathic)	5	5	10
Hypospadias	10	–	–
Pyloric stenosis:			
Male proband	2	4	13
Female proband	10	17	38
Renal agenesis	3	–	–
Spina bifida (see text also)	4–5	4	–
Talipes (club foot)	3	3	10

CL ± P, cleft lip with or without palate.

Management NTD can be diagnosed prenatally by ultrasound scanning and elevation of α-fetoprotein (**AFP**) in maternal serum, or amniotic fluid if the lesion is open (see Chapters 72 and 73). It is claimed that 50–70% of NTDs could be avoided if women trying to conceive took 0.4 mg of folic acid daily, or 4–5 mg before and during early pregnancy if there is already an affected child.

Aetiology In Britain incidence is highest in Celtic people and correlates with multiparity, poor socioeconomic status, valproic acid exposure and folic acid deficiency.

Crohn disease

Crohn disease is one of two main clinical subtypes of **inflammatory bowel disease** (the other being **ulcerative colitis**).

Frequency 1–2% in Western countries.

Genetics Maps to 16p12, 16q, 12q, 6p and 3p; λs: 25. Relative risk for heterozygous and homozygous genotypes: 2.5 and 40.0.

Aetiology The receptor product of the *NOD2* (or *CARD15*) gene at 16p12 normally activates the cytoplasmic transcription factor, NF-κβ, making it responsive to the surface lipopolysaccharides of potentially harmful bacteria. This property is deficient in Crohn disease.

Management The most effective drugs target the NF-κβ complex.

Congenital heart defects (CHDs) (see also Chapters 45, 47 and 48)

Frequency 7/1000 live births.

Features Abnormalities include ventricular septal defect (VSD: 1/400), atrial septal defect (ASD: 1/1000), patent ductus arteriosus (PDA: 1/800), pulmonary stenosis (1/2500), coarctation (constriction) of the aorta (1/1600) and aortic stenosis (constriction of the aortic valve; 1/2000).

Complex anomalies include **tetralogy of Fallot** in about 1/1000 and **transposition of the great arteries**, in 1/16000 (see Chapter 48). CHDs can result in inadequate oxygenation of blood and/or poor perfusion of tissues.

Genetics 90% are multifactorial, others chromosomal or monogenic.

Insulin-dependent or Type 1 diabetes mellitus (IDDM; T1DM)

Features **Diabetes mellitus** is characterized by **hyperglycaemia**, causative of serious renal, retinal and vascular problems and ultimately coma and death. There are several forms (see Chapter 59). Insulin-dependent or **juvenile-onset diabetes** affects possibly 3–7% of Western adults, its peak age of onset being 12 years. The annual incidence of new cases varies from around 1/100000 in Japan and China, to 8–17 in northern Europe, to 35/100000 in Scandinavia.

Genetics MZ concordance: 50%; DZ: 12% indicating a penetrance of 0.5 (see Chapter 53); λs: 15. Two loci are especially important: *IDDM-1* and *IDDM-2*, that together account for 40–50% of genetic predisposition. There is strong association (95%) with HLA-B8 and B15, c.f. 50% of the general population. (See also Tables 50.2 and 66.2.)

Aetiology There is a range of predisposing environmental factors and susceptibility is enhanced by >20 other gene loci.

Atopic diathesis

Atopic diathesis constitutes an exuberant IgE response to low levels of antigen (see Chapter 65). One in four of the population shares an AD allele that is possibly imprinted, as incidence is highest in offspring of affected mothers. Patients develop 'hay fever', eczema and asthma.

Infantile autism

Frequency 4–10%; 4 ♂:1♀.

Features There is severe impairment in development of social responsiveness, very poor verbal and non-verbal communication and repetitive, stereotypic behaviour and interests, often associated with developmental delay. Onset is usually before the age of 4 years. It can be associated with chromosome imbalance, fragile X syndrome and **tuberous sclerosis** (an AD tendency toward **hamartomas** caused by growth of blood vessels, especially in the brain).

Genetics MZ concordance: 80%; DZ concordance 20%. There are susceptibility loci on Chromosomes 7q, 17q, 5p, 11, 4 and 9.

Combined recurrence risk for sibs of male probands is 3.5%, that for sibs of female probands, 7%.

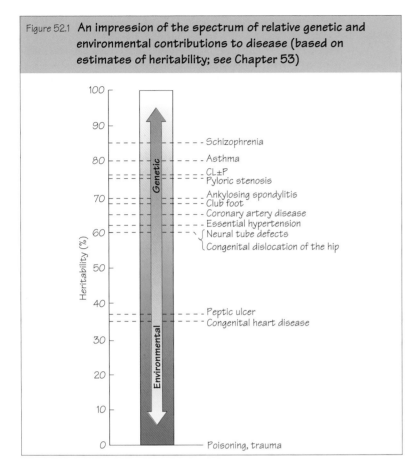

Figure 52.1 **An impression of the spectrum of relative genetic and environmental contributions to disease (based on estimates of heritability; see Chapter 53)**

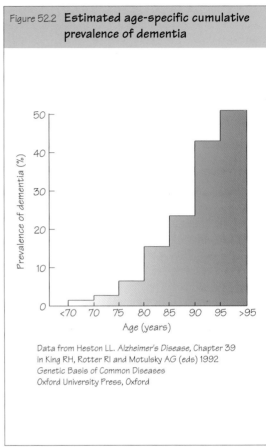

Figure 52.2 **Estimated age-specific cumulative prevalence of dementia**

Data from Heston LL. *Alzheimer's Disease*, Chapter 39 in King RH, Rotter RI and Motulsky AG (eds) 1992 *Genetic Basis of Common Diseases* Oxford University Press, Oxford

Overview

Disease frequencies vary between populations, for example, **Type 2 diabetes (T2DM)** is 20 times as prevalent in North America as in China (see also Table 29.1). Such variation probably has underlying genetic predispositions, but in some cases it also relates to lifestyle. For example the genome of the Pima Indians of the American Southwest has been naturally selected for survival through severe food shortages, but when regular and richer food is available its associated frugal metabolism creates a tendency to T2DM.

Among the leading causes of death in economically developed countries are **stroke**, **coronary artery disease** and **cardiomyopathy**, linked through obesity, T2DM, **hypertension**, indolence, smoking, alcohol consumption, bad nutrition and other aspects of an economically privileged lifestyle. Schizophrenia, affective psychosis, mental retardation and Alzheimer dementia are also very common health problems of adult life, with multifactorial origins.

Odds ratios

Assessment of the probability that an individual will develop disease can be facilitated by identification of disease-associated genetic markers, but with multifactorial conditions the strength of association is frequently nowhere near 100%. Prediction is therefore sometimes best indicated by an '**odds ratio**'. Odds ratios provide an indication of how much more frequently the disease occurs in individuals with a specific marker than in those without it.

However, many markers are characterized by only modest disease associations, with odds ratios as low as 1.2–1.5. In one study with T2DM the highest odds ratio for the markers studied was only 1.36. Individuals with that marker would on average have a 36% increased chance of developing T2DM.

Calculation of the odds ratio for disease association with a putative marker allele:

	Freq. of Allele 1	Combined freq. of all other alleles
Patients	a	b
Controls	c	d

Odds ratio for Allele 1 = a/c ÷ b/d = **ad/bc**

Coronary artery disease (CAD)

Features CAD can account for up to 50% of deaths in developed countries.

Aetiology Lipid deposition in the coronary arteries causes fibrous conversion (**atherosclerosis**), failure of blood supply (**ischaemia**) and death of heart muscle (**myocardial infarction**). Predisposing

Medical Genetics at a Glance, Third Edition. Dorian J. Pritchard and Bruce R. Korf.
© 2013 John Wiley & Sons, Ltd. Published 2013 by John Wiley & Sons, Ltd.

conditions include **familial combined hyperlipidaemia (FCH)**, **familial hypercholesterolaemia (FH)** and point mutations in **apo B-100** (all AD), diabetes mellitus and hypertension.

Genetics Fifteen per cent of cases show AD inheritance at >12 loci, including the gene for the **low density lipoprotein receptor (LDLR)** (see Chapter 5).

Risk increases several-fold if a first-degree relative is affected, especially if female, if onset was before 55 years, or if additional relatives are affected.

Management Incidence is dramatically reduced by non-smoking, control of hypertension and fat intake, exercise and slimming.

Cardiomyopathy (see Chapters 47 and 48)

About half of **cardiomyopathy** cases are familial, involving hypertrophy of the left ventricle wall and caused by AD mutations in any of 10 genes that encode various components of the cardiac sarcomere. The most common are mutations in the genes for the **β-myosin heavy chain** (35%), **myosin-binding protein C** (20%) and **troponin T** (15%).

Dilated cardiomyopathy involves increase in size, with impaired contraction of the ventricles and circulation. There are AD, X-linked and mitochondrial defects and the proteins affected include **actin**, **cardiac troponin T**, **desmin** and components of the **destroglycan–sarcoglycan complex**.

In the **long QT (LQT) syndrome** there is elongation of the electrocardiogram QT interval, with potentially fatal cardiac arrhythmia. It shows familial patterns, but is also induced by drugs that block potassium channels. **Romano–Ward syndrome** is inherited as AD, **Jervell–Lange–Nielsen syndrome**, as AR.

Hypertension

High blood pressure affects 25% of adults of most developed countries and promotes heart disease, stroke and kidney disease. With no obvious cause it is called **essential hypertension**; when induced by pregnancy, **pre-eclampsia**.

Frequency Up to 40% of 70 year olds are hypertensive.

Genetics Essential hypertension shows heritability of 20–40%. Monogenic AD inheritance is suggested in rare families.

Biochemical studies implicate the **sodium–potassium transmembrane pump**, the **angiotensin I converting enzyme (ACE)**, the **angiotensin II type I receptor** and the gene coding for **angiotensinogen** involved in sodium reabsorption and vasoconstriction. At least eight rare mutations concerned are indicated.

Management Recommendations include avoidance of sodium intake, reduction of body weight and stress.

Stroke

Stroke, or **apoplexy**, refers to brain damage caused by sudden and sustained loss of blood flow to the brain. **Ischaemic stroke** arises from **embolism**, or arterial obstruction. **Haemorrhagic stroke** is due to rupture of a blood vessel in the brain. It may include loss of consciousness and **hemiplegia** (paralysis of one side of the body) and is the third leading cause of death in Americans. It is associated with hypertension, obesity, atherosclerosis, diabetes and smoking tobacco.

MZ concordance is 10%, DZ 5% (see Chapter 53). It can be a consequence of sickle cell disease (see Chapter 29) and cerebral autosomal dominant arteriopathy with subcortical infarcts and leucoencephalopathy (**CADASIL**).

Type 2 diabetes mellitus and MODY

Type 2 (T2DM), **late-onset** or **non-insulin-dependent diabetes mellitus (NIDDM)** is a genetically heterogeneous group of disorders of glucose intolerance. It occurs at a frequency of 4–10% of adults, 10 times that of T1DM, with over 200 million sufferers worldwide (see above and Chapter 51). **Maturity-onset diabetes of the young (MODY)** is a subset that affects 1–2% of diabetic subjects in early adulthood.

Genetics MODY has an AD monogenic basis, affecting glucokinase activity in pancreatic β-cells, where it controls the rate-limiting step in glucose metabolism. A few mutations are in the structural gene, but at least five others encode essential transcription factors. One of these, **hepatocyte nuclear factor 1α (hnf1α)**, is responsible for 65% of British cases of MODY.

There are no major predisposing alleles for other forms of T2DM although several predisposing indicators are known (see also Table 50.2). The *SNP43* allele of the **calpain 10 gene** is of particular significance in Mexican-Americans. Calpain 10 is a cysteine protease coded on 2q, its pathogenic sequences being located in its introns. Certain heterozygous combinations lead to disease though all are non-pathogenic in the homozygous state.

Low intelligence (Table 52.1)

IQ (mental age/chronological age) is inherited as a polygenic trait (see Chapter 50). An IQ of 50–70 is shown by 3% of the population, at the lower end of the 'normal' range. **Severe non-specific intellectual disability** (IQ <50) usually has a single cause, with an overall risk of recurrence of about 3%. This is increased to 15% if the parents are related, or 25% after the birth of two affected children (see Table 52.1). Some male cases are XR, predicting an increased risk for subsequent male births.

Schizophrenia (Table 52.2)

Schizophrenia is a seriously disabling psychosis affecting 1% of the population. Twin concordance rates, family and adoption studies support a monogenic AD basis, with low penetrance, although this interpretation is by no means widely accepted. Gene mapping indicates genetic heterogeneity.

Suggested environmental triggers include prenatal viral infection, recreational drugs and social stress.

Affective disorder (Table 52.2)

Affective disorders include purely **depressive** or **unipolar**, and **manic depressive** or **bipolar illness**. The average lifetime risk for

Table 52.1 Risk of recurrence of severe non-specific mental retardation in affected families.

Family category	Recurrence risk
One male offspring affected	1/25
One female offspring affected	1/50
Two offspring affected	1/4
Parents consanguineous	1/7

Table 52.2 Empiric risks of recurrence of schizophrenia and affective psychosis in relatives.

	Population incidence (%)	Sibling (first-degree relative) (%)	Offspring of one affected parent (first-degree relative) (%)	Offspring of two affected parents (first-degree relative) (%)	Second-degree relative (%)	Third-degree relative (%)
Schizophrenia	1	9	13	45	3	1–2
Affective psychosis (unipolar + bipolar)	2–3	13	15	50	5	2–3

bipolar is about 1%, for unipolar 2–25% depending on cultural background. In women it is associated with adjustment of reproductive hormone regimes.

Twin, family and adoption studies point to a genetic basis. Mapping studies indicate genetic heterogeneity and there is evidence of anticipation (see Chapter 28).

Alzheimer disease

Alzheimer disease involves progressive **dementia** and memory loss and affects 40–50% of Americans in their 90s. It is less common in Hispanics and Africans than Europeans and Japanese.

There is defective cleavage of **amyloid-β precursor protein (APP)**, causing **β-amyloid plaques** and neurofibrillary tangles in the brain, with progressive loss of neurons.

In the 3–5% of families with early-onset dementia AD inheritance is indicated, with at least seven susceptibility loci, including those for **presenilins-1** and **-2**. Another codes for a defect in the cleavage site within APP coded on Chromosome 21 (c.f. Down syndrome, Chapter 36). Late-onset cases fit a multifactorial model best with the **epsilon 4 (ε4)** allele of **apolipoprotein E**, involved in clearance of cleaved amyloid protein, the best characterized risk factor.

Obesity

Body Mass Index (BMI) is defined as: (weight in kilograms)/(height in metres)^2. An 'obese' person has a BMI > 30, for example a person of height 5′8″ (173 cm) who weighs 90 kg, or 14 stone (156 lbs) has a BMI of $90/[1.73]^2 = 30$, at the borderline of obesity. About 30% of American adults are classed as obese, providing an exacerbating factor for heart disease, stroke, hypertension and T2DM.

A serum protein called **leptin** is closely involved with the pathogenesis of eating disorders. Leptin is secreted by adipocytes and its concentration in the serum reflects the amount of lipid in store. It regulates food intake and energy expenditure by binding to specific receptors in the hypothalamus, thereby modifying its expression of neuropeptides. Congenital deficiency of leptin is associated with early-onset obesity.

Genetics Twin and adoption studies indicate a heritability of 0.6–0.8, but the genetics is obscure.

Alcoholism

Frequency 10% of (American) males, 4% of females.

Features Type 1 alcoholism is a feature of introverted, solitary behaviour. Age of onset is usually over 25 years and it is relatively easily cured. Type 2 is associated with extraversion and thrill-seeking; it usually begins before 25 and is less easily treated.

Genetics Risk of becoming an alcoholic is increased fourfold if there is an affected parent. The heritability of Type 1 is 0.2, that for Type 2, 0.9.

Unpleasant consequences of alcohol consumption due to hereditary metabolic deficiencies reduce heavy drinking and alcoholism in some ethnic groups (see Chapter 29).

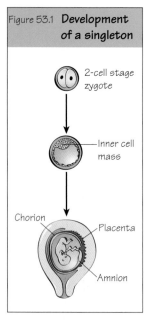

Figure 53.1 **Development of a singleton**

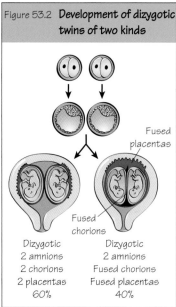

Figure 53.2 **Development of dizygotic twins of two kinds**

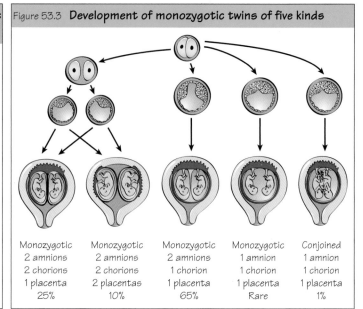

Figure 53.3 **Development of monozygotic twins of five kinds**

Overview

The main value of twins in genetic analysis is that they can reveal the relative importance of genotype ('nature') and environment ('nurture') in multifactorial disease.

There are two major categories of twins, **monozygotic (MZ)** or **identical**, and **dizygotic (DZ)** or **fraternal**. DZ twins originate from two eggs and two sperm; like ordinary sibs they share 50% of their alleles. MZ twins originate from a single zygote that divided into two embryos during the first 2 weeks of development. MZ twins are always of the same sex and their genomes are (initially) 100% identical.

Sixty-five per cent of MZ twins share a placenta and chorion, around 25% have separate chorions and almost all have separate amnions. They have non-identical, but very similar fingerprints. Their '**DNA fingerprints**' are essentially identical, although recent comparisons of MZ twins revealed unexpected **gene copy number variation** (**CNV**; see below and Chapter 70).

Frequency of multiple births

Around 1/80 British pregnancies yield twins, about 1/260 births of MZ, 1/125 of DZ. Up to 1/20 births are of DZ in some African populations, but less than 1/500 in Chinese and Japanese. Multiple births involve various combinations of DZ- and MZ-like twinning events. Triplets occur in 1/7500 and quadruplets in 1/658 000 European births.

DZ twinning is increased at late births and greater maternal age, the peak being at age 35–40 years, possibly related to levels of **follicle stimulating hormone** (**FSH**). Women treated with ovulation-inducing agents like *clomiphene citrate* and *gonadotrophins* are at increased risk of multiple pregnancy. There is probably no familial tendency toward MZ twinning but there is for DZ, with up to three times the normal rate in some families.

Analysis of discontinuous multifactorial traits

Concordance ratio

If both twins are affected by a condition they are said to be **concordant** for that condition. If only one is affected they are **discordant**. The **pair-wise concordance rate** is given by

$$C / (C + D)$$

where C = the number of concordant pairs and D = the number of discordant pairs.

Since MZ twins are virtually genetically identical, whereas DZ share only around 50% of their genomes, the ratio of their concordances for a condition gives a rough indication of the relative importance of genotype in its causation.

If $C_{MZ} : C_{DZ} = 3–6 : 1$, the genome is the major determinant, e.g. schizophrenia, CL ± P;

If $C_{MZ} : C_{DZ} = 2–3 : 1$, both genetic and environmental factors are significant, e.g. blood pressure, mental deficiency;

If $C_{MZ} : C_{DZ} = 1–2 : 1$, the main determinant is environmental, e.g. measles, tobacco smoking.

The Holzinger statistic

The Holzinger (*H*) statistic provides values from close to zero, for minimal genetic involvement, to close to unity for almost entirely genetic causation:

$$H = \frac{C_{MZ} - C_{DZ}}{1 - C_{DZ}}$$

Estimation of penetrance and gene counting

MZ concordance relates to penetrance (*P*) by the expression:

$$C_{MZ} = \frac{P}{2 - P}$$

Medical Genetics at a Glance, Third Edition. Dorian J. Pritchard and Bruce R. Korf.

Table 53.1 Twin concordances and derived values for some complex traits.*

Disorder	Population frequency /1000	MZ conc. (%)	DZ conc. (%)	n	P
Atopic diathesis	250	50	4	3	0.7
Autism	40–100	80	20	1 or 2	0.9
Bipolar affective disorder	4	79	24	1	0.9
CL ± P	1	30	5	2	0.5
Cleft palate	0.5	26	5	2	0.4
Congenital dislocation of hip	1	41	3	3 or 4	0.6
Coronary artery disease	Up to 500	46	12	1 or 2	0.6
Epilepsy	10	37	10	1 or 2	0.5
Essential hypertension	100	30	10	1	0.5
T1DM	2	30–40	6	2	0.5
Leprosy	Varies	60	20	1	0.75
Measles	Varies	97	94	0	–
Multiple sclerosis	1	20–30	6	2	0.4
T2DM	30–70	100	10	2	1.0
Psoriasis	10	61	13	1 or 2	0.75
Pyloric stenosis	3	15	2	3	0.3
Rheumatoid arthritis	20	30	5	2	0.5
Schizophrenia	10	45	13	1	0.6
Spina bifida	5	6	3	1	0.1
Talipes equinovarus	5	32	3	3	0.5
Tuberculosis	Varies	87	26	1	0.9
Unipolar affective disorder	20–250	54	19	1	0.7

n, number of major genes acting in a monogenic or together in an oligogenic system, estimated from DZ concordance; P, approximate penetrance estimated from MZ concordance. (These data give no indication of genetic heterogeneity.)

*This table is meant to present only a general picture, actual frequencies and concordances vary in published reports.

From which penetrance can be calculated.

When P is known the number of major causative alleles can be derived from DZ concordance:

$$C_{DZ} = \frac{P}{4 - P}, \text{ for ONE major autosomal dominant;}$$

$$C_{DZ} = \frac{P}{8 - P}, \text{ for TWO dominants, or a pair of recessives;}$$

$$C_{DZ} = \frac{P}{16 - P}, \text{ for THREE dominants; or one dominant}$$

and a pair of recessives.

Analysis of continuously variable multifactorial traits

The most widely used estimate of genetic involvement is **heritability** (**h^2**), defined as *the fraction of variation in a quantitative character that can be ascribed to genotypic variation*. It can furnish information on, for example, the effectiveness of a nutritional regime. It varies

between populations and is derivable from (1) the standard deviations of the differences between co-twins, or (2) the coefficients of correlation (r) between them.

$$h^2 = \frac{V_{DZ} - V_{MZ}}{V_{DZ}}$$

V stands for 'variance', the square of the standard deviation of the differences between members of twin pairs.

$$h^2 = \frac{r_{MZ} - r_{DZ}}{1 - r_{DZ}}$$

Health risks in twins

Twin pregnancies have a 5 to 10-fold increased incidence of perinatal mortality and a tendency toward premature birth. Deformations occur in both kinds of twins, but MZ also have twice the normal risk of malformation (see Chapter 45).

Monochorionic MZ twins often (~15%) share a blood supply. This can lead to **twin-to-twin transfusion syndrome** when one twin becomes severely undernourished while the other develops an enlarged heart and liver and **polyhydramnios**. There are marked differences in birth weights and both twins are at great risk of morbidity and mortality.

Conjoined and parasitic twins

Conjoined or 'Siamese' twins develop from incompletely separated inner-cell masses and represent about 1% of MZ pairs. They may be united at the same position of any part of the head or trunk.

A **parasitic twin** is a portion of a body protruding from an otherwise normal host. Common attachment sites are the oral region, the pelvis and the **mediastinum** (the wall dividing the thoracic cavity).

Copy number variation (CNV)

Healthy diploid individuals are generally believed to have just two copies of every gene, but recent comparison of the DNA of MZ twins revealed considerable, unexpected variation in gene copy number, caused probably by DNA replication errors during individual development. One study found 12% of the genomes of healthy people to be subject to CNV. Variant sequences are typically in tandem clusters and average 250kb long. This observation suggests new approaches to disease gene mapping, forensic study and explanation of discordance among family members (see Chapter 70).

Weaknesses of the twin study approach

1 Concordant pairs can be **ascertained** (i.e. recognized) through both individuals, discordant through only one, leading to **bias of ascertainment**.

2 The first two blastomeres may be fertilized by separate sperms.

3 Separate eggs may be fertilized by different fathers.

4 MZ discordance can arise from somatic mutation, transfusion syndrome and CNV, rather than incomplete penetrance.

54 | The signal transduction cascade

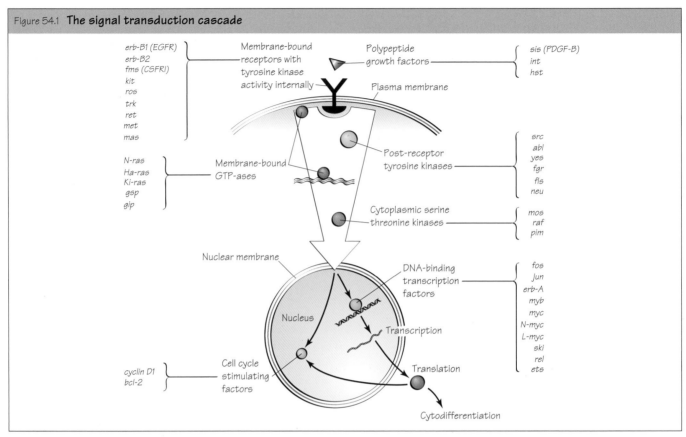

Figure 54.1 **The signal transduction cascade**

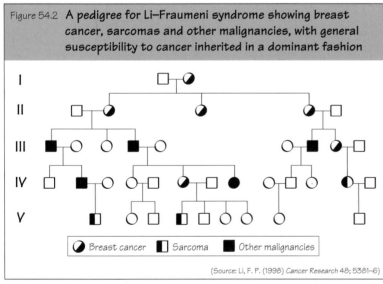

Figure 54.2 **A pedigree for Li–Fraumeni syndrome showing breast cancer, sarcomas and other malignancies, with general susceptibility to cancer inherited in a dominant fashion**

Breast cancer ◑   Sarcoma ◧   Other malignancies ■

(Source: Li, F. P. (1998) *Cancer Research* 48; 5381–6)

Table 54.1 **Comparison of the properties of oncogenes and tumour suppressor genes**

Oncogenes

(Over-) active in tumour
(Over-) activity associated with translocation or substitution
Abnormality rarely inherited
Dominant at cellular level
Broad tissue specificity
Frequently causative of leukaemia and lymphoma

Tumour suppressor genes

Normal allele inactive in tumour
Abnormality due to deletion or specific mutation of normal allele
Abnormality can be inherited
Recessive at cellular level
Considerable tumour specificity
Causative of solid tumours

Overview

Normal progress through the cell cycle (Chapters 16 and 17) is promoted by polypeptide **growth factors** that bind to specific receptors on the cell surface. Their presence is conveyed to the nucleus by a series of phosphorylations of **kinases** (themselves phosphate-attaching enzymes) that constitute the **signal transduction cascade (STC)**. Phosphorylated **DNA-binding proteins** then bind to specific sites in the DNA and promote transition to the next phase of the cycle. The genes that code for the (normal) proteins involved in the STC are **proto-oncogenes**. Cancer-causing derivatives are called **oncogenes**.

Progress through the cycle is moderated by the protein products of the **mitosis suppressor genes**, known to cancer biologists as '**tumour suppressor genes**' (see Chapter 17) and cancers are frequently initiated by their failure, sometimes indicated by **loss of heterozygosity**

Medical Genetics at a Glance, Third Edition. Dorian J. Pritchard and Bruce R. Korf.

at that locus. The properties of tumour suppressor genes and onco-genes are compared in Table 54.1.

Environmental triggers

Most mutagens (see Chapter 26) can trigger **carcinogenesis**; non-mutagenic cancer-promoting chemicals generally operate by activation of kinases.

Viruses

Viruses can '**transform**' normal cells into cancer cells by insertion of a viral promoter beside a host proto-oncogene (as with **Epstein–Barr virus** in some cases of Burkitt lymphoma), or by introduction of a viral genome that already carries an oncogene. Other DNA viruses implicated in human cancer include **papilloma** and **hepatitis B**) (see Chapter 17). Oncogenic RNA retroviruses include **T-cell leukaemia virus** and **Kaposi sarcoma associated herpes virus**.

Tumour suppressor proteins

The cell cycle is interrupted by checkpoints in G1 and G2 (see Chapter 16). At the G1 checkpoint, if the nuclear DNA is found to be damaged, a protein called **p53** increases in activity and stimulates transcription of protein **p21** (see Chapter 17). Protein p21 binds to the specific cyclin–Cdk complex responsible for driving the cell into S-phase, so inactivating it and arresting the cell in G1. This allows sufficient time for the DNA repair enzymes to make good the damage to the DNA. For this and related reasons, p53 is known affectionately as the '**Guardian of the Genome**' (see below and Chapter 17).

If no appropriate growth factors are present the cell is held at the 'G0' block, which is reinforced by other tumour suppressor proteins such as the **retinoblastoma (Rb) protein** encoded by the *normal* allele of the Rb gene and *CDKN2A* (Chapter 17). These bind to specific regulatory proteins preventing them from stimulating the transcription of genes required for cell proliferation.

The signal transduction cascade

1 Growth factors. Extracellular growth factors destroy the G0 block by activating other G1-specific cyclin–Cdk complexes (see Chapter 17), which phosphorylate the Rb protein, altering its conformation and causing it to release the bound regulatory protein E2F. The latter is then free to activate transcription of target genes and cell proliferation ensues. The best-known growth factor is *c-sis*, identical to the B subunit of platelet derived growth factor (PDGF). Two others, *hst* and *int-2*, have been found amplified in stomach cancers and malignant melanomas, respectively.

2 Growth factor receptors. Growth factor receptors span the cell membrane and have tyrosine kinase properties at their cytoplasmic ends. An example is *c-erb-B*, which encodes **epidermal growth factor receptor** (EGF-R, or *erbB*). Activation of *erb-B2* independently of growth factor stimulation, or its over-expression, are associated with cancer of the stomach, pancreas, ovary, brain and breast (Chapters 55 and 56). **Glioblastomas** produce their own **platelet-derived growth factor** (PDGF) and sarcomas, **tumour growth factor α** (TGF-α).

3 Postreceptor tyrosine kinases. The target of kinase activity of the growth factor receptor is characteristically a **postreceptor tyrosine kinase**, which in turn phosphorylates another cytoplasmic kinase that phosphorylates a third, and so on.

4 Serine threonine kinases. Some steps in the STC involve phosphorylation of serine or threonine residues by, for example, the *raf* protein. Mutant versions of *raf* maintain continuous transmission of the growth-promoting signal.

5 GTPases. Phosphate for kinase activity is largely supplied by ATP, but the intracellular membranes carry GTPases also, including multiple *ras* proteins. Mutations resulting in increased or sustained GTPase activity lead to continuous growth. In ~25% of cancers mutant *ras* proteins release mitogenic signals spontaneously.

6 DNA binding proteins and cell cycle factors. DNA-binding oncoproteins control expression of genes concerned with the cell cycle. Over-production of *myc* and *myb*, which stimulate transition from G1 to S-phase, prevents cells from entering G0.

Conversion of proto-oncogenes to oncogenes

1 Point mutation. Thirty per cent of tumours contain mutated versions of a *ras* protein that is unable to adopt the inactive form.

2 Translocation. Examples are the Philadelphia chromosome (see Chapters 39, 56 and 57) and translocations of *myc* on Chromosome 8, to alongside the promoters of the Ig heavy chain on Chromosome 14, the κ light chain on 2 or the λ light chain on 22 (see Chapter 64). These are found in at least 90% of cases of Burkitt lymphoma (see Chapter 56).

3 Insertional mutagenesis. See 'Viruses' above.

4 Amplification. In 10% of tumours are tiny, supernumerary pieces of DNA called **double-minute chromatin bodies**, composed of amplified copies of a proto-oncogene, for example of *N-myc* in some neuroblastomas and *erb-B2* in breast cancers. If inserted into chromosomes they are detectable as **homogeneously staining regions**, or **HSRs**.

Enabling characteristics

While defining the 'hallmarks of cancer' (Chapter 55) Hanahan and Weinberg also described some characteristics that enable its development. The most prominent is **genomic instability**, which enables generation of random mutations and chromosomal rearrangements. A key player here is the Guardian of the Genome, tumour suppressor protein, p53. If p53 is defective the unrestrained replication that ensues allows that line of cells to accumulate mutations and a cancer can develop. Point mutations or deletions of its structural gene *TP53* occur in 70% of all tumours. p53 not only enforces the G1 block, but also mediates commitment to apoptosis in response to DNA damage and release of angiogenesis inhibition (Chapters 17 and 54). A germline defect in TP53 causes **Li–Fraumeni syndrome**, notable for its assortment of tumours (see Figure 54.2 and Chapter 56).

The second enabling characteristic is an **inflammatory microenvironment**. Tumours are densely infiltrated by cells of the immune system, mirroring inflammation in non-neoplastic tissues. These contribute growth factors, survival factors that limit apoptosis, pro-angiogenic factors, ECM modifying enzymes and inductive signals that help activate the epithelial–mesenchymal transition (see Chapter 55).

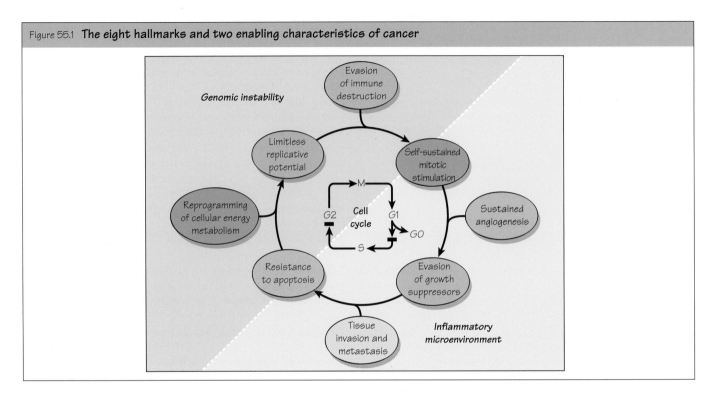

Figure 55.1 **The eight hallmarks and two enabling characteristics of cancer**

Overview

Normal cells can divide only a limited number of times and do so only when stimulated by polypeptide growth factors (GFs; see Chapters 17 and 54). If cells get damaged their replication is arrested while repairs are carried out; if the damage is irreparable, **apoptosis** ('cell suicide') takes place. Healthy tissues also generally remain at locations where they 'ought' to be.

Cancers disobey these rules. As they progress individual cells acquire and retain defects in a random, multistep progression. They develop extraordinary survival skills and evasion tactics and become subject to natural selection, so that malignant cancers display a characteristic set of abnormalities. Malignant tumours of epidermal origin are called **carcinomas**, mesodermal ones, **sarcomas**.

Six acquired functional capabilities of malignant tumours were defined by Hanahan and Weinberg in 2000 and in 2011 the same authors proposed two more, plus two 'enabling characteristics' (see Chapter 54). Below are their 8 'hallmark' abnormalities common to the 100 or more kinds of malignant cancer:

1 self-sufficiency in mitotic stimulation;
2 evasion of growth suppressors;
3 resistance to apoptosis;
4 limitless replicative potential;
5 sustained angiogenesis;
6 tissue invasion and metastasis;
7 reprogramming of cellular energy metabolism;
8 evasion of immune destruction.

1 Self-sufficiency in mitotic stimulation

GFs are normally required for mitosis and these engage with specific receptors (GFRs) on cell surfaces. Cancer cells however can grow and divide without external signals, utilizing three unusual capacities: production of self-stimulatory GFs, hyperexpression of GFRs and spontaneous transmission of intracellular mitotic signals by unstimulated GFRs.

2 Evasion of growth suppressors

Cancer cells generally resist growth inhibitory signals from the ECM and neighbouring cell surfaces. Normally such signals are transmitted internally, ultimately through the retinoblastoma protein (pRB) and others, preventing inappropriate transition from G1 to S (see Chapter 16). This transition is blocked by under-phosphorylated pRB, which sequesters the necessary E2F transcription factors. Normally TGFβ inhibits the phosphorylation that would inactivate pRB.

If the action of pRB is harmed by mutation, or upset by intervention of papilloma virus in uterine cervical cells, uncontrolled cell division can lead to cancer.

3 Resistance to apoptosis

Accumulation of tumour cells depends also on their rate of attrition. In normal cells 'sensor' molecules check for metabolic abnormalities before 'effectors' activate 'the death pathway'. The sensors include IGF-1/IGF2 and its receptor IGF-1R. These monitor DNA damage, proto-oncogene expression levels, hypoxia and signals from the ECM and cell neighbours. The effectors include Fas ligand (FasL) and TNF-α and their receptors. Apoptosis is normally triggered by overexpression of a proto-oncogene (Chapter 54) and a cancer can progress to malignancy only if that is overcome.

4 Limitless replicative potential

With human cells the 'Hayflick limit' restricts their multiplication to ~80 doublings, but cancer cells ignore this restriction. The limit is normally imposed by proteins pRB and p53 (see Chapters 17 and 54), but when they are disabled, as in typical cancer cells, mitosis continues until a stage called 'crisis' is reached, resulting usually in death of the cell. However, in about 1/10 000 000 mitoses an 'immortalized' cell emerges that can divide without limit.

The mitotic count is recorded by the telomeres (Chapter 20) from each of which 50–100 bp of DNA is lost at each cycle. Close to 90% of cancers up-regulate the enzyme **telomerase** that reinstates telomere structure. The rest achieve a similar outcome by interchromosomal exchange.

5 Sustained angiogenesis

Tissues need capillaries within a range of 100 μm and initiation of growth of capillaries, **angiogenesis**, requires both inducers and inhibitors. Inducers include **vascular endothelial growth factor (VEGF)**, and **acetic and basic fibroblast growth factor (FGF 1/2)**, which bind to tyrosine kinase receptors on endothelial cell surfaces. **Thrombospondin-1** is an angiogenesis inhibitor regulated by p53. VEGF expression is activated by the *ras* oncogene, or loss of VHL tumour suppressor.

6 Tissue invasion and metastasis

When cancer causes death this usually results from invasion of neighbouring tissues, frequently following dispersal to distant sites. However, most tumours are 'benign'. These rarely present a threat to their hosts, whereas 'malignant' cancers can kill, most often by pressure or occlusion. Tumours of both types are found in the same organs, can be derived from the same cell types, can grow to the same size, be induced by the same agents or inherited mutations, or arise spontaneously. The major distinction of malignant tumours is their ability to invade other tissues and to metastasize, that is to fragment and be transported in the blood or lymph streams (see also 'Enabling characteristics', Chapter 54).

The **invasion-metastasis cascade (IMC)** envisions the following progression: **local invasion → 'intravasion' of adjacent blood and lymph vessels → transit through blood and lymphatic systems → 'extravasion' into parenchyma of distant tissue → formation of micrometastases → 'colonization' as macroscopic tumours**.

The **epithelial–mesenchymal transition (EMT)** seems to exploit normal steps in embryogenesis and wound healing, the various transcription factors involved orchestrating events up to colonization.

Cell adhesion involves molecular links between ligands and complementary receptors on other cell surfaces or the ECM. **Cell adhesion molecules (CAMs)** typically span the phospholipid bilayer, with an extracellular domain responsible for external binding and an intracellular domain that interacts with the cytoskeleton.

There are four major classes of CAM: **cadherins**, which participate in binding cells of similar type, **integrins** concerned mainly with ECM

interactions and substrate preferences, **selectins** involved in transient cell adhesions and **Ig-CAMs** related to the immunoglobulins.

E-cadherin normally transmits antigrowth signals, helping assembly of epithelial cells in sheets and maintaining quiescence; loss of E-cadherin leads to carcinomas. N-cadherin is normally expressed in migrating neurons and mesenchymal cells during organogenesis, but is frequently up-regulated in invasive carcinomas.

N-CAM (an Ig-CAM) also suppresses metastasis, but in Wilms tumour, neuroblastoma and small cell lung cancer it is modified to a poorly adhesive or repulsive isoform. Its expression is reduced in invasive pancreatic and colorectal cancer.

Migrating cancer cells also characteristically switch off integrin expression, while carcinoma cells facilitate invasion by shifting integrin expression from types that adhere to ECM to those that bond with protease-degraded components of the stroma.

Colonization requires adaptation to new microenvironments and micrometastases sometimes remain dormant for decades, perhaps unable to initiate angiogenesis. In some cases, when removed from the original EMT-inducing signals they revert to a non-invasive state.

7 Reprogramming of cellular energy metabolism

Under aerobic conditions normal cells process glucose to pyruvate through **glycolysis** and thereafter to CO_2 in the oxygen-consuming mitochondria. Under anaerobic conditions glycolysis is normally favoured and relatively little pyruvate is dispatched to the mitochondria. However, even in well-oxygenated cancer cells glucose metabolism is restricted largely to glycolysis. This involves an 18-fold reduction in ATP production, but this is compensated by up-regulation of glucose transporters (notably GLUT1) and multiple enzymes of the glycolytic pathway.

Some tumours also contain subpopulations of cells that metabolize lactate by the citric acid cycle, as in muscle.

8 Evasion of immune destruction

Our immune system eliminates possibly 100 000 potential cancer cells every day, but 'successful' cancer cells have found ways to evade immune surveillance and destruction. They flourish best in immunocompromised hosts, including HIV and pharmacologically suppressed patients deficient in T and B cells (see Chapter 64).

Cancer cells paralyse infiltrating immune cells by secreting TGF-β and other immunosuppressive factors and recruit immunosuppressive regulatory T cells and myeloid suppressor cells, both of which can suppress cytotoxic lymphocytes.

Cancer stem cells

It is believed that some, if not all, cancers include stem cells (CSCs), which despite having become tumorigenic, retain the capacity to differentiate into all the cell types of that tumour, causing relapse and post-therapeutic metastasis.

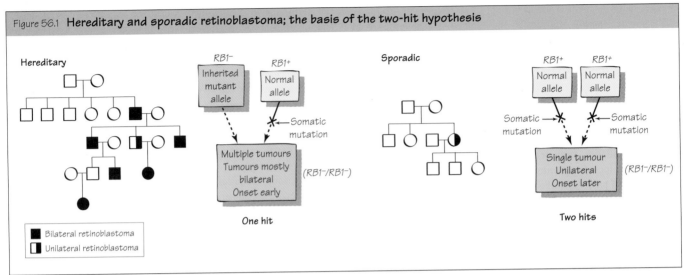

Figure 56.1 **Hereditary and sporadic retinoblastoma; the basis of the two-hit hypothesis**

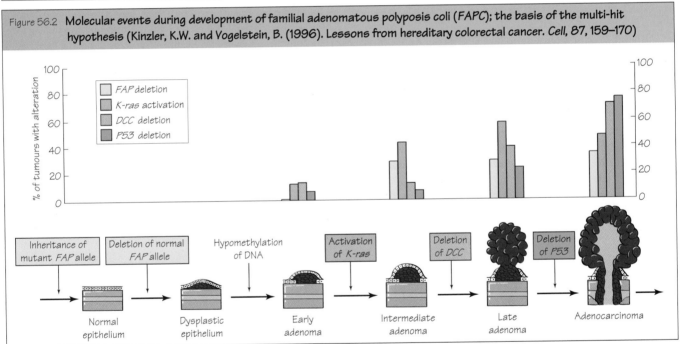

Figure 56.2 **Molecular events during development of familial adenomatous polyposis coli (FAPC); the basis of the multi-hit hypothesis (Kinzler, K.W. and Vogelstein, B. (1996). Lessons from hereditary colorectal cancer. Cell, 87, 159–170)**

Overview

Oncogenesis, that is cancer development, is a multistage process during which a cell accumulates damage in several critical genes related to mitosis and/or cell differentiation (see Chapters 17 and 55). **Oncogenes** are mutated derivatives of proto-oncogene participants in the signal transduction cascade (Chapter 54). Dominant inheritance patterns are often ascribed to defective 'tumour suppressor' genes and some of these code for mitosis suppressor proteins (see Chapters 17 and 54). Knudson's **Two-hit Hypothesis** was an early explanation correlating familial and sporadic incidences of similar cancers.

A more recent concept is the **Gatekeeper Hypothesis** (Kinzler and Vogelstein, 1996), in which one particular gene plays a pivotal role in maintaining a constant cell number in a given tissue type. Examples are *RB1* for retinal progenitor cells and *NF2* for Schwann cells.

Indicators of inherited cancer

Familial disease clusters can be caused by shared environments; the following are pointers to *genetic* causation of cancer.

• several close relatives with the same or genetically associated cancers;
• two family members with the same rare cancer;
• unusually early age of onset;
• bilateral tumours in paired organs;
• non-clonal tumours that are multifocal, or in different organ systems of the same individual.

The two-hit hypothesis

Familial retinoblastoma is inherited as an AD, with 90% penetrance, and a frequency of 1/18000. It can be: (a) sporadic, unilateral, with

Medical Genetics at a Glance, Third Edition. Dorian J. Pritchard and Bruce R. Korf.

average age of onset 30 months; or (b) familial, bilateral, with average age of onset 14 months and accompanied by other cancers.

The product of the normal allele for retinoblastoma blocks mitosis of retinal cells at the G1 checkpoint (see Chapter 17). Knudson's **two-hit hypothesis** proposed that cancer develops only if *both RB* alleles are inactive; in familial cases one *RB* lesion is inherited and only one further mutation of the *RB* gene *in any retinal cell* is therefore necessary. Hence a tumour arises much earlier within affected families than in normal homozygotes and may develop independently at multiple sites.

Li–Fraumeni syndrome (AD) is also caused by a defect at the G1 checkpoint, in the gene for protein P53 (see Figure 54.2 and Chapter 17). Patients have a wide range of tumours.

The multi-hit hypothesis
Cancer of the colon
Familial adenomatous polyposis coli (FAP, FAPC; AD) has a frequency of 1/10 000. There are multiple benign polyps of the colon, with 90% risk of malignancy by the 5th decade and **retinal hypertrophy** in 80% of families. The *APC* gene product is concerned with cell adhesion and cytoskeletal organization. Inheritance of a single mutant allele is associated with multiple benign polyps (**adenomas**) of the colon lining and progression toward an **adenocarcinoma** begins with deletion of the normal allele. Subsequent steps involve abnormal activation of the *K-ras* GTPase and deletion of *P53*. The **deleted in colorectal carcinoma** (*DCC*) gene is involved in axon guidance and apoptosis. Its deletion initiates cell surface changes and further mutation leads to metastasis. The specific mutations described are characteristic but can occur in any order.

Recessive DNA repair defects
See Chapter 26 also.

Damage detection errors
Ataxia telangiectasia AR; frequency: 1/50 000. There is hypersensitivity to X-rays, rearrangement of Chromosomes 7 and 14, cerebellar degeneration and enlargement of capillaries (**telangiectasis**) in the conjunctivae and facial skin. A 35% risk of lymphoreticular malignancy leads to early death in 30% of cases.
Fanconi anaemia AR; 1/350 000. There is undue sensitivity to DNA cross-linking agents, with chromosome breakage, and a 5–10% risk of leukaemia and carcinomas.

Nucleotide excision repair defects
Xeroderma pigmentosum (XP) AR, at least seven types; 1/250 000. Errors in pyrimidine dimer excision lead to multiple skin cancers, with corneal scarring and early death.

Postreplication repair errors
Bloom syndrome AR; there is a 10-fold increased rate of sister chromatid exchange typically associated with short stature and increased risk of leukaemia, lymphoma and carcinoma. The defective gene is a **DNA helicase**.

Dominant DNA repair defects
Damage detection errors
Basal cell naevus (Gorlin) syndrome AD; 1/57 000. There are skin naevi from puberty and a predisposition to basal cell carcinoma in sun-exposed skin, medulloblastoma and ovarian fibromas, etc. Patients are unduly sensitive to UV and X-radiation.

DNA mismatch repair
Hereditary non-polyposis colon cancer (HNPCC) AD; **HNPCC** accounts for 2–5% of cases of inherited colorectal cancer, germline mutations being associated with an 85% risk. Affected women also have a 40–60% risk of endometrial cancer. At least five genes encode proteins that are involved in the detection of single-base mismatch loops within DNA. Defects in any of these result in HNPCC.

Postreplication repair
Familial breast cancer, BRCA1, BRCA2 AD; ~1/200. One in eight British women develop breast and/or ovarian cancer, about 5% of these having inherited susceptibility. *BRCA1* and *2* account for well over half of these. The age-related penetrance for ovarian cancer is 40–65% for *BRCA1*, 10–37% for *BRCA2*. Quoted values for penetrance of breast cancer are confused by its reduction following bilateral **oophorectomy** (removal of the ovaries), but are up to 80% for *BRCA1* and 88% for *BRCA2* by age 80.
Prostate cancer Possibly AD. This is the second most common cancer in white males (after skin cancer), with a lifetime risk of 10% and a median onset age of 72 years. Five to 10% of cases are probably inherited. Men carrying *BRCA1* have a 7% risk and those carrying *BRCA2* a 16% risk by age 70 years (c.f. 4% of the general population). There are several additional susceptibility loci.

Oncogenes
Growth factor reception
Multiple endocrine neoplasia, Type 2 (MEN 2) There are three subtypes: **MEN2A** (representing 90%), **MEN2B** and **familial medullary thyroid carcinoma** (MTC). All three carry a high risk of thyroid cancer and are associated with gain-of-function mutations, typically involving constitutive activation of the *c-ret* proto-oncogene (*ret* = *re*arranged during *t*ransfection).

Signal transduction
Chronic myeloid (or myelogenous) leukaemia (CML) Translocation of *c-abl* (a postreceptor tyrosine kinase), normally on 9q, to a position beside the '**breakpoint cluster region**' (*BCR*) on 22q initiates synthesis of a chimaeric '**fusion protein**' with increased tyrosine kinase activity. Reciprocal exchange of the 22q telomere leaves a characteristic modified version of 22, the '**Philadelphia chromosome**', in the affected cell line (see Chapters 39 and 57).
Neurofibromatosis Type 1 (NF1; von Recklinghausen disease) AD; 1/3000; 50% are new mutations. Loss of the NF1 normal protein allows accumulation of **ras-GTP** (a membrane-bound GTPase) with increased cell turnover. There are numerous prominent benign neurofibromas and malignant tumours of the CNS.
Neurofibromatosis Type 2 (NF2) AD; 1/35 000. There are bilateral Schwann cell tumours (**schwannomas**) of vestibular, cranial and spinal nerves and intracranial and spinal meningiomas. The normal gene product is the cytoskeletal merlin which is a cytoskeletal protein.

Transcription factors
Burkitt lymphoma This is a B-lymphocyte tumour of the jaw, the most common childhood cancer of equatorial Africa. The DNA-binding proto-oncogene *c-myc* at 8q24 becomes activated by translocation adjacent to an immunoglobulin enhancer at 14q32, 2p11 or 22q11 (see Chapter 39).

Dominant transcriptional control defects
Von Hippel–Lindau syndrome AD; 1/36 000. There are **haemangioblastomas** of the retina and cerebellum, early onset renal carcinomas and **phaeochromocytomas** (tumours of sympathetic nervous tissue).
Wilms tumour (nephroblastoma) AD; 1/10 000. This is a highly malignant kidney tumour; 1% of cases are familial. It forms part of the **contiguous gene syndrome WAGR** (**W**ilms tumour, **A**niridia, **G**enitourinary anomalies and mental **R**etardation) caused by a major deletion (see Chapter 40).

57 Genomic approaches to cancer management

Figure 57.1 **Use of 'array comparative/competitive hybridization' for categorization of tumours with respect to gene expression and potential response to treatment**

The figure depicts clustering of tumours showing high or low levels of expression of groups of genes to form a 'heat map'. There is a subset with a pattern of high expression of some genes and low expression of others that respond well to treatment and another subset with the opposite pattern that exhibits a poor response.

- ■ – Increased expression in tumour
- ■ – Decreased expression in tumour

Expression data displayed as 'heat map'
Each column is a different tumour

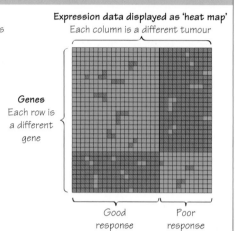

Genes
Each row is a different gene

Good response   Poor response

Figure 57.3 **FISH analysis of HER2 amplification**

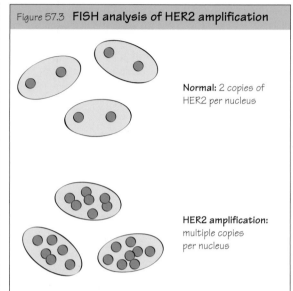

Normal: 2 copies of HER2 per nucleus

HER2 amplification: multiple copies per nucleus

Figure 57.2 **The Philadelphia chromosome, Ph1**

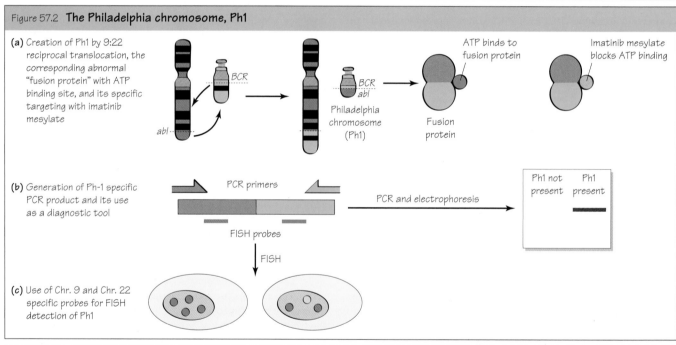

(a) Creation of Ph1 by 9:22 reciprocal translocation, the corresponding abnormal "fusion protein" with ATP binding site, and its specific targeting with imatinib mesylate

BCR

abl

Philadelphia chromosome (Ph1)

BCR / abl

Fusion protein

ATP binds to fusion protein

Imatinib mesylate blocks ATP binding

(b) Generation of Ph-1 specific PCR product and its use as a diagnostic tool

PCR primers

FISH probes

FISH

PCR and electrophoresis

Ph1 not present   Ph1 present

(c) Use of Chr. 9 and Chr. 22 specific probes for FISH detection of Ph1

Figure 57.4 **Targeting of the V600E mutation in the BRAF oncogene by the specific BRAF inhibitor, vemurafenib**

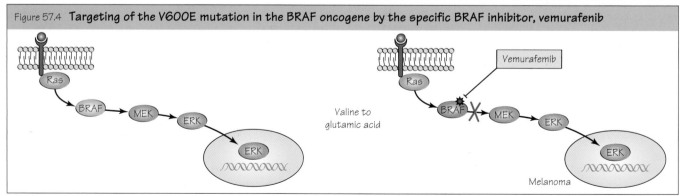

Ras

BRAF

MEK

ERK

ERK

Vemurafemib

Ras

BRAF

MEK

ERK

ERK

Valine to glutamic acid

Melanoma

Medical Genetics at a Glance, Third Edition. Dorian J. Pritchard and Bruce R. Korf.

Overview

Genomics is the study of all the nuclear DNA, together with its mRNA (**transcriptome**) and protein (**proteome**) products. Genomic analysis typically begins with a comprehensive data set that is sequentially refined toward a much smaller set of significant features.

Initiation and progression of cancer involves acquisition of multiple genetic changes that convey selective advantages on cells and leads to progressive loss of growth control, combined with the ability to grow at distant sites (see Chapter 55). There is a long history of study of tumours at the genetic level and well-established genetic tests used routinely in the diagnosis of cancer. Genomic approaches are now being used to catalogue these changes comprehensively. It is hoped that genomically guided therapeutics will allow for more precise targeting of drugs, with improved outcomes and reduction of side effects.

Analysis of tumour gene expression

Genomic technologies can be used to assess overall patterns of gene expression in tumour tissues, by means of competitive hybridization to DNA microarrays (Chapter 67) or by sequencing of cDNA (RNA-seq, see Chapter 68). Both approaches begin with isolation of RNA from the tumour and synthesis of cDNA copies using the enzyme **reverse transcriptase**.

A typical microarray-based approach would involve hybridization of cDNA from tumour tissue labelled red, in competition with cDNA from a normal standard labelled green, to a microarray of oligonucleotides corresponding to thousands of human genes bound onto a solid substrate (Chapter 67). RNA-seq involves **next-generation sequencing** (see Chapter 68) of cDNAs made from the entire population of mRNAs in the tumour and analysis of the sequences detected.

In either case the result is a profile of genes that are expressed at higher or lower levels in tumours, as compared to normal tissues. In some cases these expression patterns correlate with sensitivity of the tumours to treatment, permitting them to be grouped according to responsiveness (Figure 57.1). Gene expression profiling has been a valuable research tool in categorizing cancers and predicting responsiveness, though it is unclear whether this approach yet provides a practical basis for clinical management of individual patients.

Analysis of cancer genomes

Rapid sequencing of entire genomes (Chapter 68) offers the possibility of characterizing those specifically of cancer cells. The goal is to provide an inventory of the various kinds of mutation that accumulate in cancer cells and contribute to their abnormal behaviour. This is done by extracting the DNA of both cancerous tissues and normal (usually blood), from a group of patients with a particular type of cancer and sequencing both samples from each patient. Any individual genome will have millions of genetic variants, as compared to a standard reference human genome, but the majority of these will be the same in a tumour and the normal DNA from the same individual. Any differences between the latter indicate genetic abnormalities in the tumour, and may play a role in contributing to the tumour phenotype. It is hoped that this approach will lead to discovery of new genetic markers that will eventually shed light on tumourigenesis, as well as identify new diagnostic and prognostic tools, and new drug targets.

Genetic testing in cancer diagnosis

Chromosomal studies of cancer cells typically reveal multiple abnormalities in chromosome number and structure. Structural changes include deletions, duplications, translocations and gene amplification; all of which may alter patterns of gene expression, including activation of oncogenes and inactivation of tumour suppressors (see Chapters 17, 54 and 55).

Some chromosomal rearrangements are highly characteristic of particular malignancies. The first discovered and best known example is the Philadelphia chromosome, resulting from reciprocal translocation between Chromosomes 9 and 22, causing fusion of the *ABL* oncogene on Chromosome 9 with the *BCR* gene on 22, and leading to production of an abnormal 'fusion protein' (Chapter 39; Figure 57.2). Presence of the Philadelphia chromosome is highly characteristic of leukaemia, especially chronic myeloid leukaemia (CML), and can be a valuable aid in diagnosis. Finding cells with the Philadelphia chromosome following treatment of CML is an indication of relapse.

Performing cytogenetic studies is especially difficult for solid tumours and can be time consuming and expensive. It also has low sensitivity, since it is difficult to examine a sufficiently large number of cells to detect a very small number of tumour cells following treatment. Molecular testing offers a simpler, less expensive and more sensitive solution. This can include use of FISH probes to detect gene amplification events or translocations (see Chapter 35; Figures 57.2 and 57.3), as well as PCR-based systems (Chapter 69) to detect translocations. The high sensitivity of these molecular techniques following treatment allows detection of small populations of tumour cells, predicting relapse, long before any clinical indication.

Genetic testing and treatment of cancer

Tumours that look the same microscopically may be very different in their growth patterns and response to treatment. In some cases, genetic tests are helpful in predicting their probable response, allowing therapeutic agents to be targeted more precisely toward the tumours most likely to be controllable. Some such differences are attributable to certain genetic changes themselves, so that discovery of a tumour-specific genetic change can suggest new treatments.

The Philadelphia chromosome again provides an illuminating example. The fusion protein of BCR and ABL functions as a kinase (a phosphate-attaching enzyme), albeit one expressed at higher levels than normal. The kinase inhibitor **imatinib mesylate** was developed to inhibit this function by occupying the ATP attachment site and now has a significant role in the treatment of CML as well as other tumours driven by genetic changes that activate specific kinases (Figure 57.2).

HER2 is a growth factor receptor tyrosine kinase coded by the *erb-B2* oncogene (Chapter 54). Amplification of *erb-B2*, and hence of HER2, in breast cancers predicts response to the drug **trastuzumab**, an antibody designed to inhibit HER2. Its amplification is readily detectable in breast cancer specimens by FISH or other molecular approaches, so identifying potentially responsive patients. Detection by FISH is feasible because amplified copies of *erb-B2* exist as separate double-minute chromatin bodies (see Figure 57.3).

Melanomas found to have a mutation in the *BRAF* oncogene that substitutes a glutamic acid for valine at codon 600 (mutation designated V600E) are more prone than those with the wild type sequence to respond to specific BRAF inhibitors such as **vemurafenib**, which are directed at the modified protein component (Figure 57.4). Genetic testing of tumour specimens is now commonly carried out prior to initiation of therapy with these drugs.

These examples are all now part of routine care of patients with these tumours and it is highly likely additional examples will be developed in the coming years.

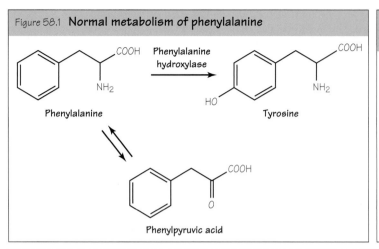

Figure 58.1 Normal metabolism of phenylalanine

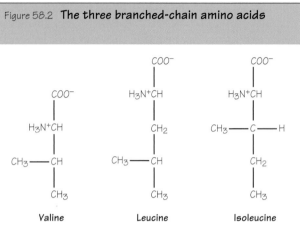

Figure 58.2 The three branched-chain amino acids

Valine Leucine Isoleucine

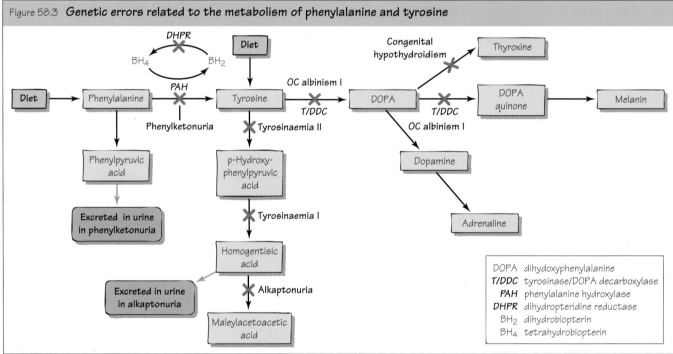

Figure 58.3 Genetic errors related to the metabolism of phenylalanine and tyrosine

DOPA dihydoxyphenylalanine
T/DDC tyrosinase/DOPA decarboxylase
PAH phenylalanine hydroxylase
DHPR dihydropteridine reductase
BH₂ dihydrobiopterin
BH₄ tetrahydrobiopterin

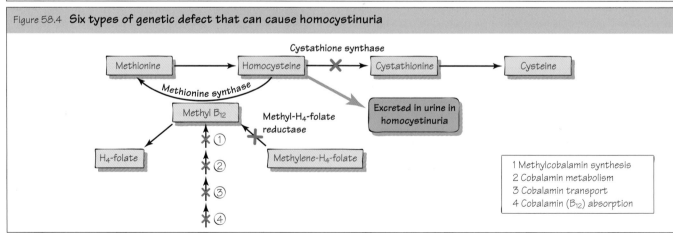

Figure 58.4 Six types of genetic defect that can cause homocystinuria

1 Methylcobalamin synthesis
2 Cobalamin metabolism
3 Cobalamin transport
4 Cobalamin (B₁₂) absorption

Table 58.1 Inherited disorders of amino acid metabolism.

Disorder	Prevalence	Inheritance	Defective biomolecule
Phenylketonuria	1/10 000	AR	Phenylalanine hydroxylase
Tyrosinaemia Type 1	1/100 000	AR	Fumarylacetoacetate hydrolase
Tyrosinaemia Type 2		AR	Tyrosine aminotransferase
Oculocutaneous albinism	1/35 000	AR	Tyrosinase; P protein
Maple syrup urine disease	1/180 000	AR	Branched-chain α-ketoacid decarboxylase
Cystinuria	1/7000	AR	SLC3A1 / SLC7A9
Homocystinuria	1/340 000	AR	Cystathione β-synthetase
Alkaptonuria	1/250 000	AR	Homogentisic acid oxidase

Inborn errors of metabolism

Gregor Mendel published his paper on experiments in plant hybridization (Chapter 3) in 1866, but his deductions were ignored until their rediscovery in 1900. However, only 9 years later Archibald Garrod published *Inborn Errors in Metabolism*, proposing a relationship between human inheritance and metabolic disease and thereby laying the foundations of human biochemical genetics.

Garrod's first interest was in **alkaptonuria**, a familial disorder involving black urine and arthritis. He proposed that such patients lack activity of a specific enzyme necessary to carry out a specific biochemical reaction. Noting that 60% of affected individuals were the offspring of unaffected first cousins, he proposed the defect would be inherited as a recessive. The black pigment turned out to be oxidized **homogentisic acid**, a derivative of tyrosine; its breakdown is affected in these patients and the condition is indeed inherited as a recessive.

Of the 20 amino acids required as constituents of human proteins, 11 can be synthesized in the body, but the remaining nine are **essential** dietary constituents. These are: **histidine, isoleucine, leucine, lysine, methionine, phenylalanine, threonine, tryptophan** and **valine**.

Some enzymes acquire biological activity only after association with cofactors and in some cases (e.g. **homocystinuria**) administration of cofactor can boost their reduced activity. Defects in this category are among the most responsive to biochemical therapy.

▶ Problems requiring immediate attention

As a general rule, if any of the disorders described in this chapter are suspected, the recommendation is diagnostic testing and a management plan.

Enzyme deficiencies and disease
Generality of recessive status

Most of our 200 or so currently recognized inborn errors of metabolism are inherited as recessives, because most enzymes are produced in considerable excess and the 50% deficiency in a mutant heterozygote goes unnoticed. However, if the reaction is a rate-limiting step, or the product of the defective gene is part of a multimeric complex, the disorder can manifest in the heterozygous state and be classed as dominant. Some of the enzymes involved in porphyrin synthesis are examples of this principle (see Chapter 61).

Product efficiency and substrate accumulation

The pathological consequences of an enzymopathy generally arise from accumulation of the substrate or its derivatives, as in phenylke-

tonuria (PKU; see below), or to deficiency of a product, as in albinism, or some combination of the two.

Effect of molecular size

Enzyme defects in which the substrate is a readily diffusible, small molecule, can affect parts of the body distant from the site of action of the enzyme. Amino acid metabolic defects are typically revealed in the urine. When the substrate or product is a non-diffusible macromolecule such as a mucopolysaccharide, pathological changes are generally restricted to the site of action of the enzyme (Chapter 62).

Pleiotropic effects

A single-gene defect can have multiple phenotypic outcomes (known as **pleiotropy**) when the substrate and/or product of the enzyme for which that gene codes contributes to multiple functions. A single-gene defect may also cause malfunction of more than one pathway if several enzymes require the same cofactor, or share a common subunit, or the same activating, processing or stabilizing protein (e.g. the **GM2 gangliosidoses**; Chapter 62).

In some cases organelle uptake of different enzymes involves a common mechanism. In **I-cell disease**, the failure to add mannose 6-phosphate to several enzymes blocks lysosomal uptake of them all.

Phenotypic homology

The pathological features due to a defect in one enzyme may be shown by other diseases if they function in the same area of metabolism, as with the **mucopolysaccharidoses** (Chapter 62). Partial enzyme deficiencies can also be confusing when their consequences represent subsets of full clinical phenotypes. For example, partial deficiency of hypoxanthine guanine phosphoribosyl transferase (HGPRT) causes only hyperuricaemia, as found in several conditions, whereas complete deficiency causes full-blown Lesch–Nyhan disease (see Chapter 61).

Errors in amino acid metabolism
Alkaptonuria

Alkaptonuria is caused by a failure in conversion of homogentisic acid (HA), a derivative of tyrosine, to maleylacetoacetic acid (Figure 58.3) due to deficiency in **homogentisic acid oxidase**. HA is excreted in the urine, to which it gives a dark colour on exposure to air. Dark pigment is deposited in the earwax, cartilage, including the pinna, and joints (**ochronosis**), causing arthritis. It is usually detected by black staining of babies' nappies (diapers).

Oculocutaneous albinism

See Chapters 6 and 30.

There are multiple forms of albinism. **Oculocutaneous albinism Type I (OCA1)** affecting both the skin and eyes is caused by a defect in '**tyrosinase**', or **dihydroxyphenylalanine oxidase (DOPA oxidase**; Figure 58.3). This enzyme controls the two-step conversion of tyrosine into **DOPA quinone**, a precursor of melanin. However, the most common form of OCA is **OCA2**, caused by faulty **P protein**, a component of the external membrane of the **melanosomes**, the defect preventing melanin accumulation.

Phenylketonuria

See Chapters 8 and 63.

Phenylketonuria (PKU) is caused by a block in conversion of phenylalanine to tyrosine (Figures 58.1 and 58.3), in most cases due to homozygosity, or **compound heterozygosity**, among the 450 defective versions of the gene coding for **phenylalanine hydroxylase (PAH)**. Rarely (1–3%), it may instead be due to deficiency in **dihydropteridine reductase (DHPR**; Figure 58.3), which is responsible for recycling the PAH cofactor, tetrahydrobiopterin (**BH$_4$**). Either way, phenylalanine and its derivatives, mainly phenylpyruvic acid, build up to toxic levels, with irreversible damage to the CNS, possibly by inhibition of pyruvate carboxylase causing defects in myelin production.

The deficiency of tyrosine in PKU also depresses production of downstream products, including **melanin**, resulting in hypopigmentation, and DOPA, possibly contributing to hormonal dysfunction.

Phenylacetic acid in patients' urine gives it the smell of mice.

Tyrosinaemia

Hereditary **tyrosinaemia Type 1** is relatively common (1/700) in French-Canadians in the Saguenay-Lac Saint Jean region of Quebec (rare elsewhere), caused by a splice donor site mutation in intron 12 of **fumarylacetoacetate hydrolase**. It is detectable in infants, whose urine has the odour of cabbages, due to their excretion of **succinylacetone**, a mitochondrial toxin. Accumulation of substrates causes neurological, kidney and liver dysfunction. **Tyrosinaemia Type 2** is characterized by herpetiform corneal ulcers, thickening of the palms and soles and mental retardation (Figure 58.3).

Maple syrup urine disease

The essential **branched chain amino acids (BCAAs) valine**, **leucine** and **isoleucine** (Figure 58.2) share a part of their metabolic pathways.

Deficiencies in the common enzyme **branched chain α-ketoacid dehydrogenase** results in maple syrup urine disease, which owes its name to the odour of α-ketoacids derived from these BCAAs. Accumulation of the BCAAs and their ketoacids in the blood is neurotoxic, causing severe neurological symptoms, cerebral oedema and mental retardation. Newborns present with vomiting and abnormal muscle tone, proceeding to death within a few weeks.

Management Treatment involves dietary restriction of the BCAAs.

Cystinuria

Cystinurea is very common (1/7000) and involves failure of renal tubule reabsorption of **c**ystine, **o**rnithine, **a**rginine and **l**ysine (**COAL**) causing **cystine urolithiasis**, or **renal calculi** (kidney stones) due to the low solubility of cystine. There is sometimes also infection, hypertension and renal failure.

Management Consumption of large volumes of water, alkalinization of the urine and use of cystine chelating agents such as penicillamine.

Homocystinuria

The sulphur-containing amino acid, cysteine can be synthesized in the body from methionine, via intermediates **homocysteine (HC)** and **cystathione** (Figure 58.4). The latter conversion is performed by **cystathione synthase** (or **cystathione β-synthetase**), deficiency of which is the main cause of homocystinuria, with prior elevation of serum homocysteine.

Methionine synthase re-methylates HC to methionine, so loss of this enzyme also causes build up of HC. Methionine synthase requires a methyl derivative of vitamin B$_{12}$ (**methylcobalamin**) as cofactor. Several defects in the uptake, transport and processing of B$_{12}$ are also pathogenic (see Figure 58.4).

Homocystinuria is associated with seizures, thromboembolic episodes and osteoporosis. The further combination of scoliosis, pectus excavatum, arachnodactyly and lens dislocation can cause confusion with Marfan syndrome (AD; see Chapter 5), though mental retardation in homocystinuria provides a distinction.

Management Cystathione synthase requires **pyridoxal phosphate** as a cofactor and administration of pyridoxine can often ameliorate the condition Most are partially or completely treatable with high doses of vitamin B$_{12}$. A vegan diet can create phenocopies of homocystinuria due to dietary deficiency of vitamin B$_{12}$.

Figure 59.1 Digestion of lactose

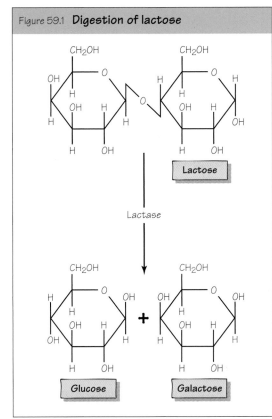

Figure 59.3 Digestion of sucrose

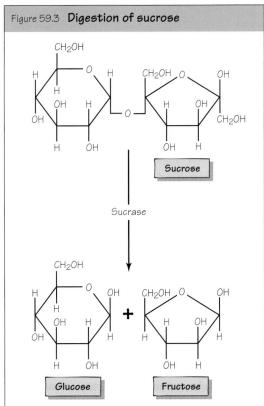

Figure 59.2 Metabolism of lactose and galactose

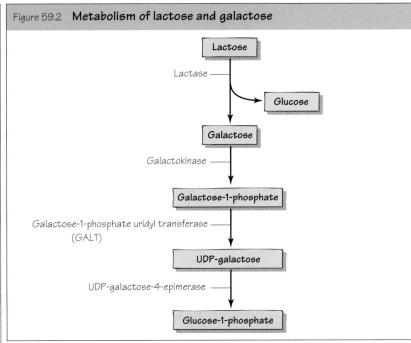

Figure 59.4 Glycation of protein

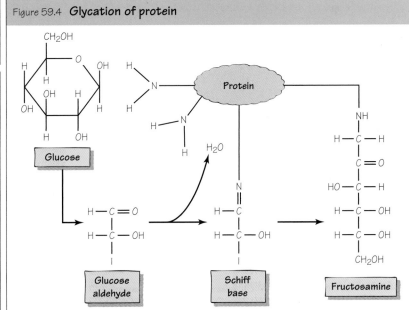

Table 59.1 GALT genotypes in relation to enzyme levels and phenotype

Genotype	Enzyme activity (%)	Phenotype
G^+/G^+	100	Normal
G^+/G^D	75	Normal
G^D/G^D	50	Normal
G^+/g	50	Normal
G^D/g	25	Borderline
g/g	0	Galactosaemia

Medical Genetics at a Glance, Third Edition. Dorian J. Pritchard and Bruce R. Korf.
© 2013 John Wiley & Sons, Ltd. Published 2013 by John Wiley & Sons, Ltd.

Table 59.2 Main inherited defects of carbohydrate metabolism.

Name	Prevalence	Inheritance	Age of onset	No. of genes	Defective molecule	Pathophysiology
Classical galactosaemia	1/35 000–1/60 000	AR	<2 days	3	GALT	Enzyme deficiency
Hereditary fructose intolerance	1/20 000	AR	<6 months	1	Aldolase B	Enzyme deficiency
Diabetes mellitus, Type 1	1/400 (Caucasians)	Polygenic	Childhood/ adolescence	>40	Unknown	Autoimmunity
Diabetes mellitus, Type 2	1/10	Polygenic	Middle/old age	~30	Various	Insulin resistance
MODY	1/400	AD	Adolescence/early adulthood	>8	Various	β-cell dysfunction
Neonatal diabetes	1/100 000	Imprinting	<6 months	>14	ZFP57	β-cell dysfunction
Lactose intolerance	1/10 (Caucasians), 9/10 in others	AD	<2 days	1	Lactase	Enzyme deficiency

Overview

Carbohydrates account for the major part of the human diet. All are eventually broken down by glycolysis, following conversion to the monosaccharides, glucose, galactose and fructose, or stored as glycogen. The failure to utilize these three sugars effectively accounts for most defects of carbohydrate metabolism. The glycogen storage disorders are all rare and are detailed in Chapter 62.

Some 20 mitochondrial (Chapter 12) and several AR nuclear (Chapters 6–8) disorders of oxidative phosphorylation are known. All are rare and their management is generally aimed at promoting alternative pathways of energy generation.

Lactose intolerance

Lactose is a disaccharide comprised of one molecule of glucose and one of galactose. It constitutes 7% of human milk and is the principal energy source for infants. In babies it is metabolized largely by the intestinal brush-border enzyme **lactase** (or **lactose-phlorizin hydrolase**), which splits it into its monosaccharide components (Figure 59.1).

In North European and African populations with traditional consumption of animal milk, lactase activity persists in most adults. Adult lactose utilization is inherited as an AD trait and provides a selective advantage in the derivation of nutrition from milk. **Primary lactase deficiency** (AR) occurs in 15% of European adults, causing **lactose intolerance**, but is common (50–100%) in adults of most tropical and subtropical populations. Dietary lactose accumulation causes flatulence, bloating, cramps, diarrhoea and nausea, as undigested lactose is metabolized by bacteria in the colon. Milk products can however be consumed by lactase-deficient individuals after processing, for example by *Lactobacillus* fermentation.

Galactosaemia

Features Galactosaemia is one of the most common monogenic disorders of carbohydrate metabolism, caused by deficiency in any of three enzymes involved in the elaboration of galactose (see Figure 59.2).

Newborn infants present with vomiting, lethargy, failure to thrive, sepsis and jaundice. It can progress to fatality within a few months. Hepatic insufficiency, developmental delay, poor growth, mental retardation, lens cataract and ovarian failure may later become apparent.

Genetics There are three alleles of *GALT*: *G+*, *g* and *G_D* (the Duarte allele), G_D/G_D homozygotes have 50% of normal levels of the enzyme (see Table 59.2).

Aetiology The main initial source of galactose is lactose in milk. Galactose is converted into galactose-1-phosphate by **galactokinase**, to UDP-galactose by **GALT** and to glucose-1-phosphate by **UDP-galactose-4-epimerase**. Defects in GALT are responsible for the most common form.

Management Newborn screening is by enzyme direct assay on a drop of dried blood, by a modified bacterial inhibition (Guthrie) test.

▶ Problems requiring immediate attention

A lactose- and galactose-free diet is required within the first 2 days after birth, although this does not necessarily prevent later problems with balance, impaired motor skills, liver cirrhosis and ovarian failure.

Fructose intolerance

Symptoms of **hereditary fructose intolerance** (**HFI**) usually become apparent within 20 minutes of first feeding on food containing fructose, with violent vomiting and hypoglycaemia, followed by jaundice, lethal hepatic and renal insufficiency and convulsions. Diagnosis is confirmed by demonstration of fructosuria and enzyme assay on intestinal mucosa or liver biopsy specimens. Lactic acid accumulates, causing metabolic acidosis with compensatory hyperventilation.

Aetiology there is a basic deficiency in **fructose-1-phosphate aldolase** (or **aldolase B**). Dietary fructose is present in honey, fruit and some vegetables and as a component of sucrose (white sugar) and sorbitol (see Figure 59.3). Accumulation of fructose-1-phosphate in the liver blocks glucose metabolism and depletes inorganic phosphate stores, inhibiting both glycogen phosphorylase and ATP synthesis. Outcomes include lactic acidosis and hyperuricaemia.

Management Dietary exclusion of fructose provides good prognosis, but if left untreated, failure to thrive progresses to **cachexia** (serious debility) and continuing liver damage to cirrhosis.

Diabetes mellitus

There are many errors of glucose metabolism, notably several forms of **diabetes mellitus** (**DM**; see Chapters 46, 51, 52 and 66. The term 'diabetes' relates to excessive production of urine, 'mellitus' to its sweet taste (c.f. in **diabetes insipidus**). There are >20 monogenic forms and it is also a feature of several syndromes (Prader–Willi, Bardet–Biedl and Friedreich ataxia, etc.). It is characterized by **hyperglycaemia** due to defective insulin secretion and/or defects in its action. The global prevalence of DM is >200 million cases.

Hypertonic effects of hyperglycaemia include dehydration and excessive urination. High concentrations of glucose in the pancreatic β-cells cause enhanced oxidative phosphorylation, oxidative stress and further loss of β-cell function, thereby creating a vicious cycle exacerbating the initial defect.

Prolonged exposure of body proteins to high concentrations of glucose also results in damage called **glycation** (Figure 59.4). This involves formation of Schiff bases between glucose aldehyde and the N-terminal α-amino groups of proteins and the ε-amino groups of their lysines. The result is **fructosamine** attachments to protein molecules and crosslinks between them. Glycation is responsible for vascular stiffening, hypertension, neuropathy and retinopathy in diabetes. The degree of glycation can be monitored by examination of serum albumin and glycated A1C haemoglobin.

Type 1 or insulin-dependent diabetes mellitus (T1DM; IDDM)

Overview The basic function of insulin is to maintain low blood glucose levels, by promoting conversion of excess free glucose into glycogen. **T1DM** involves a deficiency of insulin.

Features See Chapter 51.

Aetiology T1DM is usually of sudden onset during adolescence, with weight loss, as insulin secretion ceases. The β-cells of the pancreatic islets are destroyed by autoimmune attack following viral infection, probably due to 'molecular mimicry' of viral antigens (Chapter 65). Known exacerbating factors include diet, viral exposure in early childhood and certain drugs.

Genetics (see also Chapter 51) PCR analysis (Chapter 69) has shown that the HLA allele contribution to susceptibility (Chapter 66) is determined by the 57th amino acid at the *DQ* locus where aspartic acid confers protection whereas others enhance susceptibility. Susceptibility is also influenced by the number of tandem repeats of a 14-bp sequence upstream of the insulin gene at 11p15. Many repeats of *INS VNTR* confer protection. More than 40 additional susceptibility loci are suggested.

Type 2 or non-insulin-dependent diabetes mellitus (T2DM; NIDDM)

T2DM currently occurs in up to 10% of many populations, but its prevalence is increasing and has been predicted to reach 300 million worldwide by the year 2025. It is often associated with obesity and presents with slow, insidious onset until diagnosis in middle age. Patients are prone to macrovascular and microvascular complications, increased morbidity and mortality.

Genetics There are no major predisposing loci, but around 30 susceptibility loci that show overlap with those for MODY (e.g. *HNF1A* and B), but not T1DM. The risk of developing disease is virtually directly proportional to the number of inherited risk alleles (see Chapter 50).

Aetiology Insulin is present in the blood at supranormal concentrations, but does not work effectively, termed '**insulin resistance**'. There are very many different causes, for example structural abnormalities of the insulin molecule, or of the insulin receptor, the signalling proteins and the enzymes involved in glucose uptake and metabolism.

Management T2DM frequently responds to dietary restriction of carbohydrate and oral hypoglycaemic medication; some require insulin.

Maturity onset diabetes of the young (MODY)

This represents 1–2% of people with diabetes. It shows affinities with T2DM, but is characterized by early onset. It differs from T1DM in that some insulin is secreted, although insufficient to control hyperglycaemia.

Genetics AD. Six gene defects account for 87% of MODY cases in the UK: **glucokinase** (*MODY2*), **transcription factor HNF4-α** (**hepatic nuclear factor 4-α**; *MODY1*), **HNF1-α** (*MODY3*), **IPF** (**insulin promoter factor**; *MODY4*), **HNF1-β** (*MODY5*) and **NeuroD1** (**neurogenic differentiation 1**; *MODY6*).

Aetiology The rate-limiting step of glucose metabolism in the pancreatic β cells is phosphate attachment by **glucokinase**, deficiency of which causes mild hyperglycaemia. Mutations of HNF1-α account for 65% of British cases.

Management The condition generally responds to sulphonylurea.

Gestational diabetes mellitus (GDM)

In about 4% of pregnancies normal, transient 'insulin resistance' becomes severe causing hyperglycaemia and GDM. Raised levels of maternal oestrogen and placental lactogen, and low levels of **adiponectin** have been implicated as causative. Affected women usually revert to normality after pregnancy, but rather more than half later develop T1DM.

Neonatal diabetes

This is a rare complication of childbirth affecting ~1/100 000 births. It has a monogenic inheritance pattern of β-cell dysfunction. From a genetic viewpoint its main interest is that most cases arise as a rare consequence of paternal imprinting of the zinc finger transcription factor ZFP57 at 6q27 (see Chapter 22).

Glycogen storage disorders (GSDs)

Errors in the synthesis or breakdown of the glucose polymer, **glycogen**, cause **glycogen storage disorders** (**GSDs**) primarily affecting either the liver or skeletal muscle. Apart from DM, all such conditions are rare. Their management is typically aimed at maintenance of blood sugar levels.

60 Metal transport, lipid metabolism and amino acid catabolism defects

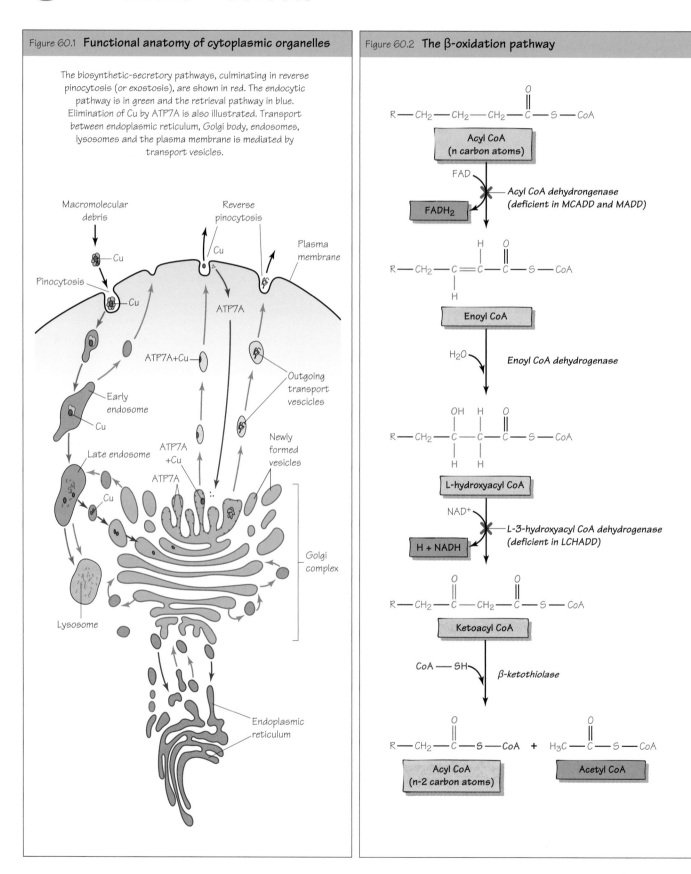

Figure 60.1 **Functional anatomy of cytoplasmic organelles**

The biosynthetic-secretory pathways, culminating in reverse pinocytosis (or exostosis), are shown in red. The endocytic pathway is in green and the retrieval pathway in blue. Elimination of Cu by ATP7A is also illustrated. Transport between endoplasmic reticulum, Golgi body, endosomes, lysosomes and the plasma membrane is mediated by transport vesicles.

Macromolecular debris
Reverse pinocytosis
Cu
Plasma membrane
Cu
Pinocytosis
Cu
ATP7A
ATP7A+Cu
Outgoing transport vescicles
Early endosome
Cu
ATP7A +Cu
Newly formed vesicles
Late endosome
ATP7A
Cu
Golgi complex
Lysosome
Endoplasmic reticulum

Figure 60.2 **The β-oxidation pathway**

$R-CH_2-CH_2-CH_2-\overset{\overset{O}{\|}}{C}-S-CoA$

Acyl CoA (n carbon atoms)

FAD — Acyl CoA dehydrongenase (deficient in MCADD and MADD)
FADH$_2$

$R-CH_2-\overset{\overset{H}{|}}{C}=\overset{\overset{H}{|}}{C}-\overset{\overset{O}{\|}}{C}-S-CoA$

Enoyl CoA

H$_2$O — Enoyl CoA dehydrogenase

$R-CH_2-\overset{\overset{OH}{|}}{\underset{H}{C}}-\overset{\overset{H}{|}}{\underset{H}{C}}-\overset{\overset{O}{\|}}{C}-S-CoA$

L-hydroxyacyl CoA

NAD$^+$ — L-3-hydroxyacyl CoA dehydrogenase (deficient in LCHADD)
H + NADH

$R-CH_2-\overset{\overset{O}{\|}}{C}-CH_2-\overset{\overset{O}{\|}}{C}-S-CoA$

Ketoacyl CoA

CoA — SH — β-ketothiolase

$R-CH_2-\overset{\overset{O}{\|}}{C}-S-CoA$ + $H_3C-\overset{\overset{O}{\|}}{C}-S-CoA$

Acyl CoA (n-2 carbon atoms)   **Acetyl CoA**

Table 60.1 Disorders of metal transport.

Disorder	Prevalence	Inheritance	Defective biomolecule
Menkes disease	1/250 000	XR	General Cu transport protein ATP7A
Wilson disease	1/50 000	AR	Liver Cu transport protein ATP7B
Acrodermatitis enteropathica	Rare	AR; 31 alleles	Zinc transporter protein
Haemochromatosis	~1/300 Caucasians; low in others	AR, 4 loci	HFE, transferring receptor 2, ferroportin

Metal transport defects

Copper: Menkes disease (MND); kinky hair disease

Copper is absorbed by intestinal epithelial cells and transported away for use largely as an enzyme cofactor. The Cu transport protein **ATP7A**, located in the Golgi body in many tissues except liver, binds the Cu ion at its aspartyl phosphate groups and carries it to the plasma membrane for release into the bloodstream, before returning to the Golgi body (see Figure 60.1).

Menkes disease (MND) is characterized by mental retardation, seizures, hypothermia, twisted and hypopigmented hair, loose skin, scurvy-like symptoms of the long bones and arterial rupture. Male infants typically die by 2–3 years, but carrier females may have only hair shaft abnormality (**pili torti**). Cultured fibroblasts of males have grossly elevated Cu content and Cu export by the gastrointestinal epithelium into the bloodstream is ineffective, leading to overall Cu deficiency. The liver is virtually unaffected (c.f. Wilson disease, see below).

Aetiology The basic fault is in ATP7A, much of the phenotype being explicable as failure of five enzymes that require Cu as a cofactor:
• **tyrosinase** failure: amelanogenesis;
• **lysyl oxidase** failure: lack of crosslink formation in elastin and collagen and slackness of connective tissue;
• **monoamine oxidase** failure: pili torti, due to deficient disulphide bonding of keratin;
• **ascorbate oxidase** failure: skeletal demineralization and scurvy;
• **cytochrome oxidase** inefficiency: poor energy metabolism and hypothermia.

Management Subcutaneous administration of copper histinate (in which form Cu can cross the blood–brain barrier).

Copper: Wilson disease

In **Wilson disease** there is cirrhosis (hardening) of the liver, with fibrous discoloration and destruction of parenchyma cells, also neurological abnormalities, such as **dysarthria** (inability to articulate words correctly), **dysphagia** (difficulty in swallowing) and diminished coordination. It commonly presents in childhood or early adolescence, with fits, deteriorating coordination, abnormal muscle tone, involuntary movements, changes in behaviour or frank psychiatric disturbance. Adults develop arthritis, cardiomyopathy, kidney damage and hypoparathyroidism.

Diagnostic signs are increased urinary copper and incorporation of Cu isotopes into cultured cells and the **Kayser–Fleischer ring** caused by deposition of copper in Descemet's membrane at the corneal margin.

Aetiology Wilson disease results from an abnormality in ATP7B, which plays a similar role in liver to ATP7A elsewhere, controlling excretion of Cu into the biliary tract.

Management Copper chelating agents such as **D-penicillamine** and **trientine**.

Zinc: Acrodermatitis enteropathica

Acrodermatitis enteropathica (**AE**) is characterized by failure to thrive, with intermittent diarrhoea and scaly dermatitis of the genitals, buttocks, limbs and face. Before weaning, maternal milk is generally protective, but thereafter AE can be rapidly fatal, patients showing growth retardation and immune dysfunction.

Aetiology AE is caused by a defect in the uptake of zinc by the intestinal epithelial cells, due to absence of functional pancreatic **zinc-transporter protein**.

Management Supplemental zinc and/or **diodoquin** (**diiodohydroxy-quinoline**).

Iron: Hereditary haemochromatosis

Hereditary haemochromatosis is a disease of iron overload and one of the commonest recessive disorders in Caucasians.

Inheritance AR, with incomplete penetrance. The major mutation is substitution of cysteine by tyrosine at position 282 (Cys282Tyr) in the *HFE* gene. This maps within the HLA cluster at 6p21 and for reasons of linkage disequilibrium (Chapter 66), 75% of patients are HLA-A*0301, compared to 13% of controls. An additional three unlinked AR genes have been implicated, including that for **transferrin receptor 2** and one AD, for **ferroportin**, conferring a range of ages of onset.

Frequency 1/200–1/400 North Europeans; 1/8 are carriers, much less common in non-Europeans. Most (90–95%) of patients are homozygous for the Cys282Tyr mutation, the remainder being compound heterozygotes of this and substitution His63Asp.

Aetiology Both iron absorption from foodstuffs and its release by phagocytosis of old red blood cells are regulated by the hormone **hepcidin**. Mutant *HFE* alleles interfere with hepcidin signalling and excess iron accumulation in liver, kidney, heart, joints and pancreas. Reduced incidence in women relates to menstrual blood loss.

Features Fatigue, joint pain, diminished libido, diabetes, increased skin pigmentation, cardiomyopathy, liver enlargement and cirrhosis. Males are symptomatic at 40–60 years, females at 10–50% of the rate in men and only after the menopause.

Management Diagnosis is by abnormal serum **ferritin** and **transferrin** saturation levels and liver biopsy histochemistry; confirmation is by DNA test. Treatment is by serial **phlebotomy** to reduce iron stores.

Metal transport, lipid metabolism and amino acid catabolism defects – continued

Figure 60.3 **The β-oxidation degradative spiral**

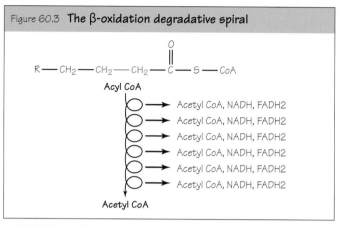

Figure 60.5 **Glutaric acid**

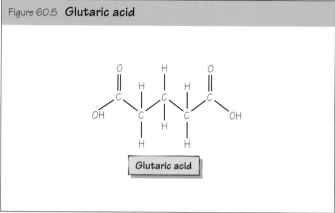

Figure 60.4 **Breakdown of succinogenic amino acids**

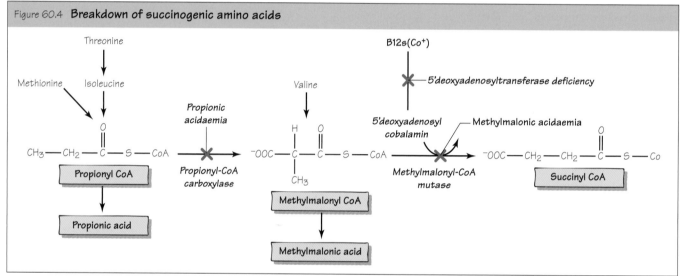

Lipid metabolism

Table 60.2 Inherited disorders of lipid metabolism.

Lipid metabolism defect	Prevalence	Genetics	Defective biomolecule
Familial hypercholesterolaemia	1/500	AD	Low-density lipoprotein receptor
Smith–Lemli–Opitz syndrome	1/10 000	AR	δ-7-sterol reductase
MCAD deficiency	1/20 000	AR	Medium-chain acyl-CoA dehydrogenase
LCAD deficiency	Rare	AR	Long-chain acyl-CoA dehydrogenase

Familial hypercholesterolaemia

This is one of the commonest monogenic AD disorders in Western society, responsible for **coronary artery disease** due to defective LDLR action during uptake of cholesterol (see Chapters 5 and 52).

Smith–Lemli–Opitz (SLO) syndrome

An AR defect in **7-dehydrocholesterol reductase** (**7DHCR**), catalysing the final step in *de novo* cholesterol biosynthesis causes SLO syndrome, characterized by congenital abnormalities of the brain and heart, hypospadias or ambiguous genitalia, polydactyly and syndactyly (see Chapters 7, 42 and 44).

Management Cholesterol supplementation of the diet.

Fatty acid catabolism by β-oxidation

Fatty acids are important substrates for mitochondrial respiration. Their carboxyl groups are 'activated' on the mitochondrial surface by combination with the sulphydryl group of CoA, catalysed by **acyl-CoA synthetase**. Their internalization then involves creation of **carnitine-acyl-SCoA complexes**, catalysed by **carnitine acetyltransferase I**. Within the mitochondrial matrix, the carnitine is released for re-export. Saturated acyl-SCoAs are then degraded by a recurring sequence of four reactions known as **the β-oxidation pathway** (Figure 60.2):

- oxidation by an **acyl-CoA dehydrogenase** linked to FAD;
- hydration by **enoyl-CoA hydratase**;

- oxidation by **L-3-hydroxyacyl-CoA dehydrogenase***, linked to NAD;
- thiolysis by **β-ketothiolase** and CoA.

(*There are several species of **L**-3-hydroxyacyl-CoA dehydrogenase, of different chain length specificities.)

At the end of this sequence the fatty acyl chain is shortened by two carbon atoms and $FADH_2$, NADH and acetyl-CoA are generated. The shortened acyl-CoA then undergoes further cycles of β-oxidation known as the **β-oxidation degradative spiral** (Figure 60.3).

Medium-chain acyl co-enzyme A dehydrogenase (MCAD) deficiency

MCAD deficiency is the most common disorder of lipid metabolism, most patients being of north-west European origin. Patients present with episodic hypoglycaemia, often provoked by fasting that causes accumulation of fatty acid intermediates. There is failure to produce ketones and exhaustion of glucose supplies, causing potentially lethal cerebral oedema and encephalopathy.

Aetiology The defect is in **acyl-CoA dehydrogenase**, at the first step of β-oxidation (see also Figure 60.2; MADD, below).

Management Maintenance of caloric intake is of vital importance.

Long-chain L-3-hydroxyacyl co-enzyme A dehydrogenase (LCHAD) deficiency

LCHAD deficiency is one of the most severe, although rare, disorders of fatty acid oxidation, causing severe liver disease, cardiomyopathy, peripheral neuropathy, etc., culminating in **sudden infant death**. Mothers can develop 'fatty liver of pregnancy' and related disorders.

Aetiology The defect is in the third step of the β-oxidation pathway (Figure 60.2).

Acidaemia and aciduria due to defective amino acid catabolism

Table 60.3 Disorders of amino acid catabolism.

Defect	Prevalence	Genetics	Defective biomolecule
Glutaryl-CoA dehydrogenase deficiency	1/35 000; 1/300 in Ojibway and Amish	AR >50 alleles	Mitochondrial glutaryl-CoA dehydrogenase
Multiple acetyl-CoA dehydrogenase deficiency	Very rare	Mainly AR	>9 mitochondrial dehydrogenases
Propionic acidaemia	1/35 000– 1/75 000	AR, several alleles	Propionyl-CoA carboxylase
Methyl malonic acidaemia	1/25 000– 1/48 000	AR	Methylmalonyl-CoA mutase; or cobalamin

Glutaryl-CoA dehydrogenase deficiency (GCDHD)

Features Macrocephaly at birth, episodes of encephalopathy with spasticity, dystonia, seizures and developmental delay; reduced blood pH due to glutaric acidaemia (Figure 60.5).

Aetiology Defects in the decarboxylation of glutaryl-CoA to crotonyl-CoA in the degradative pathway of the **glutarigenic amino acids**, lysine, hydroxylysine and tryptophan, cause secondary deficiency of carnitine.

Management Dietary restriction of glutarigenic amino acids; administration of carnitine.

Multiple acetyl-CoA dehydrogenase deficiency (MADD)

Genetics Associated with enzymes that utilize FAD as a cofactor, *including* the acyl-CoA dehydrogenase of β-oxidation (see above and Figure 60.2).

Features Two severe neonatal forms, one with congenital anomalies. Both have hepatomegaly, metabolic acidosis and hypoketotic hypoglycaemia. A third form presents in late childhood with failure to thrive, metabolic acidosis, hypoglycaemia and encephalopathy.

Management Mild forms: riboflavin, carnitine and diets low in protein and fat.

Propionic acidaemia

Features Early onset: presentation in the first week, with mental retardation, median lifespan 3 years; late onset (>6 weeks): severe movement disorders, dystonia and usually permanent neurologic damage.

Aetiology Metabolism of the amino acids isoleucine, threonine and methionine and some fatty acids produces propionyl-CoA. **Propionyl-CoA carboxylase** catalyses its conversion to methylmalonyl-CoA, using **biotin** as a cofactor (Figure 60.4). Defects cause propionic acidosis, vomiting, dehydration, lethargy, encephalopathy and bilateral damage to basal ganglia.

Management Administration of biotin.

Methylmalonic acidaemia

Features Appears in early infancy, variable in severity. Poor feeding, vomiting, hypotonia and lethargy, low white blood cell and platelet counts, hypoglycaemia, hyperammonaemia and chronic nephritis. Can lead to coma and death.

Aetiology Deficiency of **methylmalonyl-CoA mutase** or the **cobalamin** coenzyme in the breakdown of methionine, threonine, isoleucine and valine causes failure in formation of **succinyl-CoA**, with accumulation of toxic methylmalonic acid (Figure 60.4).

Management Fluid replacement, correction of metabolic acidosis and cessation of protein intake; vitamin B_{12} for selected patients; combined liver–kidney transplantation (see Chapter 63).

61 Disorders of porphyrin and purine metabolism and the urea/ornithine cycle

Figure 61.1 **The synthesis of haem and causation of porphyria**

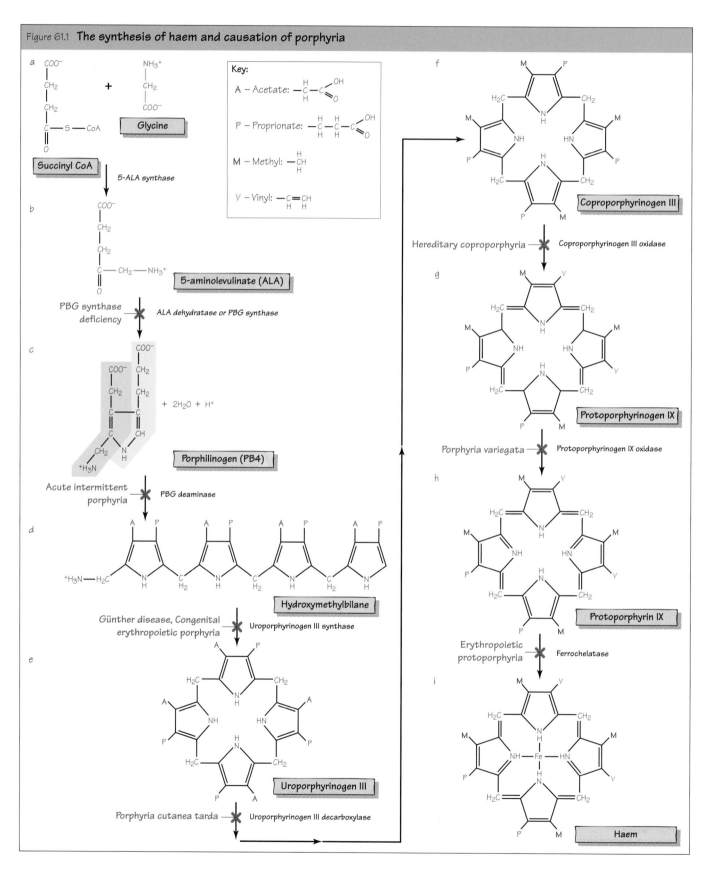

Medical Genetics at a Glance, Third Edition. Dorian J. Pritchard and Bruce R. Korf.

© 2013 John Wiley & Sons, Ltd. Published 2013 by John Wiley & Sons, Ltd.

Table 61.1 Disorders of porphyrin and purine metabolism.

Disorder	Prevalence	Inheritance	Defective biomolecule
Hepatic porphyrias			
Acute intermittent porphyria	Rare	AD	Porphobilinogen deaminase (Figure 61.1c,d)
Porphyria cutanea tarda	Rare	AD	Uroporphyrinogen III decarboxylase (Figure 61.1e,f)
Hereditary coproporphyria	Rare	AD	Coproporphyrinogen III oxidase (Figure 61.1f,g)
Porphyria variegata	Common in South Africa	AD	Protoporphyrinogen oxidase (Figure 61.1g,h)
Erythropoietic porphyrias			
PBG synthase deficiency	Rare	AD	Porphobilinogen synthase (5-aminolevulinate dehydratase) (Figure 61.1b,c)
Congenital erythropoietic porphyria; Günther disease	Rare	AR	Uroporphyrinogen-III synthase (Figure 61.1d,e)
Erythropoietic protoporphyria	Rare	AD	Ferrochelatase (Figure 61.1h,i)
Purine metabolism disorders			
Lesch–Nyhan syndrome	Rare	XR	Hypoxanthine-guanine phosphoribosyl transferase
Severe combined immunodeficiency; adenosine deaminase deficiency	1/70 000	AR	Adenosine deaminase
Purine nucleoside phosphorylase deficiency		AR	Purine nucleoside phosphorylase

Overview

Haemoglobin, myoglobin, cytochrome C, peroxidase and catalase all have **haem** as a prosthetic group. This consists of a tetravalent atom of iron surrounded by four **porphyrin rings** (Figure 61.1i). The latter are derived initially from a simple condensation reaction between the amino acid glycine and succinyl-CoA catalysed by **5-ALA synthase** (Figure 61.1a,b). There are genetic errors in all subsequent steps, which cause the class of diseases known as **porphyria**. All the porphyrias are AD except **congenital erythropoietic porphyria** (Figure 61.1h,i, which is AR), as they are rate-limiting in their pathways. All have neurological or visceral involvement and all except **acute intermittent porphyria** (Figure 61.1c,d) have cutaneous photosensitivity.

Porphyrins are normally present in all body tissues at small concentrations but in the porphyrias urinary excretion of porphyrins is greatly increased.

Biosynthesis of haem

The product of the first reaction is **5- (or δ-) aminolevulinate (5-ALA,** Figure 61.1b), a reaction catalysed by mitochondrial **5- (or δ-) ALA synthase**. In the liver this is an important control step, subject to feedback inhibition by the end product, haem, but promoted by ethanol, sex steroids, barbiturates, sulphonamides and anticonvulsants, with a general knock-on effect on downstream metabolite pools. Two molecules of 5-ALA then condense to form **porphobilinogen (PBG)** under the action of **ALA dehydratase** (or **PBG synthase**).

A linear tetrapyrrole called **hydroxymethylbilane** (Figure 61.1d) is then created from four PBG molecules, through the agency of **PBG deaminase**, which then cyclizes under the joint action of **uroporphyrinogen III synthase** and **cosynthase**, to create the tetrapyrrole ring structure, **uroporphyrinogen III (UPG III**; Figure 61.1e).

Coproporphyrinogen III (Figure 61.1f) is formed from this by decarboxylation of the acetate side chains to methyl groups, by **UPG III decarboxylase**, then **protoporphyrinogen IX** (Figure 61.1g) by oxidation of two propionate side chains to vinyl groups. Chelation of a molecule of ferrous iron finally yields haem (Figure 61.1i), under the action of **ferrochelatase**.

Nomenclature In porphyrins the pyrrole rings are joined by methane (–CH=) bridges, in porphyrinogens by methyline (–CH2–). In proto-porphyrins the side chains contain carboxyl (–COOH) groups. The Roman numerals refer to specific isomers of that molecule.

Disease causation

Deficiency of enzymes downstream of hydroxymethylbilane (Figure 61.1d) causes accumulation of intermediates that are diverted by non-enzymic oxidation to form several porphyrins which when exposed to light form singlet oxygen ($O_2^{\cdot}$). The latter is cytotoxic, causing photosensitivity on exposure to sunlight.

The reason why all the porphyrias except **congenital erythropoietic porphyria** follow AD inheritance is that all the relevant enzymes are rate limiting, so that haploinsufficiency generally results in clinical disease. The different types are variably associated with neurological or visceral involvement and cutaneous photosensitivity from accumulation of the different precursors in those organs. They are divisible into two groups depending on whether excess production occurs predominantly in the liver or erythropoietic system (see Table 61.1).

Porphyria

Acute intermittent porphyria (AIP)

Features Hepatic involvement, abdominal pain, weakness, vomiting, confusion, emotional upset and hallucinations; episodic, frequently affects women in relation to the menstrual cycle. Can be precipitated by steroids, anticonvulsants, barbiturates, oral contraceptives, etc. and is fatal in 5%. AIP is notable in not causing a photosensitive rash. The urine turns the colour of port wine on standing

Aetiology Partial deficiency of **PBG deaminase** (Figure 61.1c,d) leads to liver accumulation and urinary excretion of precursors PBG and 5-ALA.

AIP heterozygotes fall into two classes: in 90% the condition is in a latent state, in 10% it is clinically expressed, but all have a 50% reduction in activity of PGB deaminase. The condition is therefore considered to be dominant, but of only 10% penetrance (see Chapter 9).

Chemical expression occurs in response to factors that decrease the concentration of haem in liver cells. These include barbiturates, some steroid hormones, reducing diets, illness and surgery. These increase the synthesis of cytochrome P450, decreasing the body store of haem and reducing its feedback inhibition on 5-ALA synthase, the first, rate

Disorders of porphyrin and purine metabolism and the urea/ornithine cycle – continued

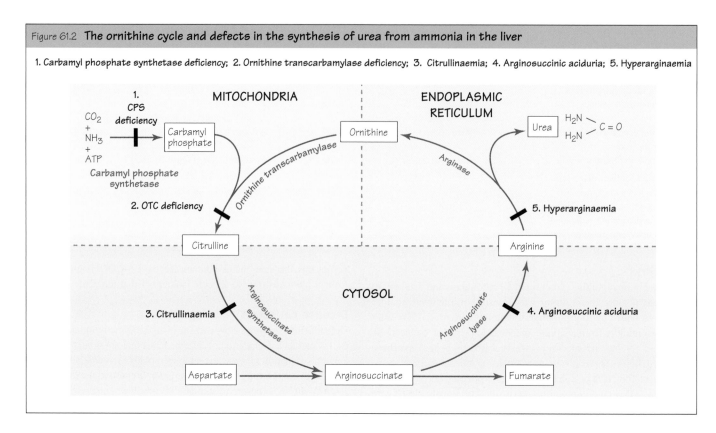

Figure 61.2 **The ornithine cycle and defects in the synthesis of urea from ammonia in the liver**

1. Carbamyl phosphate synthetase deficiency; 2. Ornithine transcarbamylase deficiency; 3. Citrullinaemia; 4. Arginosuccinic aciduria; 5. Hyperarginaemia

limiting step in the pathway. The result is increased expression of this enzyme at both transcriptional and translational levels and because PBG deaminase is deficient, PBG accumulates. Pathogenesis of neurological symptoms may be due to increased levels of 5-ALA and PBG. Peripheral, autonomic and CN systems are all affected, with diverse manifestations from acute abdominal pain to psychosis.

Management Treatment is aimed at reducing 5-ALA synthase activity by intravenous infusion of haematin.

Congenital erythropoietic porphyria, Günther disease

Features AR, non-acute, seen in children. Extreme photosensitivity with blistering of the skin and extensive scarring, nail abnormalities, haemolytic anaemia, red coloration of teeth which fluoresce red under ultraviolet light, marrow hyperplasia, splenomegaly.

Aetiology Defect in UPG III synthase (Figure 61.1d,e).

Management Protection from sunlight, blood transfusion, splenectomy.

Hereditary coproporphyria

Features Similar to AIP, but a third of patients also have photosensitive skin.

Aetiology Partial deficiency of CPG III oxidase (Figure 61.1f,g).

Porphyria variegata

Features Hepatic involvement, particularly prevalent in white South Africans; neurological and visceral illness triggered by drugs, variable skin photosensitivity, increased faecal excretion of protoporphyrin and coproporphyrin. King George III (1738–1820), the British king whose irrational behaviour may have helped trigger the American Revolution (1775), is thought to have suffered from this condition.

Aetiology Deficiency in protoporphyrin oxidase (Figure 61.1g,h).

Erythropoietic protoporphyria

Features Non-acute, usually AD, seen in children. Photosensitivity, chronic liver disease. There is accumulation of protoporphyrin in erythrocytes causing them to fluoresce.

Aetiology The basic defect is in ferrochelatase (Figure 61.1h,i).

Management Treatment of photosensitivity with β-carotene.

Porphyria cutanea tarda

Features Non-acute, hepatic, mostly acquired in association with alcohol abuse or oestrogen administration. There is photosensitivity and hepatomegaly.

Hepatic coproporphyria

Features Acute, AD, hepatic, neurological with photosensitivity.

Errors of purine metabolism
Lesch–Nyhan and Kelley–Seegmiller syndromes

Features The bizarre behavioural abnormality of **Lesch–Nyhan syndrome** involves compulsive self-mutilation, uncontrolled movements, spasticity, intellectual disability and aggressive behaviour.

Genetics XR

Aetiology LNS is associated with virtually complete deficiency of **hypothanxanthine guanine phosphoribosyl transferase (HGPRT)** involved in the **hypoxanthine salvage pathway**, causing high levels of phosphoribosyl pyrophosphate and accumulation of uric acid, etc. Partial HGPRT deficiency causes **Kelley–Seegmiller syndrome,** of which the only clinical manifestations are excessive purine production, renal stones, uric acid nephropathy, renal obstruction and gout following puberty.

Diagnosis In LNS, uric acid in urine revealed by 'orange sand' in nappies (diapers); lack of HGPRT activity in skin fibroblasts.

Management Allopurinol alleviates symptoms.

Severe combined immunodeficiency disease (SCID); adenosine deaminase deficiency (ADA deficiency)
See Chapter 65.

Features Presentation in infancy, with recurrent infections that can rapidly prove fatal.

Inheritance AR

Frequency Very rare.

Aetiology **Adenosine deaminase deficiency** causes ATP and dATP to accumulate, which feed back to inhibit **ribonucleotide reductase** in thymocytes and peripheral RBCs. This in turn restricts their DNA synthesis and hence production of T and B cells.

▶ Problems requiring immediate attention

Urgent need for control of actual and potential fatal infections.

Purine nucleoside phosphorylase deficiency (PNP deficiency)
Inheritance AR

Features Severe recurrent and potentially fatal viral infections due to impaired T-cell function.

Management Treatment by injection of irradiated red blood cells

Disorders of the urea/ornithine cycle
Catabolism of surplus dietary amino acids generates highly toxic ammonium ions. The essential biochemical task of the urea pathway is to dispose of these by their conversion to urea through the agency of ornithine (Figure 61.2), for excretion by the kidneys. The penultimate product is arginine, which when hydrolysed to urea regenerates ornithine, ready for repetition of the cycle. Defects in the cycle cause high concentrations of ammonia in the blood, which is toxic to the CNS and can lead to coma and death.

The cycle consists of five major chemical reactions, which take place primarily in the liver cells. Deficiency of any of these can lead to progressive neurological impairment, lethargy, coma and death from build-up of ammonium ions and glutamine. These operate in the mitochondria, endoplasmic reticulum and cytosol (see Figure 61.2). Consequences of defects in the cycle include deficiencies of **carbamoyl synthetase** and **ornithine transcarbamylase (OTC)**, **citrullinaemia, arginosuccinic aciduria** and **hyperargininaemia**.

The most common defect is mitochondrial **ornithine transcarbamylase** deficiency (X-LR).

Management Largely dietary.

Table 61.2 Urea cycle disorders.

Disorder	Prevalence	Genetics	Defective biomolecule
Ornithine transcarbamylase deficiency	1/70 000–1/100 000	XR	Ornithine transcarbamyl transferase
Carbamoyl phosphate synthetase deficiency	1/70 000–1/100 000	AR	Carbamoyl phosphate synthetase
Arginosuccinic aciduria	1/70 000–1/100 000	AR	Arginosuccinic lyase
Citrullinaemia	1/100 000	AR	Arginosuccinate synthetase
Hyperargininaemia	1/300 000	AR	Arginase

62 Lysosomal, glycogen storage and peroxisomal diseases

Figure 62.1 Enzymatic defects in lysosomal lipid storage disorders
The activities of the indicated enzymes are measured in screening for disease

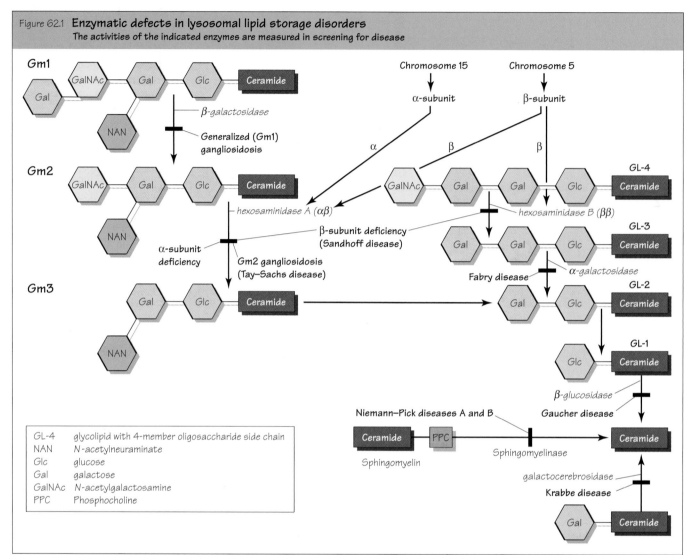

GL-4   glycolipid with 4-member oligosaccharide side chain
NAN   N-acetylneuraminate
Glc   glucose
Gal   galactose
GalNAc   N-acetylgalactosamine
PPC   Phosphocholine

Figure 62.2 (a) α-D-glucose, carbon atom numbering scheme

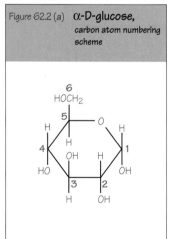

Figure 62.2 (b) α-14, linkage

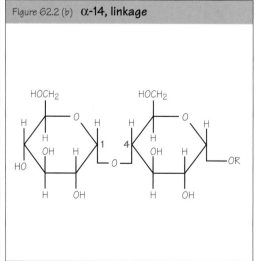

Figure 62.2 (c) α-1,6 linkage

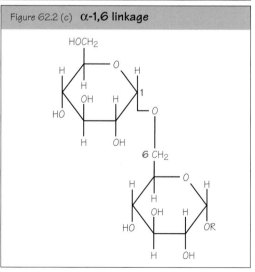

Medical Genetics at a Glance, Third Edition. Dorian J. Pritchard and Bruce R. Korf.

Overview

Lysosomes are membrane-bound organelles with a large complement of hydrolytic enzymes (**lysozymes**), all with acidic optimal pH (4.0–5.0). They are in effect recycling centres, where waste proteins, fats and carbohydrates, damaged mitochondria, viruses and bacteria are sent for breakdown. The lysozymes are synthesized in the ER and conveyed to the Golgi apparatus for packaging into vesicles that are budded off as **primary lysosomes** (see Figure 60.1). Early endosomes containing newly pinocytosed foreign or unwanted materials fuse with these to form **secondary lysosomes** (or **late endosomes**) and their digested contents are released into the cytosol. Indigestible components are expelled by the now **tertiary lysosome** undergoing reverse pinocytosis at the plasma membrane, or else they remain in the lysosomes, causing them to swell and distort.

The **lysosomal storage diseases** are a group of about 50 rare recessive disorders that result when the lysosomes malfunction, usually as a consequence of deficiency in a single enzyme required for breakdown of a complex lipid, glycoprotein or mucopolysaccharide. Affected children are usually normal at birth, but with time, commence a downhill course, due to accumulation of one or more specific macromolecules.

In the nervous system **gangliosides,** constitute 6% of the lipids in grey matter. These are membrane glycolipids derived from sphingosine, which carry branched chains of several sugar residues. They are continually synthesized and degraded by sequential removal of terminal sugars and their breakdown occurs within the lysosomes. The **sphingolipidoses** are characterized by deposition of lipid or glycolipid, primarily in the brain, liver and spleen, with progressive mental deterioration, often with seizures, leading to death in childhood. There are at least 10 specific relevant enzyme deficiencies, all AR, in which parts of the brain typically become enormously swollen due to massive accumulation of partially digested waste sphingolipid material.

Infants with one of the **mucopolysaccharidoses** (**MPSs**) present with skeletal, vascular or CNS irregularities, along with coarsening of facial features. Each specific MPS has a characteristic pattern of excretion in the urine of **dermatan**, **heparan**, **keratan** or **chondroitin sulphate**.

Sphingolipidoses, lipid storage disorders (LSDs)

Tay–Sachs disease

Incidence 1/3600 in Ashkenazi Jews, ~1/62 500 in others.

Features Presents in the first 6 months with poor feeding, lethargy and poor muscle tone. Progressive neurological dysfunction leads to loss of sight and hearing and to spasticity, rigidity and death from respiratory infection in the second year.

Aetiology Defective α-subunit of **hexosaminidase-A** allows accumulation of GM2 ganglioside (Figure 62.1).

Diagnosis Cherry-red spot in macula; low hexosaminidase activity in serum.

Gaucher disease

Incidence 1/900 in Ashkenazi Jews, 1/22 000 in others (90% are Type 1).

Table 62.1 The sphingolipidoses.

	Incidence	Inheritance	Defective biomolecule
Tay–Sachs disease	1/62 500 UK; 1/3600 Ashkenazim	AR	Hexosaminidase-A
Gaucher disease Type 1	1/22 000; 1/900 Ashkenazim	AR	β-glucosidase
Gaucher disease Type 2	Rare	AR	β-glucosidase
Niemann–Pick disease	Rare	AR	Sphingomyelinase
Krabbe disease	1/100 000; 1/6000 in some Arab groups	AR	Galactocerebrosidase

Features **Type 1**: adult onset, febrile episodes, hepatosplenomegaly, bone lesions, skin pigmentation (NB. CNS is unaffected).

Type 2: infantile onset, hepatosplenomegaly, failure to thrive, neurological deterioration, with spasticity and fits; death from pulmonary infection in the second year.

Diagnosis Deficient glucosylceramide β-glucosidase (Figure 62.1).

Management Pain relief, splenectomy, enzyme replacement by intravenous infusion, enzyme augmentation, bone marrow transplantation.

Niemann–Pick disease

Features Infants fail to thrive, hepatomegaly, lethal by the age of 4 years.

Diagnosis Cherry-red spot in macula, 'foam cells' in bone marrow, **sphingomyelinase** deficiency (Figure 62.1).

Krabbe disease

Genetics AR

Features At 3–6 months, fevers, stiffness, seizures, retarded development, severe degeneration of motor skills, eating problems leading to optic atrophy, deafness, paralysis, etc., generally fatal by age 2 years.

Aetiology Defect in **galactocerebrosidase** (**GALC**) necessary for myelin synthesis causes abnormal build up of glycosphingolipid that may promote axonal degeneration (Figure 62.1).

Management Cord blood and bone marrow transplantation, physiotherapy (see Chapter 72).

Mucopolysaccharidoses (MPSs)

All the MPSs involve chronic and progressive multisystem deterioration, due to accumulation of sulphated polysaccharides (glycosaminoglycans). This causes problems with hearing, vision, joint and cardiovascular function. Affected children develop coarse facial features, short stature, skeletal deformities and joint stiffness. Hunter syndrome is X-linked, the others AR.

Bone marrow transplantation and enzyme replacement therapy are successful in some cases, though treatment of the CNS remains problematic.

Lysosomal, glycogen storage and peroxisomal diseases – continued

Figure 62.2 (d) Molecular structure of glycogen

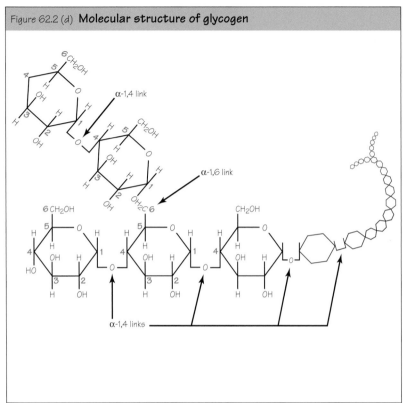

Figure 62.2 (e) Degradation of glycogen

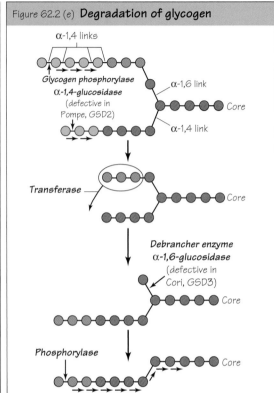

Figure 62.2 (f) Errors in the metabolism of terminal α-1→4 linked glucose from glycogen

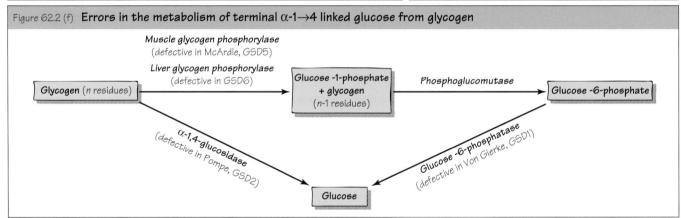

Hurler syndrome, MPS 1

This is the most severe MPS, presenting with corneal clouding and spinal curvature in the first year, with mental deterioration and death from cardiac failure or respiratory infection by the mid-teens.

Diagnosis Increased urinary excretion of dermatan and heparan sulphates, reduced activity of **α-L-iduronidase**.

Hunter syndrome, MPS 2

This usually presents at 2–5 years with a variety of problems, including hearing loss and abnormal vertebrae, progressive physical and mental deterioration and death usually in the teens.

Diagnosis Excess dermatan and heparan sulphates in the urine, decreased activity of **iduronate sulphate sulphatase** in serum or white blood cells.

Sanfilippo syndrome, MPS 3, types A, B, C and D

This is the most common MPS. Symptoms appear in the second year: intellectual loss, convulsions and death in early adulthood.

Diagnosis Increased urinary heparan chondroitin sulphate and deficiency of either one of four specific degradative enzymes (Table 62.2).

Morquio syndrome, MPS 4, types A and B

Children present in the second or third year with skeletal abnormalities that can later cause spinal cord compression. Intelligence is normal and survival long term.

Diagnosis Keratan sulphate in the urine; deficiency of **galactosamine-6-sulphatase** (type A) or **β-galactosidase** (type B).

Table 62.2 The mucopolysaccharidoses.

Hurler syndrome, MPS 1	1/10 000	AR	α-L-iduronidase
Hunter syndrome, MPS 2	1/100 000 males	XR	Iduronate sulphate suphatase
Sanfilippo syndrome			
type A, MPS 3A	1/25 000 (all types)	AR	Heparan-S-sulphaminidase
type B, MPS 3B		AR	N-acetyl-α-D-glucosaminidase
type C, MPS 3C		AR	Acetyl-CoA: α-glucosaminidase-N-acetyltransferase
type D, MPS 3D		AR	N-acetyl-glucosamine sulphatase
Morquio syndrome			
type A, MPS 4A	1/100 000 (all types)	AR	Galactosamine-6-sulphatase
type B, MPS 4B		AR	β-galactosidase
Maroteaux–Lamy syndrome, MPS 6	Rare	AR	Aryl sulphatase B
Sly syndrome, MPS 7	Rare	AR	β-glucuronidase
I-cell disease	1/640 000	AR	GlcNAc phosphotransferase

Table 62.3 Peroxisomal disorders.

Disorder	Incidence	Genetics	Defective biomolecule
Zellweger syndrome	1/40 000	AR	All peroxisomal enzymes
Adrenoleukodystrophy	1/20 000	XR	Very long chain fatty acid synthase

Maroteaux–Lamy syndrome, MPS 6

Hurler-like symptoms in early childhood, but retention of normal intelligence. Survival into adulthood or until only the third decade.
Diagnosis Increased urinary dermatan sulphate excretion, cellular **aryl sulphatase B** deficiency.

Sly syndrome, MPS 7

Diagnosis Increased urinary excretion of glycosaminoglycans; **β-glucuronidase** deficiency in serum and cells.

I-cell disease

Genetics AR

Features Features similar to Hurler syndrome, but with earlier onset, no evidence of mucopolysacchariduria and dense intracytoplasmic intrusions (I-bodies) in fibroblasts. Children often have stiff, claw shaped hands.

Aetiology Defect in **GlcNAc phosphotransferase** responsible for transfer of phosphate to mannose residues as a badge for targeting glycoproteins to lysosomes.

Management Fe and vitamin B_{12} dietary supplementation, bone marrow transplantation.

Peroxisomal disease

Peroxisomes are cytoplasmic organelles involved particularly in the metabolism of complex fatty acids and cholesterol, especially abundant in the parenchyma of the liver and kidneys. They contain more than 40 enzymes, notably those involved in β-oxidation (Chapter 60) and two in the pentose phosphate pathway.

Zellweger syndrome

Genetics AR, genetically heterogeneous.

Features Newborns present with hypotonia, weakness, persistent large anterior fontanelle and prominent forehead, sometimes also cataracts and enlarged liver. Later there are usually seizures, renal cysts, abnormal calcification of long bone epiphyses, death within the first year.

Aetiology Abnormality of one or more of the 12 *PEX* genes involved in peroxisome assembly.

Management Diagnosis is by plasma long-chain fatty acid levels.

X-linked adrenoleukodystrophy (ADA)

Genetics AR

Features Males typically present with deteriorating school performance in late childhood, some later with mild neurological features and adrenal insufficiency

Aetiology Deficiency in **peroxisome membrane protein** due to defect in the ***ABCD1* gene** causes secondary deficiency of **very long chain fatty acid CoA synthase**.

Glycogen storage disorders

Glycogen is a branched polymer of α-D-glucose residues (Figure 62.2a), a typical molecule having a molecular weight of several million (Figure 62.2d). It constitutes a largely temporary energy store, mainly in the liver and skeletal muscle.

It is constructed of numerous chains of α-(1→4) linked glucose residues (Figure 62.2b), which branch via α-(1→6) bonds (Figure 62.2c), the latter created by a '**brancher enzyme**'. During glycogen breakdown residues are sequentially cleaved off the non-reducing end either by **α-1,4-glucosidase**, yielding free glucose, or by **glycogen phosphorylase** to yield glucose-1-phosphate (Figure 62.2e). The latter is converted by **phosphoglucomutase** to glucose-6-phosphate, then by **glucose-6-phosphatase** to free glucose (Figure 62.2f).

Table 62.4 Glycogen storage disorders.

Disorder	Incidence	Genetics	Defective biomolecule
Hepatic			
Von Gierke disease, GSD1	Rare	AR	Glucose-6-phosphatase
Cori disease, GSD3	Rare	AR	Amylo-1,6-glucosidase
Anderson disease, GSD4	Rare	AR	Glycogen 'brancher enzyme'
Hepatic phosphorylase deficiency, GSD6	Rare	AR/XR	Hepatic phosphorylase
Muscular			
Pompe disease, GSD2	Rare	AR	Lysosomal α-1,4-glucosidase
McArdle disease, GSD5	Rare	AR	Muscle phosphorylase

The four closest 1→4 bonds to branch points are inaccessible to the phosphorylase, which also does not attack the 1→6 the branch. Here a **transferase** shifts a block of three glycosyl residues from one branch to the other, exposing the 1→6 link to '**debrancher enzyme'**, **amylo-1,6-glucosidase** and allowing the phosphorylase digestion to proceed (Figure 62.2e).

Errors in both the synthesis and breakdown of glycogen cause 12 **glycogen storage disorders** (**GSDs**).

Primarily hepatic disorders

Von Gierke disease, GSD 1

Features Hepatomegaly, sweating, rapid pulse, convulsions and massive liver enlargement.

Aetiology Deficiency of **glucose-6-phosphatase** (Figure 62.2f).

Management Maintenance of blood sugar.

Cori disease, GSD 3

Features Hepatomegaly and/or muscle weakness.

Aetiology Deficiency of **amylo-1,6-glucosidase**, the **debrancher enzyme** (Figure 62.2e).

Management Maintenance of blood sugar.

Anderson disease, GSD 4

Features Hypotonia and progressive liver failure.

Aetiology Deficiency of **brancher enzyme** leads to unmetabolizable, long glycogen chains.

Management Liver transplant.

Hepatic phosphorylase deficiency, GSD 6

Genetics The multimeric enzyme is coded by both XR and AR genes.

Features Hepatomegaly, hypoglycaemia, failure to thrive in the first 2 years.

Aetiology Failure of **liver glycogen phosphorylase** (Figure 62.2f).

Management Carbohydrate supplements that improve growth.

Primarily muscular disorders

Pompe disease, GSD 2

Features Hypotonia in the first few months, muscle weakness with heart enlargement and heart failure in the second year.

Aetiology **Alpha-1,4-glucosidase** deficiency affecting voluntary and cardiac muscle (Figure 62.2f).

Management Intravenous infusion of enzyme.

McArdle disease, GSD 5

Features Teenagers present with muscle cramps on exercise.

Aetiology Failure of **muscle glycogen phosphorylase** (Figure 62.2f).

Management Muscle cramps tend to decline if exercise is continued.

Figure 63.1 The basis for biochemical, chemical, bacteriological and DNA screening for phenylketonuria

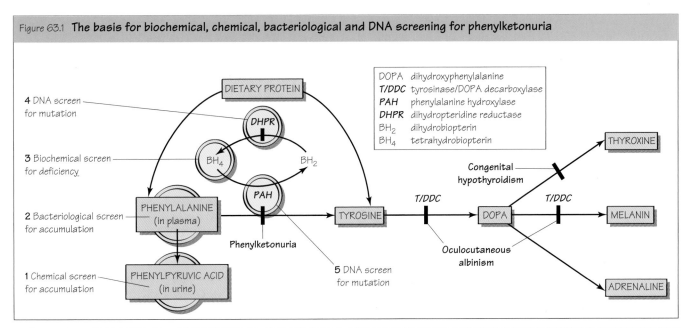

Figure 63.2 Principle of the tandem mass spectrometer used for acylcarnitine analysis

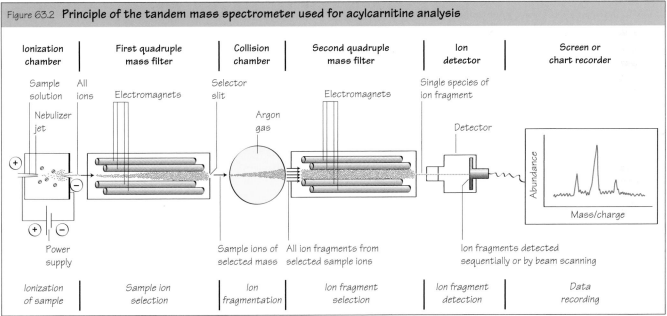

Overview

'Inborn errors of metabolism' result, directly or indirectly, mainly from either accumulation of an enzyme substrate to abnormal levels or deficiency of the product of an enzyme reaction (see Chapter 58). An example of the latter is **oculocutaneous albinism**, in which an abnormality in **tyrosinase** (**DOPA decarboxylase**) prevents synthesis of melanin pigment (see Chapters 6 and 58). Accumulated substrates can be toxic, notable examples being phenylalanine or its derivatives, methylmalonic acid and ammonia (Chapters 58, 60 and 61). Diagnosis of such conditions is usually by assay of accumulated metabolites or alternatively by enzyme assay, but more recently direct detection of mutations at the DNA level have come into favour.

Prenatal diagnosis is possible for many inborn errors. Analyses are performed on cultured amniocytes collected by mid-trimester amniocentesis, or more commonly now by biochemical or DNA testing on 12–14 week chorionic villus samples (see Chapter 72). Newborn screening and early diagnosis are performed routinely in most developed countries and recently the exceptionally rapid technique of **tandem mass spectrometry** (**MS/MS**) has come to prominence for metabolic and haematological disorders (see below).

Inborn errors of metabolism

The prototypical biochemical defect is **phenylketonuria** (**PKU**; see Figure 63.1 and Chapters 8 and 58) caused by a block in the conversion of phenylalanine to tyrosine. In most individuals this arises due to a fault in the gene coding for **phenylalanine hydroxylase** (PAH), but rarely (1–3%) it may be due to deficiency of **dihydropteridine reductase** (DHPR) responsible for the synthesis of cofactor BH_4 (Figure 58.3). Either way, phenylalanine and its derivatives accumulate.

Figure 63.1 illustrates five levels at which the likelihood of a baby developing the disease can be assessed: (1) a chemical or biochemical screen of the urine; (2) a bacteria-based screen of the plasma; (3) a biochemical screen for BH_4 deficiency; (4) a DNA screen for *DHPR* mutation; and (5) a DNA screen for *PAH* mutation. Until DNA screening became available the disorder could only be screened for postnatally, as phenylalanine does not accumulate until after birth.

Approaches to diagnosis

Detection of metabolites

Detection of metabolites is the time-honoured diagnostic approach. This offers an inexpensive, sensitive and specific means of diagnosis, and is the basis for most newborn screening methods where low cost and sensitivity are critical.

A limitation of metabolite detection is that for some disorders they accumulate only episodically. An example is **methylmalonic acidaemia** (see Chapter 60) in which mild enzyme deficiency produces episodic crises, between which blood and urine studies can be unrevealing.

The technology for metabolite detection has undergone significant evolution. In the case of PKU, newborn screening was initially based on the mouse like smell of the urine and the green colour response when ferric chloride ($FeCl_3$) is sprinkled onto the baby's wet nappy (diaper; No. 1 in Figure 63.1; Table 63.1). Following this came Guthrie's **bacterial inhibition assay** (No. 2 in Figure 63.1). Heelprick blood samples impregnated onto discs of filter paper are placed on a lawn of bacteria that cannot grow in the absence of supplemental phenylalanine. A halo of bacterial growth surrounding a disc indicates high concentration of phenylalanine in the blood.

Table 63.1 Urine signs in newborns.

Urine sign	Possible defect
Musty smell or of mice, green colour with $FeCl_3$	Phenylketonuria
Smell of burnt sugar, maple syrup	Defects in catabolism of valine, leucine or isoleucine
Smell of cabbage	Tyrosinaemia
Turns colour of port wine on standing	Acute intermittent porphyria
Turns black on exposure to air	Alkaptonuria
Contains orange sand-like granules	Lesch–Nyhan syndrome
Contains grey calculi	Cystinuria

Quantitative analysis of amino acids and organic acids can be carried out by standard biochemical techniques such as **column chromatography**, **gas chromatography** or, recently, **tandem mass spectrometry** (Figure 63.2).

Enzyme assay

Enzyme activity can be assayed *in vitro* using either synthetic or natural substrates. This approach is commonly used to diagnose lysosomal storage disorders, where metabolites are trapped within lysosomes and inaccessible to direct assay (see Chapter 62). It is, for example, used for screening for **hexosaminidase A** deficiency in white blood cells of carriers of Tay–Sachs disease (see Chapters 8 and 62).

Enzyme assay offers the advantage over substrate quantification that heterozygotes are also identifiable, although in some cases there is overlap between their levels and those in normal homozygotes.

DNA diagnosis

There are now many techniques for analysis of DNA (see Chapters 67–70). The advantages of the DNA approach include the ability to test very early in development and on any nucleated cell type, obviating the restriction to tissues that express the enzyme concerned or accumulate relevant metabolites. It is also highly specific, particularly in detecting clinically unaffected carriers, and is finding increasing use in **carrier detection schemes**, such as for **Canavan** and **Gaucher diseases** in the Ashkenazi Jewish population (see Chapter 62).

Tandem mass spectrometry (MS/MS)

Tandem mass spectrometry enables very rapid and simultaneous diagnosis of around 40 disorders of body chemistry from heel-prick blood samples of newborn babies (Table 63.2). It is especially valuable for the disorders of mitochondrial fatty acid β-oxidation associated with LCHAD and 'sudden infant death syndrome', cyclic vomiting and maternal complications of pregnancy (see Chapter 60). A general feature of these conditions is a decreased level of the mitochondrial membrane transport protein **carnitine** and an increased ratio of an **acylcarnitine** to free carnitine in the blood plasma.

In a basic MS/MS analysis, as for the acylcarnitines, the preparation is atomized by passage through a fine jet and exposed to an electric field which gives the resulting droplets an extra positive charge (Figure 63.2). The ions are then directed through selector slits and into the

Table 63.2 Some disorders detectable by tandem mass spectrometry. (Source: ACMG statement. (2000) Tandem mass spectrometry in newborn screening. *Genetics in Medicine* **2**(4).)

Disorder	Diagnostic metabolite
Amino acidaemias	
Phenylketonuria	Phenylalanine, tyrosine
Maple syrup urine disease	Leucine, isoleucine
Homocystinuria	Methionine
Citrullinaemia	Citrulline
Hepatorenal tyrosinaemia	Methionine, tyrosine
Organic acidaemias	
Propionic acidaemia	Acylcarnitine
Methylmalonic acidaemia	Acylcarnitine
Isovaleric acidaemia	Isovalerylcarnitine
Glutaric acidaemia (Type 1)	Glutarylcarnitine
Fatty acid disorders	
SCAD* deficiency	Acylcarnitine
MCAD* deficiency	Acylcarnitine
VLCAD* deficiency	Acylcarnitine
Glutaric acidaemia (Type 2)	Glutarylcarnitine

*SCAD, MCAD, VLCAD: short, medium and very long chain acyl-CoA dehydrogenases (see Chapter 60).

first quadrupole magnetic 'filter', where oscillating electromagnetic fields sort and select the ions by their mass : charge ratio. Selected ions are then transmitted into a 'collision cell' for fragmentation by collision with argon molecules. The ion fragments are passed through a second quadrupole filter, which carries out additional sorting on the basis of mass : charge ratio, to impact on a detector that converts the charges of individual species of ion fragment to electric currents. A molecular profile of the sample is displayed on a chart or computer screen, with each key metabolite represented as a peak in the 'mass spectrum'.

Diseases detectable by MS/MS include the amino acidaemias, organic acidaemias and fatty acid disorders (Table 63.2), especially disorders of fatty acid oxidation involving acyl group transport across mitochondrial membranes (e.g. **MCAD** deficiency; Chapter 60), as these involve the highly polar carnitines. The first episode of hypoketotic hypoglycaemia in MCAD deficiency is fatal in 30–50% of patients; but MS/MS allows *presymptomatic* detection.

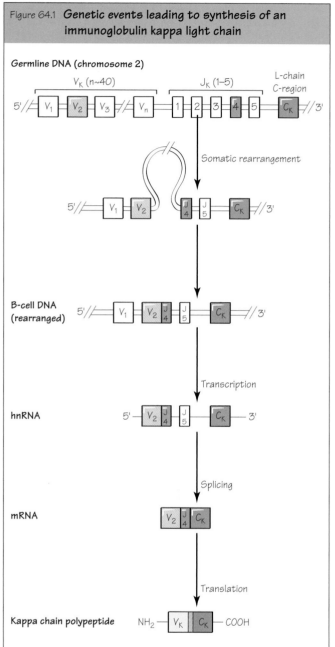

Figure 64.1 Genetic events leading to synthesis of an immunoglobulin kappa light chain

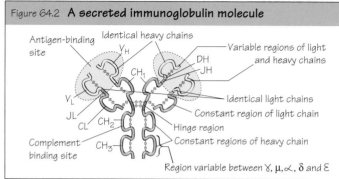

Figure 64.2 A secreted immunoglobulin molecule

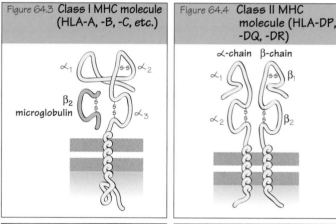

Figure 64.3 Class I MHC molecule (HLA-A, -B, -C, etc.)

Figure 64.4 Class II MHC molecule (HLA-DP, -DQ, -DR)

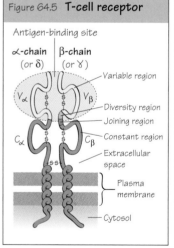

Figure 64.5 T-cell receptor

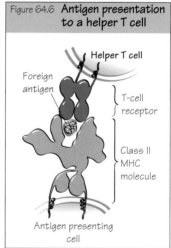

Figure 64.6 Antigen presentation to a helper T cell

Overview

Immunogenetics concerns the genetics of the **immune system**, which defends the body against invading pathogens and rejects malignant cells and incompatible tissue grafts (see also Chapters 29).

Immune defence mechanisms include **innate** and **adaptive immunity**. Both involve **humoral** and **cell-mediated** components, which combat extracellular and intracellular antigens respectively.

Three classes of bone-marrow stem cells are involved. One migrates to the spleen and lymph nodes and becomes **B lymphocytes**, or **B cells**. The second migrates to the thymus and develops into **T lymphocytes**: **T4 cells** (**helpers** and **inducers**), **T8 cells** (**cytotoxic** and **suppressor cells**)

and **natural killer cells**. T cells competent to attack the body's own components are selected and eliminated, generating **immune tolerance** to 'self antigens'. **Macrophages** move directly into the circulation.

Disorders of the immune system can result in **autoimmune disease** (Chapter 66), inflammatory disease (Chapters 55 and 65) and cancer (Chapters 55 and 56).

The innate immune system

The innate immune system attacks non-specifically, on exposure to alien macromolecules in general. It depends on the joint action of: **phagocytes**, that consume and destroy microorganisms, **natural killer**

Medical Genetics at a Glance, Third Edition. Dorian J. Pritchard and Bruce R. Korf.

cells that recognize and destroy virally infected cells, and **complement**. Complement is a complex of some 20 proteins that cooperate to attack extracellular pathogens such as microbes by 'opsonization' (coating) of their surfaces, so attracting the attention of phagocytes or generating a **membrane attack complex** that induces its lysis.

The adaptive immune system

The adaptive immune system is highly specific to the minor molecular characteristics of pathogens and depends on interaction between **B** and **T lymphocytes**. Three kinds of molecule are especially important: **MHC proteins**, **immunoglobulins** and **T-cell receptors** (**TCRs**; Figures 64.3, 64.4 and 64.5).

Mature B cells secrete soluble **antibodies**, or **immunoglobulins**, into the blood and lymph circulations. These react in a highly specific fashion with **antigens** such as peptide or polysaccharide components of invading pathogens. **Helper T cells** help other lymphocytes to respond more effectively. **Cytotoxic T cells** destroy infected cells.

The humoral component

The humoral immune response begins when phagocytes that contribute to the innate system engulf invading microbes and display their component molecules on their own surfaces. These are **antigen-presenting cells** or **APCs**. They normally display **Class II MHC molecules**, but after ingesting a foreign protein they incorporate its components into a groove in the MHC molecule (Figure 64.6). Circulating helper T cells display receptors which interlock neatly with MHC molecules, but disruption by a foreign antigen causes the T cell to respond. That the APC contains foreign molecules is advertised also by surface **co-stimulatory molecules**, which interact with other receptors on the helper T cell.

This stimulates the helper T cell to secrete **cytokine** molecules, which impact on B lymphocytes. The helper T cell detaches from the APC, but takes the MHC–peptide complex with it. Each B lymphocyte displays immunoglobulin molecules and if these are capable of binding the antigen it is stimulated to proliferate.

The very few B cells carrying antibodies with a loose, but appropriate specificity then proliferate and minor variations in the immunoglobulin coding sequences are rapidly and sequentially introduced. The process is driven by the affinity of antibody binding to antigen, so that within 5–7 days B cells are produced which bind that specific antigen with high affinity. This subset of B cells then secretes their immunoglobulin receptors into the bloodstream, as **plasma cells**. Each mature plasma cell can secrete 10 million monoclonal antibody molecules per hour.

The cellular component

Foreign peptides in infected body cells move to the surface complexed with **MHC Class I molecules** (c.f. Class II in the humoral response). Receptors on the surface of the **cytotoxic T cell** then bind to these and release chemicals capable of destroying around 50 infected body cells per hour.

One class of APCs migrates to secondary lymphoid sites in the tonsils, lymph nodes, etc., and alerts the appropriate subset of T cells. Their secretion of cytokines stimulates proliferation of T-cell subsets that bind specifically to infected cells, which then undergo selective evolutionary progression essentially similar to that of B lymphocytes.

In virally infected cells **interferon** destabilizes viral mRNA.

Memory cells

Specification for a specific response is retained by both **memory B** and **memory T cells**. **Vaccination** involves creating a bank of appropriate memory cells without exposure to harmful live pathogen.

The major histocompatibility complex (MHC)

(See Chapter 66.)

The immunoglobulins

Within each person a different species of immunoglobulin (Ig) is produced for every potential foreign antigen. *This enormous diversity is created by unique kinds of genetic rearrangement within individual B lymphocytes* (Figure 64.1).

At initial exposure to a foreign peptide, possibly one in a million B lymphocytes happens by chance to produce antibody capable of binding specifically to that peptide. Binding stimulates B-cell proliferation and hypermutation in the Ig genes, in which minor DNA sequence variations are introduced at each cell division.

An Ig molecule has two **heavy** (H) chains and a pair of **kappa** (κ) or **lambda** (λ) **light** (L) chains. The latter consist of **constant** (C), **variable** (V) and **joining** (J) **regions** (Figure 64.2).

There are five classes of heavy chain defined by their C-regions: **IgG**, **IgM**, **IgA**, **IgD** and **IgE**, with heavy chains **gamma** (γ); **mu** (μ); **alpha** (α); **delta** (δ) and **epsilon** (ϵ), respectively. There is also a 'hinge' and V, J and **diversity** (D) **regions**.

There are around 40 alternative sequences within the κ L-chain V region, five in the J, and one C gene, all on Chromosome 2. The λ light chain genes on Chromosome 22 show similar complexity. For the heavy chains, there are nine C genes (γ, μ, etc., on Chromosome 14), plus about 20 D between the arrays of V and J genes. As the V, D and J regions are assembled, slight variation occurs at the junctions. **Somatic hypermutation** also occurs, involving an increase in the mutation rate of the V, D and J genes.

The different B cells of one individual synthesize billions of different specificities of antibody by differential splicing of these alternative sequences, their transcripts being edited further at the RNA stage. Different pairs of H and L chains then link as symmetrical tetramers.

Within one B cell, antigen-binding specificity can be transferred between different species of heavy chain. This is called **class switching**. When a B cell produces both IgG and IgM of the same specificity it acquires competence to respond to antigen. Possibly as many as 10 million million distinct immunoglobulin molecular subspecies can be produced in one person.

The T-cell receptor (TCR)

The TCRs play key roles in antigen recognition and helper activity, but a T cell responds to a foreign antigen only if it is complexed with an MHC molecule.

The TCRs are dimers composed usually of a TCR α- and β-chain (or else a TCR γ- and δ-chain; Figure 64.5). Their genes also have C, V, J and D segments that are spliced alternatively to create extensive diversity, but they do not undergo hypermutation and are not secreted into the circulation.

The immune system in pregnancy

During pregnancy a particular type of antibody, IgG, is transported from the mother directly across the placenta, so babies have high levels of antibodies even at birth, with the same range of antigen specificities as their mothers. Breast milk colostrum also contains antibodies that pass through the baby's gut wall, conferring 'passive immunity' that lasts from a few days up to several months, while the baby's own immune system develops. Immune rejection of the fetus by maternal cytotoxic and natural killer cells is avoided by down-regulation of fetal MHC antigens.

65 Genetic disorders of the immune system

Figure 65.1 Phagocytosis and intracellular destruction of micro-organisms by macrophages

In normal cells hydrogen peroxide (H_2O_2) is released at phagocytosis, but not in patients with chronic granulomatous disease

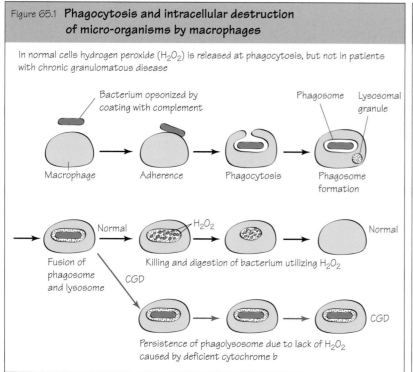

Bacterium opsonized by coating with complement — Phagosome — Lysosomal granule

Macrophage → Adherence → Phagocytosis → Phagosome formation

Fusion of phagosome and lysosome → Normal → H_2O_2 → Killing and digestion of bacterium utilizing H_2O_2 → Normal

CGD → Persistence of phagolysosome due to lack of H_2O_2 caused by deficient cytochrome b → CGD

Figure 65.2 Classification of immune phenomena and disorders of immunity

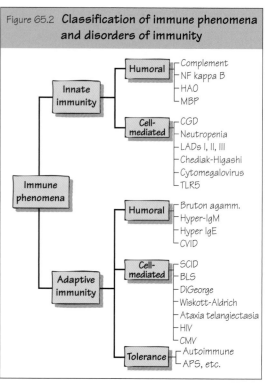

Immune phenomena

Innate immunity
- Humoral
  - Complement
  - NF kappa B
  - HAO
  - MBP
- Cell-mediated
  - CGD
  - Neutropenia
  - LADs I, II, III
  - Chediak-Higashi
  - Cytomegalovirus
  - TLR5

Adaptive immunity
- Humoral
  - Bruton agamm.
  - Hyper-IgM
  - Hyper IgE
  - CVID
- Cell-mediated
  - SCID
  - BLS
  - DiGeorge
  - Wiskott-Aldrich
  - Ataxia telangiectasia
  - HIV
  - CMV
- Tolerance
  - Autoimmune
  - APS, etc.

Figure 65.3 Points of action of inherited disorders of the immune system

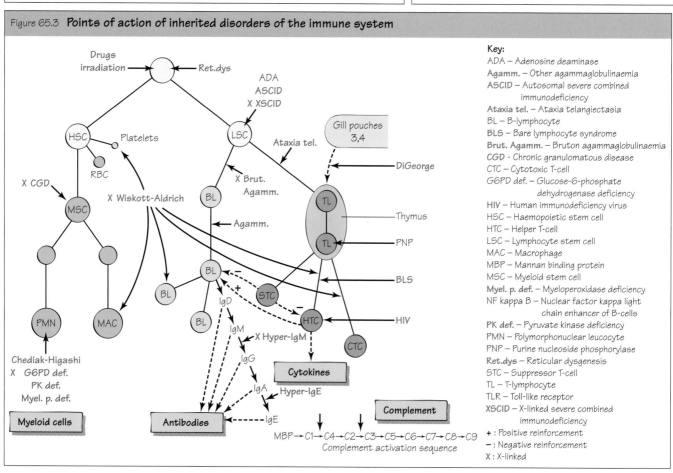

Key:
ADA – Adenosine deaminase
Agamm. – Other agammaglobulinaemia
ASCID – Autosomal severe combined immunodeficiency
Ataxia tel. – Ataxia telangiectasia
BL – B-lymphocyte
BLS – Bare lymphocyte syndrome
Brut. Agamm. – Bruton agammaglobulinaemia
CGD - Chronic granulomatous disease
CTC – Cytotoxic T-cell
G6PD def. – Glucose-6-phosphate dehydrogenase deficiency
HIV – Human immunodeficiency virus
HSC – Haemopoietic stem cell
HTC – Helper T-cell
LSC – Lymphocyte stem cell
MAC – Macrophage
MBP – Mannan binding protein
MSC – Myeloid stem cell
Myel. p. def. – Myeloperoxidase deficiency
NF kappa B – Nuclear factor kappa light chain enhancer of B-cells
PK def. – Pyruvate kinase deficiency
PMN – Polymorphonuclear leucocyte
PNP – Purine nucleoside phosphorylase
Ret.dys – Reticular dysgenesis
STC – Suppressor T-cell
TL – T-lymphocyte
TLR – Toll-like receptor
XSCID – X-linked severe combined immunodeficiency
+ : Positive reinforcement
− : Negative reinforcement
X : X-linked

Medical Genetics at a Glance, Third Edition. Dorian J. Pritchard and Bruce R. Korf.

Overview

Immunological **hypersensitivity** can cause **anaphylactic shock**, a rare and terrifying, sometimes fatal response to foreign substances, this being an exaggerated version of the more common allergic response to foreign antigens. Both involve attachment of antigen-specific IgE to **mast cells**. Physiological shock occurs when there is massive release by the mast cells of mediators such as histamine that impinge on smooth muscle, mucus glands and blood vessels. Death can occur from respiratory failure or vascular collapse. Antigens that trigger such 'atopic' responses are called **allergens**. A dominant autosomal allele that promotes **atopia** is carried by one in four northern Europeans (see Chapter 51).

Immunodeficiency results when one or more components of the immune system is missing or defective. More than 100 **primary immunodeficiency** syndromes have been described caused mainly by genetic defects affecting cells of the immune system. **Secondary immunodeficiency** can occur when the immune system is harmed by external factors such as **human immunodeficiency virus** (**HIV**). Immunodeficiency should be considered when babies have an unexplained failure to thrive, diarrhoea, recurrent or chronic infections, or unexplained **hepatosplenomegaly** (enlarged liver and spleen). Recurrent *bacterial* infection suggests humoral (B-cell) deficiency, whereas unusual susceptibility to *viral* infection is indicative of deficiency in cell-mediated immunity.

The immune system presents a serious challenge to blood transfusion and tissue/organ transplantation between individuals. **Autoimmune disease** occurs when the immune system turns against the tissues of the same individual. Both issues are dealt with in Chapter 66 (see also Chapter 29).

Hypersensitivity

Hypersensitivity is an aberrant immune response that damages the body's own tissues. There are four classes.
- Type 1: involves degranulation of mast cells and basophils cross-linked by IgE; symptoms range from mild discomfort to death.
- Type 2: IgG and IgM antibodies bind to antigens in or on the patient's own cells.
- Type 3: **immune complexes** are deposited in various tissues, these being aggregations of antigens, complement proteins, IgG and IgM.
- Type 4: usually takes 2–3 days to develop (e.g. 'contact dermatitis'), mediated by T cells, monocytes and macrophages.

Disorders of innate humoral immunity
Complement system defects
Genetics Mostly AR; HAO is AD.

Features Around 5–10% of the population has recurring respiratory tract infection, otitis media and chronic diarrhoea due to genetic defects in the **mannan binding protein** (MBP) pathway of complement activation.

Defects in complement C3 can cause failure of opsonization of bacteria, or upset the membrane attack complex (see Chapter 64), causing susceptibility to bacterial infection, especially by *Neisseria (Meningococcus)*.

Hereditary angioneurotic oedema (**HAO**) involves fluid accumulation in soft tissues and airways due to uncontrolled production of C2a, caused by deficiency of C1 inhibitor.

Management Infusion of plasma, or for HAO, C1 inhibitor, and daily therapy with attenuated androgens such as **danazol**.

Type 1 Interferon deficiency
Type 1 interferons are proteins produced by leucocytes in the frontline innate immune response against viral infection. They also play a role in induction of cytokines and stimulation of effector cells of the immune system. A common outcome of Type 1 deficiency is asthma.

Toll-like receptor deficiency
TLRs are transmembrane proteins already primed to recognize certain foreign antigens. A defect in **TLR5** predisposes to Legionnaire's disease.

Disorders of innate cell-mediated immunity
Neutropenia
The neutropenias are a heterogeneous group of disorders of innate cell-mediated immunity characterized by very low neutrophil counts.

Chronic granulomatous disease (CGD)
Genetics 1 XR, >3 AR

Features Phagocytes ingest foreign pathogens, but fail to destroy them, causing a persistent cellular immune response. **Granulomas** (nodular lesions) form containing macrophages (see Figure 65.1). Patients develop pneumonia, lymph node infections and abscesses in the skin, liver, etc.

Aetiology The XR form involves defective **Cytochrome b** that confers failure to generate hydrogen peroxide (see Figure 65.1).

Management Antibiotics, bone marrow transplantation.

Leucocyte adhesion deficiency (LAD)
Genetics AR

Features LAD I: a life-threatening, acute infection of skin and mucus membranes, with impaired pus formation. LAD II: psychomotor retardation and growth delay. LAD III: severe neonatal bleeding.

Aetiology LAD I: absence of the β2 component of the leucocyte **integrin** molecule involved in cell adhesion produces phagocytes unable to recognize and ingest microorganisms. LAD II: mutations in Golgi-specific GDP-fucose transporter. LAD III: defects in itegrin activation.

Management Antibiotics, bone marrow transplantation.

Chediak–Higashi syndrome
Genetics AR

Features Partial albinism, recurrent bacterial infections, malignant lymphoma.

Aetiology A defect in lysosome assembly causes deficiency specifically of natural killer cells.

Disorders of adaptive humoral immunity
X-linked (Bruton) agammaglobulinaemia (XLA)
Genetics XR

Features At 5–6 months boys develop multiple bacterial infections. Death can occur from chronic lung infection.

Aetiology Defective B-cell tyrosine kinase prevents maturation of B cells. Since maternal IgG crosses the placenta, infants may be unaffected for several months.

Management Prophylactic intravenous immunoglobulin.

Hyper-IgM syndrome
Genetics XR

Features Raised levels of IgM and IgD; other immunoglobulins decreased. Patients are susceptible to recurrent **pyogenic** (pus-generating) infections.

Aetiology In the most common type there is a defect in a T-cell surface ligand (CD40), preventing reception of signals, with failure of Ig class switching to IgG.

Hyper-IgE syndrome, Job syndrome
Genetics AD and AR

Features Patients have a 'coarse' facial appearance, abnormal dentition, hyperextensible joints and bone fractures, chronic eczema, recurrent infections and increased serum IgE.

Aetiology The AD form is due to a mutation in the *STAT3* (**S**ignal **T**ransducer and **A**ctivator of **T**ranscription 3) gene; AR to a mutation in *DOCK8* (**D**edicator **O**f **C**yto**K**inesis 8).

Common variable immunodeficiency (CVID)
The aetiology of the most common B-cell deficiency (1/800 Caucasians) is heterogeneous and generally unexplained. **Autosomal recessive B-cell immunodeficiency** can be caused by mutation of the Ig heavy and light chains.

Disorders of adaptive cell-mediated immunity
Severe combined immune deficiency (SCID)
(See also Chapter 61.)

Genetics 50–60% XR, AR

Features Lethal susceptibility to both viral and bacterial infections due to profound deficiency of both humoral and cell-mediated immunity.

Aetiology The XR forms have mutations in the γ-chain common to several cytokine receptors, so that T cells and natural killer cells fail to receive signals for normal maturation. This in turn upsets B-cell development, as this requires T-cell interaction.

Mutation of the intracellular signalling molecule **Jak3** (**J**anus **kinase 3**), with which the cytokine receptors interact, also causes failure of T-cell maturation, as does deficiency of **protein-tyrosine phosphatase receptor type C** (**CD45**), since CD45 normally suppresses Jak. Deficiencies in **adenosine deaminase** (**ADA**) (Chapter 61) and **purine nucleoside phosphorylase** (**PNP**) both cause accumulation of purine breakdown products that kill T cells.

SCID can also be caused by mutations in genes involving V-D-J recombination and formation of T-cell and B-cell receptors (see Chapter 64).

Management The ADA-deficient and XR forms can be treated by bone marrow transplantation and attempts are being made at gene therapy (see Chapter 74).

Bare lymphocyte syndrome (BLS)
Genetics AR

Features Lymphocytes lack surface MHC display.

Aetiology Type 1: mutations in the *TAP2* (**T**ransporter associated with **A**ntigen **P**resentation 2) gene prevent export of Class I MHC molecules to the surface. Type II has defects in MHC Class II specific transcription factors, causing deficiency of functional helper T cells.

Associated and secondary immunodeficiency
DiGeorge syndrome
Genetics AR, AD and sporadic

Features See Chapter 39.

Aetiology DiGeorge syndrome is part of a spectrum of phenotypes caused by abnormalities of the third and fourth gill pouches consequent upon contiguous gene deletion in Chromosome 22q11.2 (Chapters 39 and 40). Complete or partial absence of the thymus reduces production of T cells allowing recurrent viral infections, which however usually decrease with age. (See Chapters 42 and 64)

Wiskott–Aldrich syndrome
Genetics XR

Features Boys have eczema, diarrhoea and recurrent infections, **thrombocytopenia** (low platelet count), low IgM levels and failure of cytotoxic T-cell and helper T-cell function. Death can occur from haemorrhage or B-cell malignancy.

Aetiology The basic defect is in the lymphocyte cytoskeleton.

Management Bone marrow transplantation.

Ataxia telangiectasia
Genetics AR

Features Problems with balance and coordination, with **oculocutaneous telangiectasia** (dilated blood vessels in the conjunctivae, ears and face). There are low serum IgA and IgG levels and susceptibility to sinus and pulmonary infection. Lymphocyte chromosomes show rearrangements of Chromosomes 7 and 14 at the T-cell receptor loci (see Chapter 64).

Aetiology There is a failure of repair of DNA damage, which can lead to thymus hypoplasia and an increased risk of leukaemia and lymphoma (see Chapter 26).

Immune system subversion
Cytomegalovirus (CMV)
Some CMV strains evade T-cell detection by down-regulating expression by the host of Class I MHC protein and substituting their own non-functional versions.

Human immune deficiency virus (HIV)
See 'Resistance to HIV', Chapter 29.

A deletion within **chemokine receptor 5** (**CCR5**) causes resistance to HIV, but confers predisposition to African Nile virus infection. CCR5 is used by HIV to gain entry into macrophages.

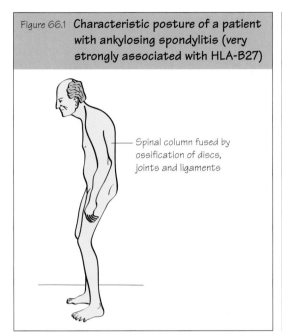

Figure 66.1 Characteristic posture of a patient with ankylosing spondylitis (very strongly associated with HLA-B27)

Spinal column fused by ossification of discs, joints and ligaments

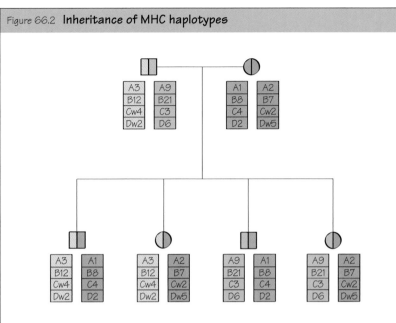

Figure 66.2 Inheritance of MHC haplotypes

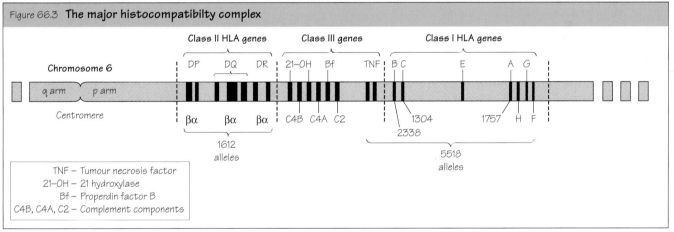

Figure 66.3 The major histocompatibilty complex

TNF – Tumour necrosis factor
21–OH – 21 hydroxylase
Bf – Properdin factor B
C4B, C4A, C2 – Complement components

Overview

The proteins of the **major histocompatibility complex (MHC)** are present on the surfaces of all nucleated cells (see Chapter 64). *They show extraordinarily wide polymorphism, but are uniform within an individual*. In the context of tissue and organ transplantation they act as antigens and are known as the **HLA** or **human leucocyte antigen** system. All the HLA genes are closely linked at 6p21.3.

MHC molecules fall into three classes. Class I (Figure 64.3) constitute an integral part of the plasma membranes of virtually all body cells and are responsible for presenting antigenic peptides to *cytotoxic T cells*. The peptides are derived by proteolytic degradation of *endogenous* antigens, derived for example from intracellular viruses, by the action of a large multifunctional protease (see Chapters 64 and 65). The Class I proteins are encoded by genes *HLA-A, -B, -C, -E, -F, -G, -H, -L, -J, -P* and *-V*, and become functional when linked with a β_2-**microglobulin** molecule.

Class II proteins are heterodimers of α and β subunits with homology to immunoglobulin (Figures 64.2 and 64.4), coded by genes *HLA-*

DP, -DQ, and *-DR* (see Figure 66.3). They occur on B cells and macrophages and are involved in presenting peptides to *helper T cells* (Figure 64.6). The antigenic material in these cases is derived from *exogenous* (i.e. extracellular) proteins that have been broken down after phagocytosis within lysosomes.

Class III includes a variety of proteins of related function, notably components of the **complement** system (Chapter 64). Functionally unrelated genes that map to the same region include those for **congenital adrenal hyperplasia** (**CAH**) (see Chapter 44) and **primary haemochromatosis**.

Some 20 loci affect cytokine levels, signalling pathways in immune cells and non-immunological steps in tissue damage.

Acquisition of tolerance

A transcription factor, the **autoimmune regulator** protein, **AIRE**, is expressed in the thymus where it controls immune tolerance (see Chapter 64). Medullary thymus epithelial cells express otherwise 'tissue-specific'

Medical Genetics at a Glance, Third Edition. Dorian J. Pritchard and Bruce R. Korf.
© 2013 John Wiley & Sons, Ltd. Published 2013 by John Wiley & Sons, Ltd.

antigens representing virtually the whole of the body. Through the agency of the AIRE, T cells capable of binding 'self-antigens' are then triggered to undergo apoptosis and are eliminated from the system. Self-recognizing B lymphocytes are likewise eliminated in the bone marrow, although some may survive if the self-antigen concentration is low.

Presentation of microbial products to T cells by immature dendritic cells lacking the full complement of co-stimulatory molecules may constitute a *negative* signal, so inducing tolerance. In addition, T cells contribute to tolerance by sometimes transmitting negative signals.

Autoimmune disease

In autoimmune disease, tolerance breaks down and cytotoxic T cells proliferate and destroy the patient's own tissues. It can be organ-specific (e.g. **Hashimoto thyroiditis)** or **systemic** (e.g. **systemic lupus erythematosus, SLE**) and is typically most common in females.

Some autoimmune diseases show association with specific HLA alleles, which can be used to predict the probability of an individual developing a disease independently of familial issues. Table 66.1 lists some important autoimmune disorders and Table 66.2 shows the relative risks of developing these diseases in relation to HLA carrier status (see also Chapter 13).

Autoimmune polyendocrinopathy syndrome, Type 1, APS-1

Features This condition is characterized by two or all three of the following conditions: **Addison disease**, **hypoparathyroidism** and **chronic mucocutaneous candidiasis**. Malabsorption and diarrhoea dominate the clinical picture.

Aetiology Mutations in the gene for AIRE.

Nuclear factor kappa B signalling

Nuclear factor kappa B (NFκ B) is a rapid response transcription factor that controls expression of cytokines, cell adhesion molecules, growth factors and immunoreceptors. Inappropriate activation of NFκ B has been linked to autoimmune arthritis, asthma, septic shock, lung fibrosis, glomerular-nephritis, atherosclerosis and AIDS. Its persistent inhibition is associated with apoptosis, abnormal immune cell development and delayed cell growth.

Ankylosing spondylitis (AS, poker spine)

AS is a chronic inflammatory condition that leads to fusion of the spine and sacroiliac junctions (see Figure 66.1). Over 90% of AS patients carry HLA-B27. Five per cent of Europeans overall carry HLA-B27 and, although only 1% of these have AS, their theoretical risk is 90 times that of those who are B27-negative. This genetic association is thought to involve interference with the normal immune response to the bacterium *Klebsiella*.

Causes of autoimmunity

1 Exposure of 'privileged sites' sequestered during acquisition of tolerance, e.g. proteins inside the eyeball or bone.
2 Mutation in the *AIRE* gene, or inappropriate activation of NFκB.
3 An invading pathogen sharing antigenic features with its host triggers anti-self response through residual self-reactive B cells.
4 First contact between self-antigens and the immune system at a late developmental stage, for example at spermatogenesis.
5 Residual self-reactive B cells stimulated to proliferate continuously by microbial polyclonal activators, for example Epstein–Barr virus.
6 Anomalous antigen presentation, for example in thyroiditis and diabetes.
7 Deficiency in suppressor T cells, for example diabetes, rheumatoid arthritis, SLE.

Explanations for HLA-disease association

1 Close genetic linkage of disease susceptibility genes to the MHC complex. For example, primary haemochromatosis and CAH due to 21-hydroxylase deficiency are caused by disease alleles that arose at 6p21.3 relatively recently and have not yet had time to segregate by chromosomal crossover from their original close neighbours in the MHC. Such disease alleles show **linkage disequilibrium** with specific **HLA haplotypes**.
2 Close similarity of structure of HLA antigens and environmental antigens ('**cross-reactivity**'). Possible examples are **ankylosing spondylitis** and Type 1 diabetes mellitus.

Tissue incompatibility in transfusion and transplantation

As a general rule a recipient will reject a tissue graft from a person who possesses a cell surface antigen absent from the recipient. The most important of these are the molecules of the HLA system.

The HLA system is very highly polymorphic, with, to date (2013), 1757 A antigens, 2338 B and 1304 C, with the other Class I loci making a total of 5518 Class I allelic variants, in addition to 1612 D in Class II. These numbers were determined by DNA sequencing. The genes are

Table 66.1 Some autoimmune diseases.

Autoimmune diseases	Causative antigen
Addison disease	Adrenal cortex components
Pernicious anaemia	Gastric intrinsic factor (vitamin B_{12} carrier)
Type 1 (insulin dependent) diabetes mellitus (T1DM)	Pancreatic β-cells
Graves disease	
Hashimoto thyroiditis	Receptor for pituitary thyroid stem hormone
Membranous glomerulonephritis	
Multiple sclerosis	Myelin
Myasthenia gravis	Postsynaptic acetylcholine receptors
Polymyositis	
Rheumatoid arthritis (RA)	'Rheumatoid factor' (IgG)
Scleroderma	
Sjögren syndrome	
Systemic lupus erythematosus (SLE)	DNA, RNA, chromosomal proteins

Table 66.2 Important HLA associations of some common diseases.

HLA group	Disease	Frequency in patients (%)	Frequency in general population	Relative risk for carriers
A3	Haemochromatosis	75	13	20
B17	Psoriasis	38	8	7
B27	Ankylosing spondylitis	>90	8	>100
	Reiter syndrome	75	8	35
B47	CAH	17	0.4	51
Cw6	Psoriasis	>50	9	>10
DR2	Narcolepsy	~100	16	>100
	Goodpasture syndrome	88	32	16
	Multiple sclerosis	57	21	5
	SLE	>70	16	>12
DR3	SLE	50	25	3
	Coeliac disease	60	12	11
	T1DM	50	12	7
DR4	T1DM	38	13	4
DR3//DR4	T1DM			33
DR5	Juvenile RA	50	16	5
	Pernicious anaemia	25	6	5

CAH, congenital adrenal hyperplasia; HLA, human leucocyte antigen; T1DM, insulin dependent diabetes mellitus; RA, rheumatoid arthritis; SLE, systemic lupus erythematosus.
Relative risk = ad/bc, where a = number of patients with the antigen, b = number of controls with the antigen, c = number of patients without the antigen, d = number of controls without the antigen.

closely linked, so alleles tend to be inherited together as a group 'haplo-type'. A1 and B8 show linkage disequilibrium of association in western Europeans, that is the A1/B8 combination is common. In north Europeans CAH due to 21-hydroxylase deficiency is associated positively with HLA haplotype A3/B47/DR7 and negatively with HLA-A1/B8/DR3.

If a parental couple has a total of four different haplotypes, each offspring has a 25% chance of inheriting the same combination as any of his/her sibs (see Figure 66.2). MZ twins have a complete antigen match and DZ twins, although sharing only 50% of their genes, may accept reciprocal grafts if they shared a placental circulation prenatally when tolerance was established (see Chapter 53).

The 10-year success rate for kidney transplantation is currently ~70% when recipient and donor are HLA-identical siblings, but <60% when they share only one haplotype. The chance of a random match between unrelated individuals is ~1/200 000 so, apart from grafts into privileged sites, successful transplantation generally requires pharmaceutical immunosuppression.

Bone marrow transplantation however introduces the additional problem of **graft-versus-host rejection** or **GVH disease**. Survival to 8 years after a bone marrow graft for chronic myelogenous leukaemia following chemotherapy is 60% with a single Class I or Class II mismatch, 25% if there is mismatch in both HLA classes.

The ABO blood groups

The ABO blood groups are a major consideration in tissue transplantation because their antigens are displayed on most body cells. As in whole blood transfusion, Group O are 'universal donors' and AB 'universal recipients' (see Chapter 29).

67 DNA hybridization-based analysis systems

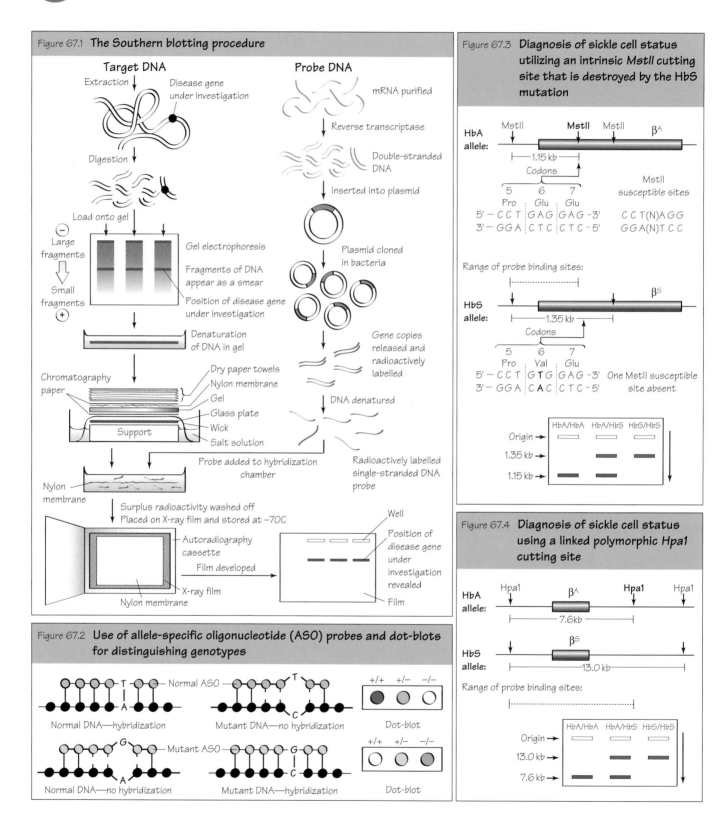

Figure 67.1 The Southern blotting procedure

Target DNA
- Extraction
- Disease gene under investigation
- Digestion
- Load onto gel
  - (−) Large fragments
  - Small fragments (+)
- Gel electrophoresis
- Fragments of DNA appear as a smear
- Position of disease gene under investigation
- Denaturation of DNA in gel
- Dry paper towels
- Nylon membrane
- Chromatography paper
- Gel
- Glass plate
- Wick
- Support
- Salt solution
- Nylon membrane
- Surplus radioactivity washed off
- Placed on X-ray film and stored at −70C
- Autoradiography cassette
- Film developed
- X-ray film
- Nylon membrane
- Well
- Position of disease gene under investigation revealed
- Film

Probe DNA
- mRNA purified
- Reverse transcriptase
- Double-stranded DNA
- Inserted into plasmid
- Plasmid cloned in bacteria
- Gene copies released and radioactively labelled
- DNA denatured
- Probe added to hybridization chamber
- Radioactively labelled single-stranded DNA probe

Figure 67.2 Use of allele-specific oligonucleotide (ASO) probes and dot-blots for distinguishing genotypes

- Normal ASO — T / A — Normal DNA—hybridization
- Mutant DNA—no hybridization — T / C
- Dot-blot: +/+ +/− −/−
- Mutant ASO — G / A — Normal DNA—no hybridization
- Mutant DNA—hybridization — G / C
- Dot-blot: +/+ +/− −/−

Figure 67.3 Diagnosis of sickle cell status utilizing an intrinsic MstII cutting site that is destroyed by the HbS mutation

HbA allele: MstII | MstII | MstII | β^A
- 1.15 kb
- Codons
- MstII susceptible sites

	5	6	7
	Pro	Glu	Glu

5' − C C T : G A G : G A G − 3'   C C T (N) A G G
3' − G G A : C T C : C T C − 5'   G G A (N) T C C

Range of probe binding sites:

HbS allele: β^S
- 1.35 kb
- Codons
- One MstII susceptible site absent

	5	6	7
	Pro	Val	Glu

5' − C C T : G **T** G : G A G − 3'
3' − G G A : C **A** C : C T C − 5'

Gel:
- Origin →
- 1.35 kb →
- 1.15 kb →
- HbA/HbA   HbA/HbS   HbS/HbS

Figure 67.4 Diagnosis of sickle cell status using a linked polymorphic Hpa1 cutting site

HbA allele: Hpa1 | β^A | Hpa1 | Hpa1
- 7.6 kb

HbS allele: β^S
- 13.0 kb

Range of probe binding sites:

Gel:
- Origin →
- 13.0 kb →
- 7.6 kb →
- HbA/HbA   HbA/HbS   HbS/HbS

Medical Genetics at a Glance, Third Edition. Dorian J. Pritchard and Bruce R. Korf.

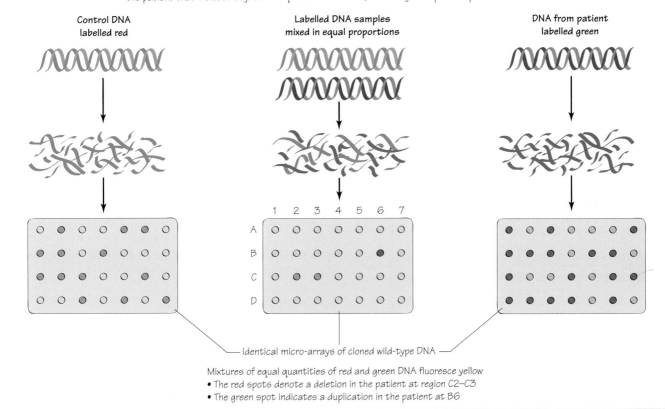

Figure 67.5 **Array comparative genome hybridization**

The array on the left illustrates a display obtained by hybridization of control DNA, labelled red, to a micro-array of wild-type (i.e. 'normal') oligonucleotide clones. The one on the right shows the equivalent for DNA from a patient, labelled green. The centre pattern is what would be obtained by competitive hybridization of the mixed red and green samples, denatured and hybridized to the same micro-array. In this the red spots identify a deletion in the DNA of the patient that includes adjacent sequences C3 and C4, and the green spot a duplication at B6.

Control DNA
labelled red

Labelled DNA samples
mixed in equal proportions

DNA from patient
labelled green

Identical micro-arrays of cloned wild-type DNA

Mixtures of equal quantities of red and green DNA fluoresce yellow
• The red spots denote a deletion in the patient at region C2–C3
• The green spot indicates a duplication in the patient at B6

Overview

A set of highly specialized molecular techniques, collectively known as 'Southern blotting', was one of the earliest effective molecular diagnostic approaches. Although largely superseded now, the components of the original method are applied in many other techniques. Five concepts are necessary to understand the Southern blotting procedure: **DNA probes**, **restriction endonucleases**, gel electrophoresis, DNA polymorphism and **DNA hybridization**.

DNA probes

A DNA probe is a short section (0.3–5.0 kb, or longer) of double-stranded DNA corresponding to part of the locus of interest. It can be prepared, for example, from the **cDNA** (complimentary DNA) copies of purified mRNA, generated with the enzyme **reverse transcriptase**, then radioactively labelled and 'denatured' into single strands. Alternatively, cloned segments of genomic DNA or synthetic oligonucleotides can be used.

Restriction endonucleases and DNA polymorphism

Restriction endonucleases are bacterial enzymes that cut double-stranded DNA at specific sequences, usually 4–8 bases in length. The sections of DNA that result are called **restriction fragments**. Variation in base sequence at the restriction enzyme recognition site can result in failure of an enzyme to cut the site, referred to as **restriction frag-**

ment length polymorphism (RFLP). These variant cutting sites provide valuable markers for disease genes that have been exploited in linkage studies (see Chapter 34), though these days, other techniques are generally used.

Gel electrophoresis

A gel is a three-dimensional mesh with pores of different sizes. They are cast as slabs of **agarose** or **polyacrylamide**, with a row of wells at one end for insertion of samples. During electrophoresis the gel is subjected to an electric current, when negatively charged DNA fragments are repelled by the negative terminal, or cathode, and migrate toward the **anode**. The smallest fragments run fastest, with the others behind them in order of size.

DNA hybridization in Southern blotting

The usual source of DNA is white blood cells, but for prenatal diagnosis samples may be taken from amniotic fluid cell cultures or chorionic villi (see Chapter 72). The DNA is digested with restriction enzymes, inserted into a well of the gel and the electric current applied.

The electrophoretically fractionated DNA is next denatured into single strands and transferred to a nylon membrane, by the Southern blotting technique (see Figure 67.1). This in effect produces a print of the DNA array in the gel, with all its bands in perfect register. The DNA is then bound to the membrane by exposure to UV light and incubated in a solution containing the denatured radioactive probe.

The probe 'hybridizes' with its complementary sequence in the sample. Unbound probe DNA is washed away and the position of the bound radioactivity is located by autoradiography or direct scanning. Alternatively, probes may be linked to molecules that can be detected through non-radioactive means.

Methodological variants

Northern blotting
Northern blotting is used to identify mRNA species in a mixture. RNA cannot be cleaved by the restriction endonucleases used for DNA analysis. However, RNA transcripts are naturally single-stranded and of different lengths so can be separated according to size by gel electrophoresis and probed in a similar way.

Dot blots and allele-specific oligonucleotides (ASOs)
When both normal and mutant sequences are known, very short 'oligonucleotide' probes can be synthesized biochemically to match each one. These are hybridized to 'dot-blots' of denatured DNA applied directly to a nylon membrane, allowing rapid identification of homozygotes and heterozygotes, and distinction between alleles.

This approach offers an inexpensive and rapid method of diagnosis, but is limited by the need for prior knowledge of mutant sequences.

Pulsed field gel electrophoresis
Standard agarose gel electrophoresis efficiently separates DNA fragments only up to 30kb in length. This modification enables resolution of DNA fragments ranging in size from 20 000 to several million base pairs.

White blood cells are embedded in agarose blocks which are exposed to proteolytic enzymes that digest away cellular materials, leaving the chromosomes intact. They are then exposed to 'rare cutter' restriction endonucleases which create very long pieces of DNA defined by the susceptible sequences at each end. These are separated electrophoretically in agarose gel, but every so often the direction of the current is changed by 90°. The DNA fragments are therefore repeatedly required to change conformation and, since the time taken for them to reorient themselves is size dependent, they end up in reverse order of size along the diagonal. This allows examination and separation of very large genes, like dystrophin, and multigenic functional units.

Diagnostic applications
One application involves selection of a restriction endonuclease for which the recognition site corresponds with either the mutant or normal version of the sequence in question. DNA is cut with the enzyme and the fragments are analysed using as a probe a DNA sequence near the site of mutation. If the mutation disrupts a normal cutting site, that segment of DNA will remain intact. Presence or absence of the mutation can then be determined by comparing fragment sizes.

An example is sickle cell disease (see Figure 25.2). In the normal β-globin allele the sixth codon is cut by the enzyme *Mst*II, but the HbS mutation destroys that site and a longer DNA fragment is produced. In most cases polymorphic cutting sites are identified outside the disease genes (see Figure 67.3).

In most laboratories the polymerase chain reaction (PCR) has replaced Southern analysis for detection of specific alterations in base sequence (see Chapter 69), but it still finds application where larger rearrangements are involved.

Very long triplet repeat expansions (see Chapter 28) cannot be reliably amplified by PCR, but Southern analysis can reveal the expanded allele by its reduced mobility. In fragile X disease (see Chapters 11 and 38) the unexpressed, expanded allele is invariably methylated; differential diagnosis can therefore be performed with a restriction endonuclease that cleaves only *non*-methylated DNA.

Array comparative genome hybridization (array CGH)
Array comparative genome hybridization is a recent method for detecting or locating chromosomal microdeletions. This approach exploits the extraordinary miniaturization and accuracy of inkjet printing and the speed of computer-based analysis.

Array CGH uses competitive hybridization between DNA from the patient and an unaffected control to detect differences in 'copy number' of chromosomal regions. A microarray of dots of cloned oligonucleotides would typically cover the whole genome, with 100 000 oligonucleotides corresponding to sites spaced <30kb apart throughout. Equal quantities of DNA from the patient and control, labelled with different fluorochromes, say green and red, are mixed and hybridized to the whole array. After washing off unbound probes, the fluorescence at both wavelengths is measured and the red : green ratio calculated for each clone. One or more adjacent red spots would indicate a deletion at that location. If the spot(s) were green, that suggests a duplication. Array CGH, or other micro-array-based methods, are becoming the test of choice for large deletions and duplications.

68 DNA sequencing

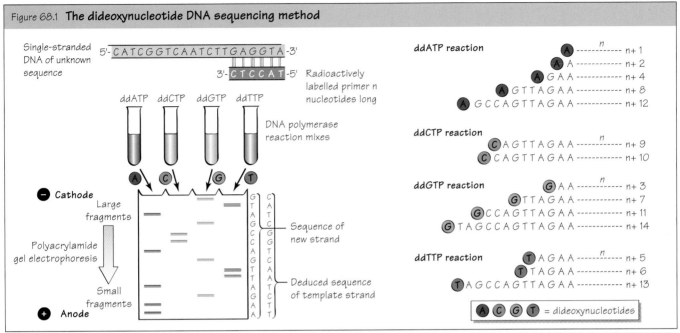

Figure 68.1 **The dideoxynucleotide DNA sequencing method**

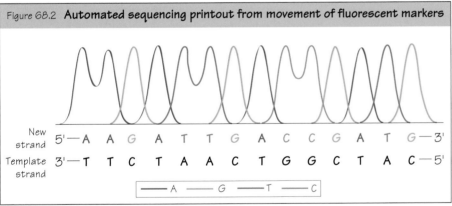

Figure 68.2 **Automated sequencing printout from movement of fluorescent markers**

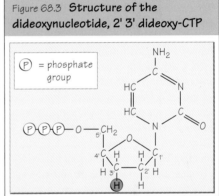

Figure 68.3 **Structure of the dideoxynucleotide, 2' 3' dideoxy-CTP**

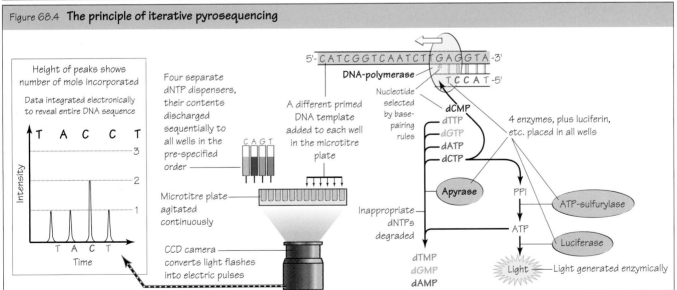

Figure 68.4 **The principle of iterative pyrosequencing**

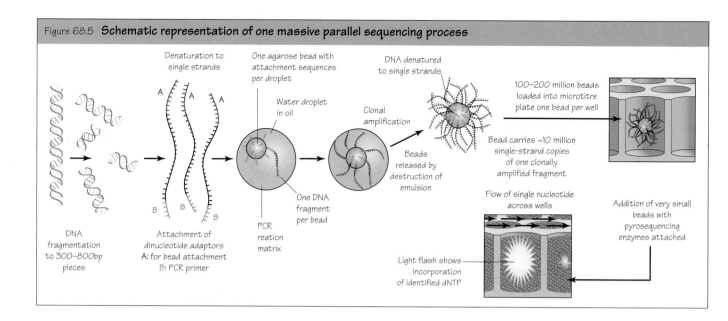

Figure 68.5 **Schematic representation of one massive parallel sequencing process**

DNA fragmentation to 300–800bp pieces

Attachment of dinucleotide adaptors
A: for bead attachment
B: PCR primer

Denaturation to single strands

One agarose bead with attachment sequences per droplet

Water droplet in oil

PCR reation matrix

One DNA fragment per bead

Clonal amplification

DNA denatured to single strands

Beads released by destruction of emulsion

100–200 million beads loaded into microtitre plate one bead per well

Bead carries ~10 million single-strand copies of one clonally amplified fragment

Flow of single nucleotide across wells

Light flash shows incorporation of identified dNTP

Addition of very small beads with pyrosequencing enzymes attached

Overview

DNA sequencing is a mainstay of current research, but can also be used in diagnostic testing, especially when the aim is to identify *specific* pathogenic mutations. To determine whether a known mutation, or the normal sequence, is present generally involves knowing the sequence for a short stretch around that site. In an individual heterozygous for a single base substitution two different bases would be present there, one on each strand. Heterozygous insertions or deletions produce a complex pattern of superimposed sequences.

DNA sequencing can also be used to scan large regions of genes for mutations. Not finding a mutation does not necessarily mean no mutation is present, as causative errors may exist in regulatory regions outside the structural gene. It should also be recognized that not all sequence variants disrupt gene function, as would be necessary for it to constitute a pathogenic mutation. Furthermore, deletion or duplication of an entire gene can remain undetected by sequencing.

Evidence that a variant is pathogenic might include inference from its likely impact on the gene product; for example, mutations that cause frameshifts are more likely to disrupt function than single base substitutions (see Chapter 25). Demonstration that a mutation is present only in affected individuals and segregates in families, together with disease, is highly suggestive of that mutation being the cause of the disorder, or else is in close linkage with it. Another important clue is recapitulation of the mutant phenotype in an animal model based on the known mutation. In some cases, computer programs can be used to model the effects of a mutation on the functioning of the protein.

Direct sequencing is currently not the method of choice for most diagnostic laboratories, when the goal is to identify the presence of a limited repertoire of mutations. In these situations techniques such as PCR followed by restriction enzyme digestion or oligonucleotide hybridization (see Chapters 67 and 69) may be most suitable.

Direct sequencing is, however, used commonly in the identification of some mutations, such as in the *BRCA1* and *BRCA2* genes (see Chapter 56). Here mutant sites are highly diverse and widely scattered, making it necessary to scan gene sequences in full.

Until recently most DNA sequencing was largely carried out by the dideoxy-DNA method of Sanger and co-workers; the end result from this technique is a ladder of bands, from which the base sequence can be read directly, or a row of peaks on a graph.

The dideoxy-DNA sequencing method

For this method the DNA to be sequenced is prepared in multiple copies of one 'template' strand. DNA polymerase is then used to synthesize multiple new complementary strands.

The enzymic reaction requires a primer complementary to the 3′ end of the sequence, DNA polymerase, co-factors, etc. and base-specific **dideoxynucleotides** (ddATP, ddTTP, ddCTP and ddGTP), in addition to the normal deoxynucleotide precursors (dATP, etc.). The dideoxynucleotides lack the hydroxyl group on the 3′ carbon atoms of deoxynucleotides which in DNA forms the link to the adjacent nucleotide. They are incorporated into growing DNA as normal, but chain extension is blocked beyond them by lack of the 3′ hydroxyl group.

Four parallel base-specific reactions are conducted using a mix of all four normal nucleotide precursors, one with a radioactive label, plus a small proportion of *one* of the four dideoxy-derivatives. If the concentration of the latter is low compared to that of its normal analogue, chain termination occurs randomly at each of the many positions containing that specific base. Each base-specific reaction generates many fragments of different lengths, with variable 3′ termini but a common 5′ end, corresponding to the primer.

In the original method the DNA fragments were then separated by electrophoresis through polyacrylamide gel, in which they migrate at speeds inversely proportional to their lengths. Following electrophoresis the gel was dried out and an autoradiographic (or X-ray) film placed in contact with it. After suitable exposure the film was developed to produce a pattern of dark bands. The sequence was then read off by simple inspection of the autoradiograph, providing the 5′-to-3′ sequence of the new strand complementary to the original template.

This process was later automated by attaching four differently coloured fluorescent markers to the four ddNTPs, instead of a radioactive label. The DNA synthesis is then performed in one vessel and the fluor-labelled reaction products are electrophoresed together through a capillary glass tube. As they migrate past a window they are excited by a beam of laser light and emit coloured fluorescence. This is captured by a digital camera, translated into an electric signal and represented as a graph, with the four dideoxynucleotides shown as peaks of different colours. The position of a mutation is then located by comparison of mutant and normal sequences. These adaptations allow sequencing to proceed at a rate of up to a million bases per day.

Iterative pyrosequencing

Iterative pyrosequencing is a very rapid process that eliminates time-consuming electrophoresis. Instead, this method monitors the sequential incorporation of nucleotides as a complementary strand of DNA is assembled by DNA polymerase along a single-strand template. Instead of adding a *mixture* of the four deoxyribonucleotide triphosphate (dNTP) precursors (C, G, A and T), these are provided sequentially. When the correct one is accepted its monophosphate derivative gets incorporated and this incorporation is revealed by release of pyrophosphate (PPi) which is used to generate light. The PPi generates ATP from ADP using **ATP sulfurylase** and the new ATP drives a **luciferase** reaction that generates a light flash which is recorded digitally. This indicates not only the identity of the dNTP species, but also the number of copies of that base that are inserted. Inappropriate dNTPs and excess ATP are degraded by **apyrase**.

Massively parallel, or next-generation, DNA sequencing

This is also currently known as 'next-generation sequencing' (NGS), with several techniques under this heading. The first to become commercially available (Roche 454 GS/FLX) is an adaptation of pyrosequencing. This involves cutting the sample DNA into fragments 300–800 bp long and splitting them into single strands. These are prepared for PCR amplification (Chapter 69) by incubating with two different single-strand DNA 'adaptors' that attach to their termini. Those that acquire *different* adaptors (A and B in Figure 68.5) are then separated out and bound to spherical agarose beads with oligonucleotide sequences on their surfaces complementary to one of the adaptors, under conditions that favour attachment of only one DNA strand per bead. The beads are then captured within an oil–water emulsion containing reagents for the PCR (Chapter 69). Clonal amplification then occurs within each emulsion droplet until 10 million copies of each segment has been produced and immobilized on that bead.

The emulsion is then 'broken', releasing the beads, which are deposited singly in tiny wells in a glass slide. The pyrosequencing reaction mix (see above), with the key enzymes attached to smaller beads is added to the wells and a controlled series of dNTP precursors (T, G, A, C; T, G, A, C; T, G . . . etc.) is then washed over the slide. Chemiluminescent light is generated with every nucleotide incorporated, according to base pairing rules. The pattern of light signals is scanned by a CCD camera and recorded for each well, indicating the nucleotide sequence of each strand. Hundreds of thousands of short sequences can be read in parallel, with an overall through-put 10 000 times that of dideoxy-sequencing. The individual sequences are then ordered by recognition of overlaps, and comparison with the 'wild-type' sequence (see Chapter 32).

More recent developments increase this rate of sequencing a further 100-fold! There are currently multiple commercial systems that employ various approaches to massively parallel sequencing, making this currently one of the most rapidly advancing areas in genomic technology.

Figure 69.1 One cycle of the PCR gene amplification procedure

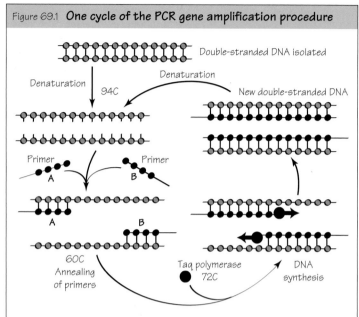

Figure 69.2 Use of quantitative PCR for testing a family with Duchenne muscular dystrophy

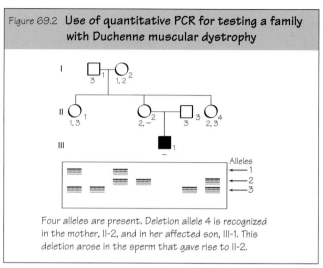

Four alleles are present. Deletion allele 4 is recognized in the mother, II-2, and in her affected son, III-1. This deletion arose in the sperm that gave rise to II-2.

Figure 69.3 Use of the ARMS test to distinguish sickle cell and normal β-globin alleles

The normal primer enables amplification of only the normal β-globin allele; the sickle cell primer amplifies only the mutant β-globin DNA

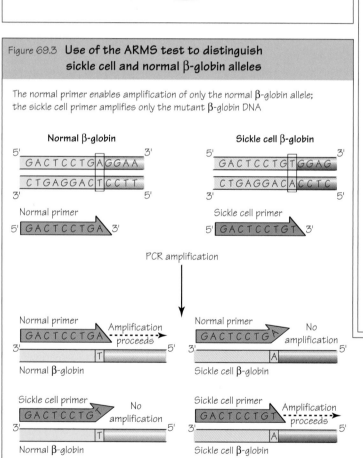

Figure 69.4 Use of PCR in testing for Huntington disease

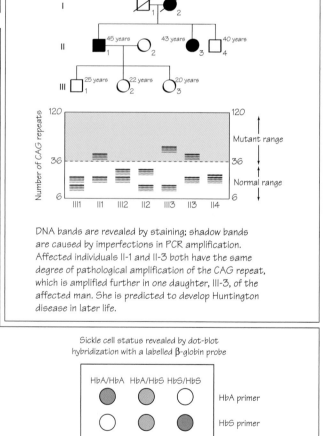

DNA bands are revealed by staining; shadow bands are caused by imperfections in PCR amplification. Affected individuals II-1 and II-3 both have the same degree of pathological amplification of the CAG repeat, which is amplified further in one daughter, III-3, of the affected man. She is predicted to develop Huntington disease in later life.

Sickle cell status revealed by dot-blot hybridization with a labelled β-globin probe

Medical Genetics at a Glance, Third Edition. Dorian J. Pritchard and Bruce R. Korf.

182 © 2013 John Wiley & Sons, Ltd. Published 2013 by John Wiley & Sons, Ltd.

Overview

The **polymerase chain reaction** (**PCR**) has utterly revolutionized the diagnosis and molecular analysis of genetic disease. Analyses can be performed on samples as minute as a single nucleus obtained from a preimplantation embryo, a mouthwash, hair root or other source. It is performed in a few hours and is cheaper than any other method. *PCR-based techniques have therefore become the most widely used methods of genetic analysis.*

The polymerase chain reaction

The reaction uses *Taq* DNA polymerase and operates on single-strand DNA, replacing the missing strand in much the same way as in DNA replication (see Chapter 20). *Taq* polymerase is isolated from *Thermus aquaticus*, a hot-spring bacterium and can withstand temperatures up to 95°C. It requires a start point of duplex DNA, which is provided by single-strand **primers** annealed one at each end of the sequence to be duplicated.

To carry out the reaction the DNA sample is first heated to 94°C to 'melt' the hydrogen bonds joining the two polynucleotide strands. The temperature is reduced to ~60° and short oligonucleotide primers are added. These are usually 15–30 nucleotides long and designed to match and anneal to complementary conserved stretches flanking the chosen sequence. In the third step, carried out at 72°, the polymerase moves down the DNA strand, away from the primers and synthesizes a complementary strand, so recreating a double-stranded molecule.

This set of three steps can be considered as one 'cycle', which is repeated by careful temperature control in the presence of excess primers. Each cycle takes only a few minutes and the amount of DNA doubles every time. After 30 cycles over 100 000 000 copies of the original sequence are created. The process is normally performed automatically in a programmed thermocycler.

PCR can also be used to amplify RNA sequences, if they are first copied into cDNA replicates by means of reverse transcriptase.

Comparative advantages of PCR

- **Sensitivity:** PCR is applicable to as little as single-genome quantities of DNA.
- **Speed:** the procedure is very fast (3–48 hours).
- **Safety:** no radioactivity is involved.
- **Molecular product:** the product is suitable for further analysis by established molecular techniques.
- **Resolution**: the process can be applied to even degraded DNA.

Disadvantages of PCR

- **Size of template:** long sequences cannot be amplified.
- **Prior knowledge:** the sequence of flanking regions must be known.
- **Contamination:** absolute purity of the sample is essential.
- **Infidelity of replication:** there is no 'proof-reading', or error correction, so that mutations that occasionally arise during the process are also propagated.

Diagnostic applications

The value of PCR in diagnosis lies in its ability to provide large quantities of specific gene sequences that can be subjected to further analysis. Primers are used that flank one specific region of a gene, or alternatively multiple regions such as several exons. Applications include the following:

1 Diagnosis of triplet repeat disorders (e.g. MD, Type 1 and Huntington disease; see Figure 69.4 and Chapters 11 and 28).

2 Direct sequencing of the gene(s) (see Chapter 68).

3 Restriction endonuclease digestion. This approach can be applied when a *specific* mutation is being sought. An endonuclease is chosen that has a recognition sequence spanning the mutant site (see Chapter 67). The enzyme will then either cut or fail to cut the DNA, depending on whether the mutation is present. Analysis of fragment sizes by agarose gel electrophoresis then indicates the genotype.

4 Single-strand conformation polymorphism (SSCP). PCR-amplified DNA is denatured and electrophoresed without renaturation, when mutant strands are detectable by their speeds of migration.

5 Allele-specific oligonucleotide (ASO) dot blots. This method, described in Chapter 67, is commonly used where analysis involves detection of a single mutation (e.g. sickle cell disease) or a limited range of *common* disease alleles (e.g. cystic fibrosis).

6 The amplification refractory mutation system (ARMS) depends on specificity of binding of PCR primers to template DNA (see Figure 69.3). A primer is designed with a 3′ end corresponding to either a mutant, or the wild-type sequence. The primer will bind only with its exact complement, so a wild-type primer permits amplification of only wild-type DNA, mutant primer only mutant DNA. Two separate PCR reactions, with either mutant or wild-type primer, together with another primer elsewhere in the gene, can be used to determine heterozygosity or homozygosity of either sequence. This approach also has been used to identify the cystic fibrosis (CFTR) mutations (see also Chapter 8).

7 Multiplex PCR. In multiplex PCR amplification is carried out simultaneously on many exons in the same reaction mix. It is particularly valuable for Duchenne muscular dystrophy, with any of many possible deletions in the very long dystrophin gene (see Chapter 10). The PCR products are designed to be of different lengths, so as to be separable by agarose gel electrophoresis on the basis of size. Simultaneous scanning reveals deletion of an exon as a missing band.

8 Multiplex amplifiable probe hybridization (MAPH). A problem with multiplex PCR (see above) is differential amplification of individual exons; MAPH is a more reliable variant. Genomic DNA from the patient is bound onto a nylon filter and a mixture of perhaps 40 DNA probes, each specific to one exon, is hybridized to it. The probes are all of different lengths and each carries common primer sequences at its ends. After careful washing, the filter is placed in a PCR reaction mix that amplifies all the bound probes uniformly. A deleted exon is then reliably indicated by gel electrophoresis.

9 Mass spectrometry. Mass spectrometry (see Chapter 63) provides an exceptionally rapid means of analysing PCR-amplified DNA. This is of great value in screening of *CFTR* and the apolipoprotein-E genes of major importance in Alzheimer disease (see Chapter 52).

10 Real-time PCR. Direct dideoxy-sequencing of the entire gene is usually too expensive to be practical even for cystic fibrosis, in which more than 1300 mutations have been described (see above and Chapter 8), Furthermore, sequencing increases sensitivity by only ~10% over dot-blot oligonucleotide hybridization for analysis of a limited number of relatively common, known mutations (see Chapter 67). However, additional opportunities become available once the nucleotide sequence of a mutation is known and specific probes can be constructed For example with CF oligonucleotides are designed corresponding to the sequences either side of each of the common mutations. For each mutation these 'probes' are labelled with one or the other components of a **fluorescence resonance energy transfer** (**FRET**) molecule of a range of colours. Multiple copies of each of the 15 *CFTR* exons are generated by multiplex PCR (see above) and challenged with these special probes. When the two probes corresponding to a mutant exon bind in close proximity, the two halves of the FRET combine and become capable of fluorescing. Emission of fluorescent light of a specific colour then indicates a specific *CFTR* mutation. This method is known as '**real-time PCR**'.

70 DNA profiling

Figure 70.1 Use of minisatellite polymorphism for DNA profiling

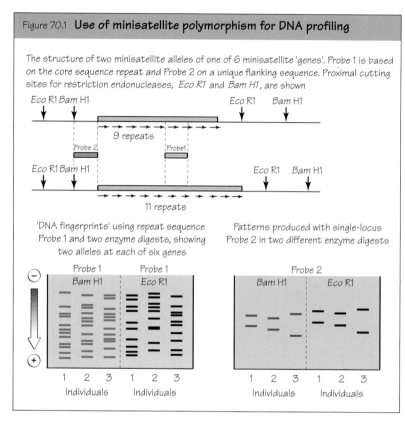

The structure of two minisatellite alleles of one of 6 minisatellite 'genes'. Probe 1 is based on the core sequence repeat and Probe 2 on a unique flanking sequence. Proximal cutting sites for restriction endonucleases, Eco R1 and Bam H1, are shown

'DNA fingerprints' using repeat sequence Probe 1 and two enzyme digests, showing two alleles at each of six genes

Patterns produced with single-locus Probe 2 in two different enzyme digests

Figure 70.2 Microsatellite repeat polymorphisms amplified by PCR

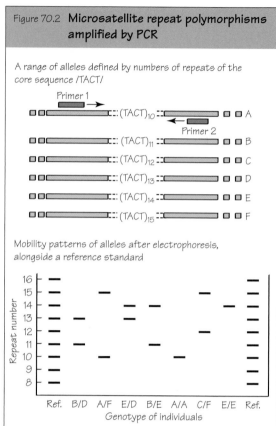

A range of alleles defined by numbers of repeats of the core sequence /TACT/

Mobility patterns of alleles after electrophoresis, alongside a reference standard

Figure 70.3 Practical applications of DNA fingerprinting

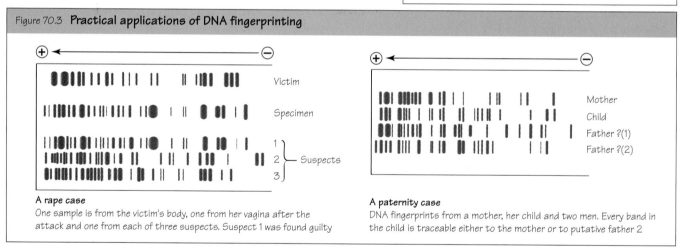

A rape case
One sample is from the victim's body, one from her vagina after the attack and one from each of three suspects. Suspect 1 was found guilty

A paternity case
DNA fingerprints from a mother, her child and two men. Every band in the child is traceable either to the mother or to putative father 2

Overview

DNA profiling is the characterization of an individual genome by DNA analysis. It includes **DNA fingerprinting**, use of **single-locus probes**, microsatellite, Y-chromosome, mitochondrial and ancestry-specific polymorphisms. It is of enormous value for identifying the father in paternity disputes, for confirming family membership in immigration cases and for identifying the perpetrators and victims of crime from traces of biological material. It is also used for confirming the zygosity of twins and for checking the progress of bone marrow transplantations.

As explained in Chapter 19, our genomes contain a large quantity of highly repetitive DNA called '**microsatellite DNA**', or **short tandem repeats** (STRs), when the sequence is short (1–4bp), and '**minisatellite DNA**', when the sequence is longer (5–64bp). Microsatellite DNA is scattered throughout the chromosomes and provides useful markers for disease genes (see Chapter 34). Minisatellite DNA is concentrated near the centromeres and telomeres and was particularly valuable for DNA profiling in the early days, although latterly STRs have become more useful in this respect.

Medical Genetics at a Glance, Third Edition. Dorian J. Pritchard and Bruce R. Korf.

Application of Southern blotting
DNA fingerprinting with minisatellite markers

The Southern blotting approach to DNA analysis (see Chapter 67) depends on the creation of **restriction fragment length polymorphisms** (**RFLPs**) due to polymorphism at restriction endonuclease cutting sites. DNA fingerprinting also depends on fragment length polymorphism, but due to variation instead in the length of repetitious sequences *between* cutting sites. These are also known as **VNTRs, or variable number tandem repeats**, as the intervening sequences are typically repetitive.

The original probe used in fingerprinting was directed against the repeated minisatellite **core sequence /GGGCAGGAXG/** (where X is any nucleotide) within the myoglobin gene. Tandem repeats of two to several hundred copies of this sequence are present at over 1000 sites, although only 8–17 are of practical value in fingerprinting.

If a sample of human DNA is digested with a restriction enzyme for which there are many cutting sites (a '**frequent cutter**'), multiple fragments are produced of many sizes and of great variation between individuals. Those fragments that contain repeats of the core sequence can be visualized on Southern blots by the core sequence probe, as a ladder of bands (see Figure 70.1). The chances of any two unrelated individuals having the same pattern are estimated at $<1/10^{11}$. The only exceptions are members of genetic clones, such as MZ twins. These patterns are known as '**DNA fingerprints**' (see Figure 70.1).

The statistical evaluation of multilocus DNA fingerprint evidence in forensic casework rests on the proportion (x) of bands that on average are shared by unrelated people. 'x' is estimated as 0.14 for each of the two most commonly used probes, irrespective of ethnicity. A conservative estimate of 0.25 would normally be used to prevent over-interpretation and to allow for possible relationship between the suspect and guilty party.

Assuming statistical independence of (i.e. no linkage between) all bands then the chance that n bands in individual A are matched by bands of precisely similar electrophoretic mobility in individual B is x to the power n (see below).

In paternity disputes germline mutation can lead to invalid exclusion of a putative father. In fact 27% of offspring show one band not present in either parent, 1.2% show two, and an estimated <0.3% show three new bands.

Repetitious regions containing multiples of other core sequences can be exploited to produce different fingerprints, using the same enzyme digest and appropriate probes. Alternatively, the same DNA sample can be digested with a different restriction enzyme and examined with the same probe or others.

Use of single-locus probes

If a fingerprinting blot is examined with a probe complementary to a sequence *flanking* one hypervariable region a much simplified pattern is revealed, derived from just that one locus (see Figure 70.1). Each such probe should reveal a maximum of two bands in any person, representing the two alleles and on average 70% of people are heterozygous at any such locus.

Statistical proof of identity requires examination of four to ten such loci and if the population frequency of each 'allele' is known, it is possible to make exact calculations of probability. However, exact numbers of repeats are not always known and fragment band positions do not always correspond precisely. So for statistical purposes the DNA track is divided into a number of 'bins' and bands are deemed to match if they fall within the same bin. Although 'binning' introduces inaccuracies it is necessary to estimate the population frequencies of fragments of specific lengths. This is always done conservatively, so that the statistical weight of evidence is biased in favour of the defend-

ant. Appropriate ethnic databases also have to be set up and when applying Hardy–Weinberg reasoning (see Chapter 30) due allowance must be made for possible population stratification based on, for example, ethnicity, religion or social class.

The Southern blotting approach to genetic profiling described above requires the DNA of about a million cells. For these reasons of scale and problems in the identification of alleles, that method is becoming obsolete.

Application of the polymerase chain reaction (PCR)

PCR amplification (see Chapter 69) dramatically increases the potential range of forensic analysis to minute samples and degraded material and enables precise identification of alleles. It can be applied to minisatellite polymorphisms by use of primers based on unique sequences flanking the tandem repeat arrays. However, the introduction of PCR also brings formidable problems of sample contamination (see Chapter 69).

The most common microsatellites are runs of bases A, AC or AG. In PCR applications they have the advantage over minisatellites in that discrete 'alleles' can be defined unambiguously by the precise number of repeats, calibrated by the mobility of standards. This avoids the requirement for some aspects of statistical proof and makes it easier to relate experimental findings to allele frequencies. The combination of data on 10–15 unlinked, highly polymorphic loci from any individual is usually unique and definitive. A computer-based analysis, called '**DNA boost**' enables discrimination of individual DNA profiles in mixed samples.

Y-chromosome and mitochondrial DNA polymorphisms are especially useful in some circumstances, such as deducing relationships to people who are deceased, because of their sex-specific modes of transmission and the fact that their genomes are transmitted complete (see Chapter 10).

Human DNA is distinguishable from non-human by testing for hybridization with a probe directed at the human-specific *Alu* repeat (Chapter 19). Probes have also been designed for population-specific polymorphisms that indicate ethnic origins.

The modern approach to proof of identification

The current basic approach to forensic identification of a DNA sample begins with establishment of which microsatellite alleles are present. The frequencies of each of these that are present in that particular population are then obtained from reference tables and multiplied together to deduce the overall probability of any member of that population inheriting that particular combination. Their product is considered to indicate the probability of an unrelated individual inheriting that specific profile. Application of this deduction must then pay regard to the consideration that family members and members of ethnic minorities are more likely to share a given profile, that DNA taken from a crime scene may be contaminated and that if the DNA is degraded an accurate profile may actually be unobtainable.

The two main standardized panels of microsatellite frequencies are CODIS in the USA, covering 13 loci and in Europe, SGM, covering 10. It is usual also to include **amelogenin** (an extracellular matrix component of dental enamel) as a sex marker, as the PCR products of the X-linked (AMELX) and Y-linked (AMELY) versions are of different sizes. Tests show this to assign sex correctly in ~98% of cases, misassignments being ascribed to a rare mutation in males.

Even MZ twins may now be distinguishable by identification of somatic copy number variants (CNVs) that have arisen during their independent development (Chapter 53).

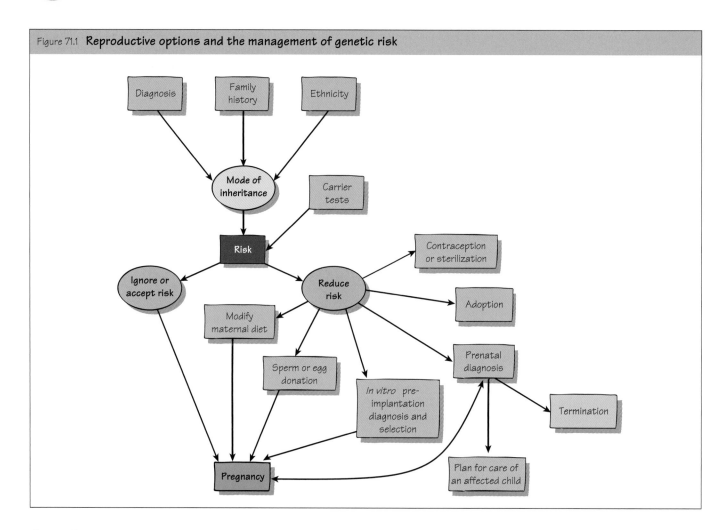

Figure 71.1 **Reproductive options and the management of genetic risk**

Overview

In essence reproductive genetic counselling involves accurate assessment of the genetic risk associated with reproduction by the couple concerned (see Chapter 13), communication of this risk to them and, if necessary, the offer of advice on reproductive options. However, genetic advice should be **non-directive**, **non-judgemental** and **supportive**. It can be summarized by three words: **communication**, **comprehension** and **care** (see also Chapters 72 and 75).

Counselling normally begins with the compilation of a family pedigree (Chapter 2). The interview at which this is drawn serves four main purposes:
• establishment of rapport between counsellor and consultand(s);
• elucidation of the mode of inheritance of the relevant trait in that family;
• collection of information on family relationships, with identification of others at risk;
• identification of the consultands' concerns and perceptions of the disease.

The counsellor should offer support in helping the family make reproductive decisions and cope with the concept of genetic risk and its associated emotional burdens. It is difficult for most people to see these in perspective, but an appreciation of their magnitude may be gained by reference to reproductive risks for the general population.

Communication

For the genetic counsellor and the health visitor good communication skills are vital, as what they convey to a family can have profound implications not only for their present happiness, but for the health of that family for ever more. When assembling information they should preserve a warm and non-judgemental attitude, take adequate time and remember to consider their own body language. It is common for people to experience fear, denial, anger or guilt, but reassurance from

Table 71.1 Reproductive hazards in the population at large.

Condition	Risk	Risk (%)
Spontaneous miscarriage	1/6	17
Perinatal death	1/30–100	1–3
Neonatal death	1/150	0.7
Major congenital malformation	1/33	3
Minor congenital malformation	1/7	14
Serious mental or physical handicap	1/50	2

Medical Genetics at a Glance, Third Edition. Dorian J. Pritchard and Bruce R. Korf.

an authoritative figure outside the family can help them come to terms with such feelings.

Family myths must be explored and disentangled before concepts such as X-linked, dominant or recessive inheritance will be accepted. Family secrets such as incestuous or extra-marital relationships may be revealed and may be critical to the assessment of genetic risk. Such problem areas must be treated with extreme discretion.

Comprehension

An important principle is that *where possible, diagnosis should precede counselling*. Physical examination for dysmorphic features can play a significant part at this stage and guidance on this is given in Chapter 49.

Chromosome examination provides a broad overview of the genome (see Chapter 35), in contrast to molecular approaches where tests are for one or a few specific mutations (see Chapters 67–69). The assessment of risks can be exceedingly complex, but instructive examples are given in Chapter 13. DNA fingerprinting, as described in Chapter 70, is of enormous value in paternity testing.

Prenatal diagnostic tests require informed consent, and consultands should be made fully aware of the limitations of such tests. 'Valid consent' requires that significant risks that would affect the judgement of a reasonable person are explained.

The counsellor's comprehension is further informed by reference to a team of experts. This generally includes additional medically trained clinical geneticists, cytogeneticists, molecular biologists and genetic nurses.

Following face-to-face consultation it is usual for the clinician to write to the family to reiterate the main points and re-address difficult aspects. This letter can become a valuable resource for the family, as it documents advice on risk. Pamphlets and booklets relating to the condition and about lay advocacy groups may also be provided and follow-up visits are appreciated.

Care

After taking family details and constructing a family tree it is necessary to assess what the consultand actually wants to know: there may be specific concerns that are not obvious to the counsellor. Individuals should, when possible, be offered the choice of more than one alternative; for example, between presymptomatic testing and medical surveillance alone.

Genetically based disease varies between ethnic groups (Table 29.1) and some knowledge of a family's educational, social and religious backgrounds is important also as these affect their reactions and decision making. Consultation can create new uncertainties and individuals may adopt a coping style known as 'functional pessimism' to protect themselves from future disappointments. Guilt and depression can arise in those who receive favourable test results when their relatives are less fortunate. Long-term emotional support should therefore be offered at the same time as any offer of predictive testing.

Concepts that conceive genetic improvement of the *population* (Chapter 75) and issues such as cost-saving or contribution to research should not be allowed to influence decisions made by consultands regarding their own lives or those of their offspring. Potential ethical problems are minimized if the *rights of individuals* are given priority.

It should be remembered that diagnosis of high liability toward genetic disease is not necessarily an irrevocable condemnation to ill health. In some cases optimal health can be maintained by avoidance of genotype-specific environmental hazards (see Chapters 73 and 74).

Reproductive options

An estimate of risk of disease for a child to be born to the couple concerned is derived from an understanding of the ethnic background of the family, the deduced mode of inheritance of the condition and the results of laboratory tests. Depending on the magnitude of the perceived risk and/or the outlook of the family, the couple may decide to ignore or accept that risk, or take steps to reduce it (see Figure 71.1).

The latter course could involve *modification of maternal diet or lifestyle*, or *aiming for prenatal diagnosis at a later stage*, with the option of termination. Other options could include *preimplantation diagnosis, artificial insemination by donor, egg donation, in vitro fertilization with embryo selection*, and *contraception or sterilization, combined with adoption of a healthy child*.

In some cases **intracytoplasmic sperm injection (ICSI)** may be considered. The main indication for this is male subfertility for a variety of reasons. There is a small (1.6%) increase in chromosome abnormalities in babies conceived by ICSI and it should be remembered that males conceived by ICSI with sperm from a naturally infertile man are likely also to be infertile.

X-linked disease

In some cultures, avoidance of X-linked recessive disease is achieved by termination of all male fetuses carried by heterozygous mothers, but this may be reducible to 50% where appropriate prenatal diagnosis is available. With *in vitro* fertilization and preimplantation diagnosis, embryo genotypes can be identified and selection introduced at that level. This is acceptable to some branches of Judaism and Islam, though abortion is forbidden. The Roman Catholic Church however disapproves of *in vitro* fertilization, pregnancy termination, sterilization and even contraception.

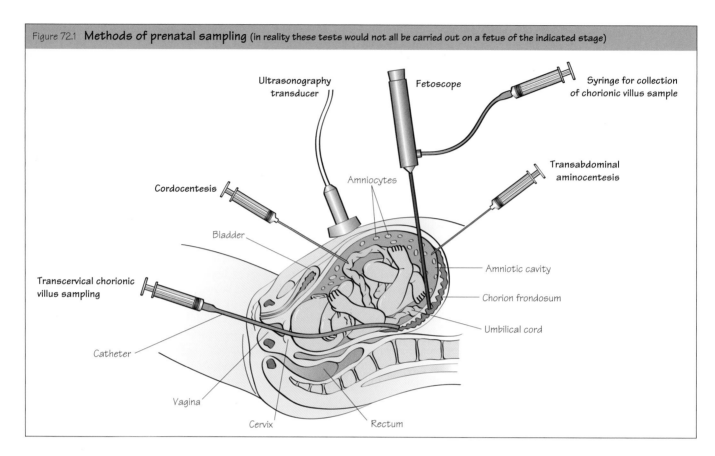

Figure 72.1 **Methods of prenatal sampling** (in reality these tests would not all be carried out on a fetus of the indicated stage)

Overview

The term '**prenatal diagnosis**' refers to the diagnosis of genetic (and other) disorders in established pregnancies. Such information can guide the family in reproductive decision-making, which may involve terminating the pregnancy, or facilitate planning of appropriate medical, surgical or psychological support. Timing, safety and accuracy are critical. It should be stressed that termination is illegal in many societies, and/or banned by religious rules. In addition many women, their partners or families find the practice ethically unacceptable (see Chapters 71 and 75). In Britain, legal grounds for termination include 'a substantial risk that if a child were born it would suffer from such physical or mental abnormality as to be seriously handicapped' (UK Abortion Act, 1967).

In North America and Western Europe most pregnant women are offered a dating scan at about 12 weeks and a fetal physical anomaly scan at 18–20 weeks. If there is to be a termination this is preferable in the first trimester (up to 13 weeks), as it can then be performed by surgery under general anaesthesia, whereas for midtrimester termination the woman must undergo labour and delivery. There is a generally applied 24-week limit for pregnancy termination in Britain, but the law permits termination for severe abnormalities up to 40 weeks.

Potential benefits of prenatal testing include:
- reassurance when results are normal;
- provision of estimates of risk for couples who would otherwise not begin a pregnancy;
- psychological preparation for the arrival of an affected baby;
- advance warning for the medical care team;
- provision of risk information for couples for whom termination is an option.

It should be emphasized that the great majority of prenatal diagnoses yield *normal* test results.

Medical Genetics at a Glance, Third Edition. Dorian J. Pritchard and Bruce R. Korf.

Non-invasive procedures

Ultrasound scanning
In **ultrasound scanning**, echoes reflected from organ boundaries are converted to images on a monitor. This identifies around 300 different malformations.

Anencephaly can be detected at 10–12 weeks, but for most abnormalities the optimum is 18–20 weeks, when the neural tube defects (NTDs), severe skeletal dysplasias, cleft lip and palate, microphthalmia and structural abnormalities of the brain, abdominal organs and heart are usually detectable (Table 72.1). By the third trimester hydrocephalus, microcephaly and duodenal atresia are also detectable.

Obstetric indications for ultrasonography include confirmation of viable or multiple pregnancy, assessment of fetal age and growth, location of the placenta and assessment of amniotic fluid volume. Ultrasonography can be used as a component of screening for fetal trisomy (see below) and is an integral aspect of invasive techniques such as **amniocentesis**, **chorionic villus** and **fetal blood sampling**.

X-rays
Because of the risk of mutagenic injury X-rays are preferably avoided altogether during pregnancy (see Chapter 26), although they are sometimes used to assess fetal skeletal dysplasia.

Magnetic resonance imaging (MRI)
New, fast MRI techniques permit prenatal imaging, useful in the diagnosis of internal anomalies such as brain malformation.

Screening of maternal blood
Maternal serum can provide useful indicators, for example of **α-fetoprotein (AFP)**, **chorionic gonadotrophin (hCG)** and **unconjugated oestriol (UE3)**, **pregnancy associated plasma protein A (PAPP-A)** and **inhibin A** in relation to trisomies 21 and 18 (see Chapters 36 and 74). Elevated levels of AFP are associated especially with NTDs (see Chapters 45 and 74) and other body wall defects such as **gastroschisis**. Addition of ultrasound markers increases the sensitivity and specificity of these screening tests. Emerging technologies are permitting maternal blood testing for fetal DNA that crosses into the maternal circulation during pregnancy.

Invasive procedures
The accepted guideline for invasive testing is that the risk of a seriously abnormal fetus must be at least as great as that of miscarriage from the procedure (Table 72.2). **Conditions considered serious include those that lead inevitably to stillbirth or early death, or to children with severe multiple or progressive handicap.** The chief indications for prenatal diagnosis are:

1 increased risk of trisomy based on maternal serum/ ultrasound screening;
2 previous child with *de novo* chromosome abnormality;
3 presence of a balanced chromosome rearrangement in a parent that predisposes to an unbalanced karyotype in the fetus;
4 family history of a detectable genetic defect;
5 elevated serum AFP or family history of NTD;
6 parental consanguinity in families with testable recessive disease;
7 maternal illness, medication or teratogen exposure;
8 abnormal amniotic fluid volume;
9 parents known to be carriers of certain disorders.

Table 72.1 Some major disorders detectable by ultrasound in the second trimester.

CNS	Skeleton	Multisystem disorders
Anencephaly	Achondroplasia	Growth retardation
Encephalocoele	Osteogenesis imperfecta	Hydrops
Holoprosencephaly	Thanatrophic dysplasia	Oligohydramnios
Hydrocephalus	Polyhydramnios	
Abdomen and pelvis	*Chest*	*Head and face*
Omphalocoele	Congenital heart disease	CL ± P
Renal agenesis	Diaphragmatic hernia	Microphthalmia
Gastroschisis		
Gastrointestinal atresia		
Renal cysts		
Hydronephrosis		

CL ± P, cleft lip and palate.

Table 72.2 Prenatal sampling and associated risks.

Stage	Optimal time	Risk of miscarriage	Availability
Preimplantation			
Embryo biopsy	6–10 cell stage	Unknown, presumed safe	Limited
First trimester (0–13 weeks)			
Chorionic villus sampling			
Transcervical	9–12 weeks	0.5–2.0%	Specialized
Transabdominal	9–13 weeks	0.5–2.0%	Specialized
Maternal circulation	From 6 weeks	Safe	Specialized
Second trimester (14–26 weeks)			
Placental biopsy, transabdominal	14–40 weeks	0.5–2.0%	Specialized
Ultrasonography	16–18 weeks	Safe	Widely available
Amniocentesis	16–18 weeks	0.5	Widely available
Cordocentesis	18–40 weeks	1%	Specialized
Fetoscopy	18–20 weeks	3%	Widely available
Fetal tissue biopsy	18–20 weeks	3%	Very specialized

When culture of embryonic tissue is necessary diagnosis is delayed by 2–4 weeks.

Induction of Rhesus iso-immunization by invasive procedures in Rh⁻ mothers is prevented by administration of anti-D immunoglobulin.

Chorionic villus sampling (CVS)

In CVS a **syncytiotrophoblast** biopsy is aspirated via a catheter through the cervix or by transabdominal puncture at 10–12 weeks' gestation, both guided by ultrasonography. The early timing allows diagnosis by about 12 weeks, but there is an associated risk 0.5–2.0% above the spontaneous abortion rate of 7%.

Since syncytiotrophoblast nuclei divide rapidly, karyotyping is possible without culturing, but cultured material provides more reliable results. DNA can be isolated directly from chorionic villi for molecular testing.

Amniocentesis

Amniocentesis is especially valuable at 16–18 weeks for estimating AFP concentration and acetylcholinesterase activity in pregnancies at risk of NTDs, or for analysis of chromosomes, DNA, or enzyme activities in cultured cells. After prior localization of the placenta by ultrasound, a needle is inserted aseptically through the mother's abdominal wall and into the amniotic cavity, and a 10–20 mL sample is withdrawn. This carries a 0.5% risk of causing miscarriage, in addition to the natural risk of 2.5% at 16 weeks, or 7% when AFP levels are high.

Cordocentesis

From week 18 onwards a fetal blood sample can be taken by inserting a fine needle transabdominally into the umbilical cord. This is carried out with guidance by fetoscopy (with a 3% extra risk of miscarriage) or ultrasonography.

Fetoscopy

Fetoscopy involves viewing the fetus through an **endoscope**. The optimum stage is 18–20 weeks and it carries a risk of fetal loss of 3%. Fetoscopy enables biopsy collection for prenatal diagnosis of serious skin and liver disorders, but its most common application is in the investigation of fetal bladder obstruction (see the Potter sequence, Chapter 45).

Preimplantation genetic diagnosis

In the context of *in vitro* fertilization, one or two cells are collected at the six to ten-cell stage for direct examination by FISH or PCR (see Chapters 35 and 69), enabling selection of healthy embryos for implantation. (Culturing of these cells would contravene the UK Human Fertilization and Embryology Act, 1990.)

Problems of prenatal sampling

True fetal **mosaicism** is found in around 0.25% of fetuses, indicated by discrepant primary cultures. About 1% have **confined placental mosaicism**. **Maternal cell contamination** is a problem in long-term CV cultures.

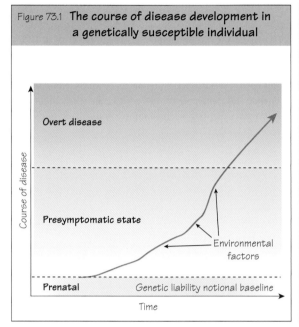

Figure 73.1 **The course of disease development in a genetically susceptible individual**

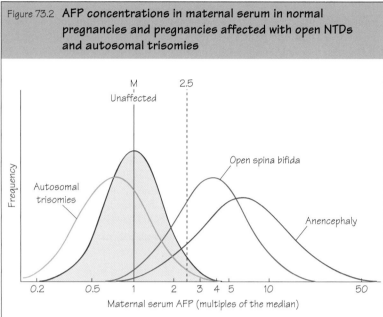

Figure 73.2 **AFP concentrations in maternal serum in normal pregnancies and pregnancies affected with open NTDs and autosomal trisomies**

Overview

More than a century ago Archibald Garrod conceived the idea of the chemical individuality of people, but it is only now that we are in a position to define exactly what that means, as we approach a new era of **personalized genetic medicine**.

Each of us inherits genes that contribute some degree of liability toward many disorders. In the case of monogenic diseases, one or a pair of defective alleles alone confers sufficient liability to cause disease. In other instances genetic liability is expressed merely as a susceptibility and manifestation of disease requires the passage of time and/or accumulation of specific environmental exposures (see Figure 73.1). **Preventative genetics** is based on testing for factors that contribute to genetic liability. This identifies persons at risk, enabling them to be educated about individually hazardous environmental factors and providing opportunities for modification of lifestyles (see Chapter 52). In some cases proactive treatment can be offered to reduce risks, or surveillance to ensure early diagnosis and the prompt institution of therapy.

There are two broadly distinct approaches to screening: **targeted**, or **family screening**, which includes **carrier** or **heterozygote screening** and **presymptomatic testing**, and **population screening**.

Population screening may be appropriate for three classes of heterozygous carrier:
- autosomal recessive diseases of high incidence;
- relatively common X-linked disorders;
- autosomal dominant disorders of late onset.

To be practical, population screening must be morally acceptable, should be widely available and preferably show a net cost benefit. A genetic disease is suitable for population screening if it is clearly defined, of appreciable frequency and if early diagnosis is actually advantageous. The test should be easily performed, be non-invasive and yield few false positives or false negatives. Appropriate information and counselling should also be available. Testing a child for a

disorder of adult onset, or carrier status should be postponed until the child is of an age to appreciate the issues and give informed consent.

Preimplantation diagnosis

Preimplantation diagnosis is valuable as an adjunct to *in vitro* fertilization and for couples who rule out termination.

Blastomere sampling One or two blastomeres are taken from embryos at the six to eight-cell stage. The DNA is tested by fluorescent *in situ* hybridization (FISH) for aneuploidy (Chapters 35–37), or amplified by PCR and analysed for a specific known genetic mutation (Chapter 69). Since PCR amplification sometimes fails for technical reasons, use of two blastomeres is recommended. Sampling at 3 days allows time to implant a healthy embryo.

Blastocyst sampling Sampling of trophectoderm at the 100-cell stage reduces the PCR failure rate, but introduces the risk of maternal contamination (see Chapter 41).

Polar body sampling This is of most value in testing for aneuploidy (see Chapter 18).

Prenatal screening
Neural tube defects

Ninety to ninety-five per cent of neural tube defect (NTD) births occur in the absence of a family history of NTDs. They are detectable at 16 weeks by assay of α-fetoprotein (AFP) concentration in amniotic fluid and in many cases also in maternal serum. However, in maternal serum there is overlap between unaffected and NTD pregnancies, so an arbitrary concentration is identified below which no further action is taken. A cut-off at 2.5 multiples of the normal median identifies >90% of fetuses with anencephaly and ~80% of those with open NTDs (see Figure 73.2).

Over 20 years, maternal serum screening with dietary improvements and preconceptional folic acid supplementation have yielded a 25-fold decrease in NTDs in England and Wales.

Medical Genetics at a Glance, Third Edition. Dorian J. Pritchard and Bruce R. Korf.
© 2013 John Wiley & Sons, Ltd. Published 2013 by John Wiley & Sons, Ltd.

Fetal trisomy

The combination of maternal age and abnormal concentrations of four biochemicals in a mother's serum can identify most pregnancies with Down syndrome. At 16 weeks, concentrations of AFP and **unconjugated oestriol (UE3)** tend to be reduced in the blood of women pregnant with babies with Down syndrome, whereas that of **human chorionic gonadotrophin (hCG)** is raised. The 'triple test', combining the three, identifies 60% of pregnancies with Down syndrome. Inclusion of **inhibin A**, increased in pregnancies with Down syndrome, raises this to 75%. Incorporation of the ultrasonographic observation of **increased fetal nuchal transparency** (abnormal accumulation of fluid behind the baby's neck) at 12 weeks, detects 80% of babies with Down syndrome.

Reduced levels of AFP, UE3 and hCG are associated with trisomy 18; reduced levels of hCG and PAPP-A*, along with consideration of maternal age, detect approximately 2 in 3 fetuses with trisomy 18. (*Pregnancy-associated plasma protein A is a metalloprotein thought to be involved in cell proliferation.) New methods based on next-generation sequencing of fetal DNA found in maternal blood are rapidly being adopted and will probably replace maternal serum screening.

Neonatal screening

All 50 US states are required by law to offer neonatal screening for **PKU, galactosaemia** and **congenital hypothyroidism** (usually non-genetic), as are offered in most developed countries. All cause intellectual disability, but screening in newborns allows prophylactic regimens to be offered. The test for galactosaemia is similar to the Guthrie test for PKU (see Chapter 63), with confirmation by enzyme assay. Screening for hypothyroidism involves assay of thyroxine and thyroid-stimulating hormone.

In some US states up to 30 diseases are screened for, including **CF, MCAAD** and the haemoglobinopathies, especially **thalassaemia** and **sickle cell disease**. In the UK consideration is currently being given also to **Pompe disease, maple syrup urine disease, tyrosinaemia, CAH, isovaleric acidaemia, glutaric aciduria Type 1** and **homocystinuria**.

Tandem mass spectrometry (Chapter 63) is providing a rapid new approach to analysis of tiny neonatal blood samples for PKU, many **amino acidurias, organic acidaemias** and **fatty acid oxidation disorders**.

If neonatal screening is to be undertaken, the consultative follow-up should be prompt and involve definitive diagnosis, prompt initiation of management and appropriate genetic counselling.

Cystic fibrosis (CF)

Currently neonatal diagnosis of CF is based on immunological quantification of trypsinogen in the blood (a consequence of blockage of the pancreatic ducts *in utero*) supplemented by DNA analysis (see Chapter 68). Up to 80% of heterozygotes of north European or Ashkenazi Jewish ancestry are detectable by tests for the Phe508del allele and a further 10% by multiplex tests for several rarer alleles, depending on ethnicity. Early use of antibiotics and physiotherapy improve long-term prognoses.

Sickle cell disease

Several techniques have been used for diagnosis of sickle cell anaemia, including electrophoresis of haemoglobin, demonstration of red cell sickling at low oxygen tensions and a range of DNA tests (see Chapters 67 and 68). Many babies die of pneumococcal infection, but prophylactic treatment can be given by administration of oral penicillin.

Thalassaemia

Populations for which thalassaemia carrier screening programmes might prove, or have proved, advantageous include China and East Asia (for α-thalassaemia) and the Indian subcontinent and Mediterranean countries (for β-thalassaemia). In Cyprus, screening led to a 95% decline in babies with β-thalassaemia in 10 years. Similar programmes in Greece and Italy have created a better than 50% reduction. Early diagnosis makes it possible to optimize transfusion and iron-chelation therapy at an early stage.

Tay–Sachs disease

Carrier screening followed by prenatal diagnosis and termination has reduced Tay–Sachs disease by 95% among American Ashkenazi Jews (see Chapter 60).

Screening for adult-onset disease

Predictive testing for inherited cancer predisposition, such as **familial adenomatous polyposis** and **breast/ovarian cancer**, can ensure inclusion in clinical surveillance programmes and the possibility of prophylactic surgery.

Occupational screening

In the workplace, genetic screening is done to monitor genetic damage due to exposure to ionizing radiation (see Chapter 26 and Table 73.1), or for susceptibility to environmental chemicals. Around 50 genetic traits are related to specific environmental agents (Table 73.2). These include **G6PD deficiency**, for which oxidants such as ozone and nitrogen dioxide are contraindicated, and the **sickle cell trait**, carriers of which are highly susceptible to carbon monoxide and cyanide.

Alpha1-antitrypsin (α1-AT) deficiency (AR) is as common as cystic fibrosis in Caucasians, but virtually absent in Chinese and Japanese. Homozygotes typically develop lung emphysema in middle age, especially tobacco smokers, in whom life expectancy in the US is reduced from 62 to 40 years. Homozygotes can be identified by dot-blots with ASO probes (see Chapter 67).

Limitations of genetic testing

1 Somatic mosaicism and operator error mean that genetic tests are never 100% reliable.
2 DNA testing can reveal mutations that are not necessarily expressed as disease because, for example, they may occur in an unimportant part of the gene, or the mutant allele is incompletely penetrant.

Table 73.1 Estimated new genetic abnormalities in one million live births in a population exposed to low-dose radiation equivalent to 0.01 Gy (1 rad) of X-rays.

Category	No. of cases
Aberrant chromosomes	38
Autosomal dominant and X-linked disease	20
Recessive lesions	30
Multifactorial diseases	5

Numbers based on atomic bomb survival statistics and animal experiments.

Table 73.2 Genetic conditions that create health risks with specific environmental agents.

Genetic susceptibility	Environmental agent	Resultant condition
G6PD deficiency	Fava beans, mothballs	Haemolytic crisis
Hypercholesterolaemia	Saturated fats	Atherosclerosis
Gluten sensitivity	Wheat protein	Coeliac disease
Defective Na/K pump	Common salt	Hypertension
Lactose intolerance	Milk sugar	Colic and diarrhoea
Deficient ADH	Alcohol	Alcoholism
Deficient ALDH	Alcohol	Flushing response
Hyperoxaluria	Oxalates*	Kidney stones
Haemochromatosis	Iron food supplement	Iron overload
α_1-antitrypsin deficiency	Tobacco smoke	Emphysema
Atopic diathesis	Pollen	Hay fever

ADH, alcohol dehydrogenase; ALDH, acetaldehyde dehydrogenase.
* e.g. in spinach and rhubarb.

3 Genetic testing may not detect all the disease alleles of a specific gene.
4 Genetic testing can introduce unwanted social and ethical problems.

Genetic registers

Genetic registers are records of local families with genetic disease. Entry to a register should be entirely voluntary and it is essential that confidentiality is never breached. Their primary purpose is to maintain two-way contact between the clinical genetics unit and relevant family members. This ensures families do not feel excluded from a source of support and allows investigation to be offered as appropriate.

They are most valuable for relatively common conditions of late onset, with potentially serious effects that are amenable to prevention or treatment. However, there are negative implications, including invasion of privacy, implied compulsion, the 'right not to know' about one's deficiencies, possible stigmatization and possible leakage of confidential data.

Prophylactic surgery

Prophylactic surgery may be appropriate for some late-acting cancer-predisposing alleles of high penetrance. These include familial adenomatous polyposis coli, breast and ovarian cancer, and thyroid cancer due to the *MEN2B* allele (see Chapter 56). The antioestrogen drug *tamoxifen* is an option for women carrying the *BRCA1* or *BRCA2* alleles (see Chapter 56), who should avoid oral contraception and hormone replacement therapy. For patients at high risk of colon cancer, non-digestible starch can slow polyposis and the anti-inflammatory *sulindac* can reduce rectal and duodenal adenomas.

Therapeutic cloning

Embryonic stem cells offer the possibility of therapy for many conditions, for example as a source of dopamine-producing neurons capable of correcting Parkinson disease.

Management of genetic disease

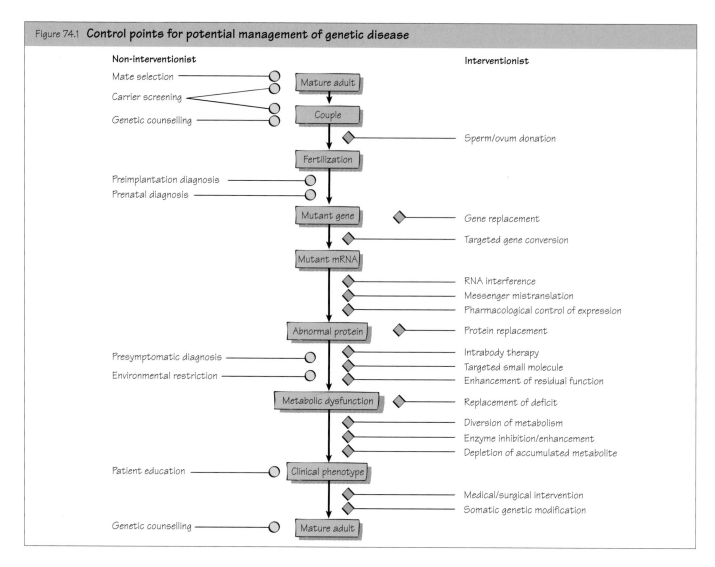

Figure 74.1 **Control points for potential management of genetic disease**

Non-interventionist
Interventionist

Mate selection
Carrier screening
Genetic counselling

Mature adult
Couple

Sperm/ovum donation

Fertilization

Preimplantation diagnosis
Prenatal diagnosis

Mutant gene

Gene replacement
Targeted gene conversion

Mutant mRNA

RNA interference
Messenger mistranslation
Pharmacological control of expression

Abnormal protein

Protein replacement

Presymptomatic diagnosis
Environmental restriction

Intrabody therapy
Targeted small molecule
Enhancement of residual function

Metabolic dysfunction

Replacement of deficit
Diversion of metabolism
Enzyme inhibition/enhancement
Depletion of accumulated metabolite

Patient education

Clinical phenotype

Medical/surgical intervention
Somatic genetic modification

Genetic counselling

Mature adult

Overview

There are many potential ways to reduce the impact of genetic disease that offer possibilities for clinical management. These include non-interventionist strategies and medical intervention. Among North American Caucasians, approximately 13% of all matings are Rh-incompatible (Chapter 29), but sensitization of an Rh⁻ mother following birth of an Rh⁺ baby is prevented by her prior injection with anti-Rh antibodies to destroy fetal erythrocytes before she mounts an immune response. Non-interventionist approaches include education and guidance of couples, and early diagnosis.

Pharmacogenomics

'Genomics' refers to the study and application of knowledge about the genome (see Chapter 57), **pharmacogenomics** with the stratification of diseases to guide selection of appropriately designed drugs and prescription of drug dosages compatible with individual metabolic rates (see Chapter 29). Microarrays are created corresponding to hundreds or thousands of cloned alleles (see Chapter 67). The amount of mRNA from a patient's tissue that hybridizes to the different clones then defines that tissue's gene expression profile. Automated analysis of genome-wide single-nucleotide polymorphisms makes it possible to identify genes involved in drug metabolism or transport, and receptors that may govern efficacy, side-effects or toxicity.

DNA microarrays can also be used to create unique genetic profiles of cancers, enabling design of individualized therapy regimens (see Chapter 57).

Another anticancer measure involves injecting a *Herpes*-virus-based vector expressing thymidine kinase, directly into brain tumours, which makes those cells uniquely susceptible to the normally non-toxic anti-*Herpes* drug, *ganciclovir*.

Medical Genetics at a Glance, Third Edition. Dorian J. Pritchard and Bruce R. Korf.

Gene therapy

Gene therapy offers exciting prospects, but there remain significant technical challenges and there is still real concern that random chromosomal integration of vectors might cause side effects as bad as or worse than the original disease.

Several methods are available to introduce genes into cells, including incubation with 'naked' DNA, or DNA enclosed within artificial lipoprotein vesicles called **liposomes**. In **receptor-mediated endocytosis** a complex is made of the DNA construct and specific polypeptide ligands for which the cell has receptors on its surface.

Other approaches utilize **retroviruses**, which have their own means for introducing genes into chromosomes. Injection of an adenovirus vector carrying the wild-type *RPE65* gene is particularly effective in relieving **Leber congenital amaurosis** (progressive loss of vision). **Lentoviruses** integrate into non-dividing cells: bone marrow cells treated with lentiviral vectors, are used to treat **X-linked adrenoleukodystrophy**.

Gene replacement

Attempts at replacement of defective genes have had mixed success. One approach in the treatment of CF (Chapter 8) involves inhalation of disabled cold virus (**adenovirus**) carrying a copy of the normal *CFTR* allele, but this has proved only temporarily effective. Replacement of the *ADA* gene in bone marrow cells of children with SCID (Chapters 61 and 65) led to leukaemia in some patients and has now been withdrawn.

Targeted gene conversion

A promising new approach is gene conversion by exploitation of normal DNA repair mechanisms (Chapter 26). It involves targeting mutant sequences with DNA–RNA double-stranded constructs containing more effective versions of those genes. A valuable application would be creation of HIV-resistant T cells from which the relevant surface receptors have been deleted.

Messenger mistranslation

Allele-specific oligonucleotides (**ASOs**) delivered into cells in liposomes can inhibit gene expression at translation. The principle is sequence-specific binding of antisense oligonucleotide to the target mRNA. ASOs can also force exon-skipping and convert reading-frame-disrupting deletions of dystrophin, causative of Duchenne MD, to in-frame deletions and the milder Becker MD (Chapter 11).

Aminoglycoside antibiotics such as gentamicin encourage ribosomes to 'skip over' translation STOP signals. A form of CF prevalent in Ashkenazi Jews involves a premature STOP at position 554 in the *CFTR* sequence (Chapter 8). In the presence of the antibiotic gentamicin, cells from such patients incorporate tyrosine at this position without cessation of translation. Nasal drops containing gentamicin offer some relief to these patients.

RNA interference

In **RNA interference** (**RNAi**), selected species of mRNA are destroyed using artificial **small interfering RNAs** (**siRNAs**). Double-stranded RNA precursors, delivered in drug form or by plasmid or viral vectors, are processed by the cell's own enzymes to produce double-stranded siRNAs about 22 nucleotides long. These bind to and activate natural **RNA induced silencing complexes** (**RISCs**) with the capacity to recognize mRNA containing the homologous 22-base sequence. This cleaves the target mRNA, reducing it to undetectable levels. SiRNAs can move between cells, so that artificial RNA duplexes introduced into one part of an embryo can cause sequence-specific messenger 'silencing' throughout the body.

Modification of the properties of proteins

Intrabody therapy

Intrabodies are genetically engineered intracellular antibodies. One used in treatment of chronic myelogenous leukaemia (CML) (Chapters 56 and 57) involves fusion of components of the dimeric enzyme, **caspase 3**, to immunoglobulin V regions specific to each of the two halves of the BCR–Abl fusion protein. The intrabodies bind in pairs to the two parts of the fusion protein, allowing the caspase to dimerize and trigger apoptosis specifically of the leukaemic cells (see also Chapter 39).

Targeted small molecules

Imatinib mesylate is another product designed to bind to the BCR–Abl fusion protein. Imatinib acts as a tyrosine kinase inhibitor (see Chapter 57).

Enhancement of residual function

Hydroxyurea or *decitabine* administered to sickle cell patients can re-stimulate synthesis of fetal haemoglobin ($\alpha 2\gamma 2$). One experimental approach to Duchenne MD is to up-regulate transcription of the homologous **utrophin** gene.

Control of cell signalling

Losartan is being tested for use to prevent or reverse aortic dilation in Marfan syndrome (see Chapter 5), by interfering with the abnormal regulation of TGF-β signalling by mutant fibrillin-1.

Correction of metabolic dysfunction

Environmental restriction

Environmental restriction includes avoidance of tobacco smoke by those with emphysema due to α_1-antitrypsin deficiency; of scuba diving and high altitude flying by sickle cell heterozygotes; of sunlight by patients with albinism, porphyria and xeroderma pigmentosa and of X-rays by those with a DNA repair disorder (see Chapters 26, 56, 58 and 61).

A diet low in phenylalanine is most effective in ensuring normal brain development in children with PKU, and early exclusion of galactose and lactose prevents serious complications in babies homozygous for galactosaemia (see Chapters 58 and 59).

Replacement of deficit

The lysosomal storage disorders include defects in the delivery of enzymes into the lysosomes (see Chapter 62). These are normally targeted by enzymes carrying mannose-6-phosphate residues that bind specifically to lysosomal surface receptors. There was dramatic recession of organomegaly in type 1 Gaucher disease after intravenous infusion of β-glucosidase to which mannose phosphate had been artificially attached.

'*Ex vivo*' gene therapy of haemophilia (Chapter 11) involves treatment of a patient's own fibroblasts with DNA coding for Factors VIII or IX, followed by their re-inoculation into the peritoneal cavity. Another approach to haemophilia is intramuscular injection of adeno-associated virus expressing the relevant factor.

In SMA (Chapter 8) the silent *SMN* genes could possibly be brought into expression to correct that deficiency.

Diversion of metabolism

This includes stimulation of alternative pathways, as in correction of ornithine/ urea cycle disorders due to OTC deficiency (see Chapter 61) by administration of sodium benzoate allowing excretion of the ammonium ions as hippurate.

Administration of **dexamethasone** to the mother from 4–5 weeks' gestation can suppress androgen production and virilization of girls with CAH (see Chapter 44). Maternal intake of biotin will correct biotin-responsive **multiple carboxylase deficiency** in the unborn baby.

Enzyme inhibition and enhancement

Competitive inhibition of rate-controlling enzymes has proved effective, for example in **familial hypercholesterolaemia** (Chapters 5 and 52).

Enzyme function can sometimes be enhanced by administration of a cofactor, such as vitamin B_6 for **homocystinuria** (Chapter 58) and B_{12} for **methylmalonic acidaemia** (Chapter 60).

Hereditary angioedema is a potentially fatal problem of the upper respiratory tract caused by an AD mutation in the gene coding for **Complement 1 esterase inhibitor**, but androgens, particularly danazol, increase abundance of its mRNA.

Depletion of accumulated metabolite

Common examples are phlebotomy to relieve haemochromatosis, and renal dialysis.

Modification of gross phenotype

Surgical correction

Surgical correction of CL ± P, cleft palate, pyloric stenosis and congenital heart defects accounts for the treatment of 20–30% of all infants with major genetically determined disorders. Spina bifida has been successfully treated by prenatal surgery.

Somatic genetic modification

Stem-cell transplantation *in utero* offers good prospects for treatment, as recipients are and remain tolerant of foreign tissues implanted at this stage. This technique could potentially cure many conditions, including SCID, thalassaemia, sickle cell disease and Fanconi anaemia. *In utero* transplantation is proving valuable for early bone marrow transfer into patients otherwise destined to develop Krabbe or Hurler disease.

Embryonic cardiomyocytes lack HLA2 and other cell surface antigens that might trigger rejection in a recipient, but they retain the ability to home in on sites of myocardial damage and contribute to heart repair. They can be obtained from the bone marrow of the patient or that of a healthy donor.

Somatic stem cells normally have restricted potential for cytodifferentiation, but can be converted to '**induced pluripotent stem cells**', with a broader differentiative range. Applications include correction of **osteogenesis imperfecta**, **retinal degeneration** and **hypophosphataemia**. Limbic stem cells from the corneal epithelium can be transplanted to the opposite eye for repair of corneal damage.

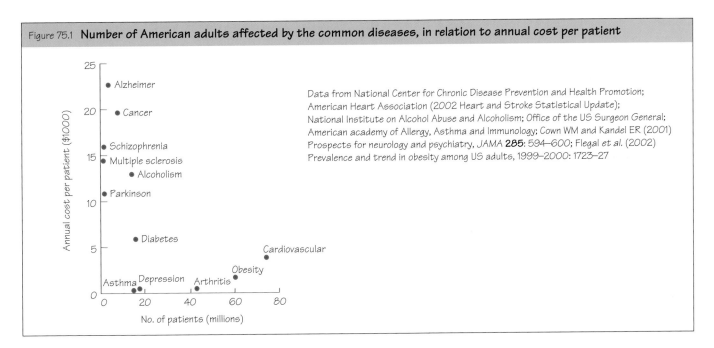

Figure 75.1 **Number of American adults affected by the common diseases, in relation to annual cost per patient**

Data from National Center for Chronic Disease Prevention and Health Promotion; American Heart Association (2002 Heart and Stroke Statistical Update); National Institute on Alcohol Abuse and Alcoholism; Office of the US Surgeon General; American academy of Allergy, Asthma and Immunology; Cown WM and Kandel ER (2001) Prospects for neurology and psychiatry, JAMA **285**: 594–600; Flegal et al. (2002) Prevalence and trend in obesity among US adults, 1999–2000: 1723–27

Overview

Ethics is the science of morals and human duty. It deals with the rules by which we should conduct our lives. In clinical ethics avoidance of conflict requires endorsement of high moral values, such as mutual respect, honesty and compassion, by both clinician and client. Ethicists talk about additional values such as beneficence and justice (see below). Occasionally there can be disagreement, or accepted values may face unexpected challenges and it is then that ethical problems can arise. For example, abortion of an affected pregnancy pits the right of choice of the parent against the right to life of the unborn child. The opportunity to terminate creates a major ethical dilemma. Optimal outcomes require that medical staff and families work constructively together to identify, analyse and resolve such dilemmas.

The Darwinian perspective

Every species shows phenotypic variation due partly to genetic variation between individuals. In accordance with Darwin's 'Theory of Evolution through Natural Selection', the assembly of alleles within the human species derives from selection by hazards faced by our ancestors and by ourselves earlier in life. Natural selection ensures that the genes of unfit or reproductively unsuccessful members of wild species are unlikely to be represented in subsequent generations, with consequent improvement in the average fitness of its members. New gene variants and combinations are constantly created by mutation and reassortment at meiosis and mating and, with the passage of generations, those that are favourable increase in frequency while the unfavourable decline. The outcome is that members of naturally selected populations are largely healthy, well adapted and fully capable of reproduction.

Goals of medicine include the restoration, maintenance, or improvement of quality of life and extension of lifespan. It helps patients survive life-threatening disease and assists reproduction of the infertile, that is it reduces or negates natural selection. In so doing it neces-

sarily allows increase in the population frequency of harmful alleles. In the long term, therefore, the practice of traditional medicine is 'dysgenic', increasing the burden of harmful alleles (the 'genetic load') our species has to carry (see Chapter 30).

By contrast, medical practices that involve healthy embryo selection (see Chapter 71) reverse the dysgenic influence and go some way toward reducing our genetic load. However, deliberate application of measures *with the aim of* changing the population frequencies of disease alleles leads us into the realm of 'eugenics', which history has taught is a dangerous path to tread (see below).

An historical perspective

The first great exposition of the ethical basis of medicine was the fifth century BC Hippocratic Oath. It notably includes the pledge: '*the regimen I adopt shall be for the benefit of my patients according to my ability and judgement, and not for their hurt or for any wrong*'. This still forms the basis of the graduation ceremony in many medical schools, although dropped by others. It strongly condemns the practice of pregnancy termination currently permitted in some societies.

In the nineteenth century Francis Galton, inspired by the evolutionary ideas of his cousin, Charles Darwin, coined the word 'eugenics' (the prefix 'eu-' denoting 'good') to describe scientific endeavours aimed at increasing the proportion of persons with better-than-average genetic endowment, through selective mating. The central idea is that human evolution could be guided toward a better future if human reproduction were to come under social guidance.

'Negative eugenics' is primarily directed toward reduction in the incidence of hereditary disease, whereas 'positive eugenics' aims to increase the frequency of superior endowments. Most medical practitioners view reduction of disease incidence as desirable but, because of unpredictable outcomes or on religious grounds, are more cautious about 'genetic enhancement'.

Medical Genetics at a Glance, Third Edition. Dorian J. Pritchard and Bruce R. Korf.
© 2013 John Wiley & Sons, Ltd. Published 2013 by John Wiley & Sons, Ltd.

Notwithstanding, most medical geneticists become distinctly uncomfortable if their practices are described as eugenic, as they view their mission as straightforward improvement of the quality of life for individuals. Furthermore, the word 'eugenics' has been irredeemably besmirched by its use in the past to justify genocidal policies and extermination atrocities, especially in Nazi Germany. To avoid misinterpretation, we believe use of the word 'eugenics' in general discussion is therefore probably best avoided.

Screening and termination of affected pregnancies are sometimes advocated as more cost-effective than caring for the affected individuals. This argument is deplored by most clinical geneticists, who generally think in terms of avoidance of health problems for individuals or families, rather than the overall health of the population.

The religious perspective

Bioethical principles derive from the societal values of the culture in which they originate. Western medical ethics derived from Judeo-Christian and classical Greek humanitarian principles sees all individuals as having equal rights, irrespective of ethnicity, social standing or caste, sex, religion or wealth. It, however, generally seems to appreciate the lives of young persons as more valuable than those of the elderly. These concepts are not necessarily recognized by members of other cultures, but Western society generally considers that they represent best practice in most medical circumstances. Should they cause conflict in any instance, attempts should be made to accommodate client values.

Contemporary Western society places a value on the gender-balanced family, but others, notably in northern India and China, have a preference for sons. The World Health Organization proposes that only disease-related criteria should be used for prenatal gender selection. Different groups view matters of genetic intervention very differently. For example, some individuals of Islamic and Jewish traditions oppose abortion, but find preimplantation gender selection acceptable. The Roman Catholic Church condemns both abortion and *in vitro* fertilization, restricting the reproductive options available.

Application of ethical principles

Important principles for the counsellor to bear in mind are:
1 One person cannot be the object of another person's 'right'.
2 Both biological parents should normally have a say in the fate of their offspring.

Some couples with what many would consider a deficiency, such as deafness or very short stature, express the wish that they would like children resembling themselves. The definition of 'deficiency' in itself is problematic, but it is a matter of serious debate whether or not medical techniques should be used deliberately to select or create such a baby, in order to satisfy parental wishes.

Texts on medical ethics generally recognize four overriding principles: (i) *respect for patient autonomy*; (ii) *beneficence* (i.e. 'being of benefit'); (iii) *non-maleficence* (i.e. avoidance of doing harm); and (iv) *justice*.

The ethical problems of clinical genetics are mainly those common throughout medicine: of conveying difficult information with adequate care; ensuring genuinely informed consent to tests and treatment; preserving confidentiality; and identifying the best available treatments. Distinctive additional problems arise with genetic tests in that they can reveal information about individuals who are not tested and about diseases of late onset. This presents ethical challenges to health professionals, the family and society at large.

A crucial distinction is between services available for pre-existing concerns of individuals or families, and population screening offered proactively to citizens who have not sought the test. Typical scenarios in the first category could involve, for example, a family seeking an explanation for a serious developmental problem in their child, a person wishing to know their risk of developing a degenerative condition, or a couple wanting to know the risk their child could develop a condition shown by an existing family member. By contrast, where the issue is of population screening, the professional, or the medical community, is actively promoting a specific course of action – that the client or patient should undergo an investigation. The offer of screening in itself may generate concerns and imply that compliance is being recommended, definitely so in newborn screening for inborn errors of metabolism.

Non-directiveness in genetic counselling

The counsellor's involvement should be both non-judgemental and non-directive. Allowing the client to reach his or her own decision has important psychological benefits for the client, but it also benefits the counsellor.
1 It helps him or her avoid emotional involvement with that decision.
2 It ensures legal responsibility for the decision lies with the client.
3 It avoids the possible implication that the counsellor is following an eugenic agenda.

The British Mental Capacity Act (2005) provides a statutory framework to empower and protect vulnerable people unable to make decisions on their own behalf.

Confidentiality

Genetic information about one individual may have implications for other family members. If a patient refuses to allow disclosure of such information his or her wish would normally be respected. Exceptionally, the genetic counsellor may decide to breach confidentiality, if the potential harm to another family member outweighs that to those first considered. However, the World Health Organization considers it to be the *counsellee* (i.e. the person who requested advice) who carries the moral obligation to inform relatives.

Medical information should never be disclosed to third parties, such as insurance companies, schools, employers or other individuals, without the subject's written consent. In the US the Health Insurance Portability and Accountability Act gives legal protection to confidentiality of medical information, etc. relating to individuals. The Genetic Information Nondiscrimination Act prevents the use of genetic information, including family history and genetic test data, in determination of eligibility for health insurance or employment. The World Medical Association Statement on Genetic Medicine (WMA 20015) makes similar recommendations and cautions that physicians should support laws offering protection from genetic discrimination. In some situations confidentiality may be protected by codification of data and anonymization of subjects.

Conflicts of interest between family members

Consider the case of a man aged 20 years whose grandfather died of Huntington disease. He wants to marry and start a family, but wishes to clarify his genetic status first. His at-risk father, aged 40 years, seems healthy, but recognizes that if his son tests positive, he himself will soon show signs of disease. Such knowledge can be very distressing and can even precipitate suicide. Should their clinician make testing available to the son, if in doing so it may have adverse consequences for the father?

This is a dilemma that requires careful consideration of the rights of all parties and usually involves many different professionals and multiple counselling sessions. Current practice in some centres in the UK supports the principle that generally, the right of (adult) offspring to know should take precedence over that of their parents *not* to know. Others simply decline such tests.

Genetic testing of children

Genetic testing of a child is appropriate: (a) if the child may have a genetic disorder requiring immediate diagnosis and management (e.g. PKU); (b) for prediction of a condition that may later manifest itself and which either requires surveillance (e.g. von Hippel–Lindau syndrome, Chapter 56); or (c) can be treated at an early stage. Some types of familial cancer, such as FAP, fall into this category, (but *not* breast and ovarian cancer). It is usually considered inappropriate to test children for untreatable conditions of adult onset, as such identification can have subtle, undesirable influences on their sense of self and well-being. Such tests are usually best deferred until the child is of an age to make his or her own informed choice.

Genetic screening

Prediction of future disability can be highly accurate but, in those who test positive, uncertainty as to *whether* an individual will develop the disease becomes replaced by worry over *when* or *how* it will manifest. Negative consequences of carrier status include the emotional impact of that knowledge, concerns about health, the burden of reproductive decisions, and potential stigmatization and discrimination in personal relationships.

In 'cascade screening' within a family, consent forms may be passed on to family members who have not been fully informed and may reveal information about family members without their consent. There can also be unexpected responses by family members given favourable predictions, such as guilt when other family members are not so favoured. Family ties strengthened from sharing concerns about the disease may weaken for those no longer personally so involved.

Additional problems in genetic counselling

Additional problems for the counsellor or client include:

1 facility with language;
2 issues of power between husband and wife;
3 religious stances and associated cultural values;
4 the sex and personal presentation of the medical contact;
5 a tradition of consanguineous marriage (especially in some South Asian and Middle Eastern groups);
6 cultural stereotyping;
7 thoughtlessly disturbing or offensive terms, like 'CATCH 22' and 'CRASH syndrome'.

Areas of ethical challenge arising from new reproductive technologies

The Ethical, Legal and Social Implications (ELSI) Program makes recommendations about how new information arising from the Human Genome Project (see Chapter 31) may be handled safely. Controversial issues that may be relevant to such considerations include the following:

1 gamete donation;
2 use of frozen sperm from a dead man;
3 creation of 'saviour siblings' for tissue donation;
4 implantation of embryos in postmenopausal women;
5 human embryo cloning;
6 gene therapy and gene patenting;
7 creation of interspecific human hybrids;
8 mitochondrial replacement therapy;
9 stem cell research;
10 life insurance and health insurance;
11 the stage at which new individuals acquire human rights;
12 molecular definition of race.

Self-assessment case studies: questions

Case 1: Unbalanced translocation

You are called to see Betsy, a 12-hour-old girl in the neonatal intensive care unit, for evaluation of multiple congenital anomalies. Betsy was born after a 37-week gestation complicated by intrauterine growth retardation. An ultrasound scan performed in the 3rd trimester was otherwise normal. Birth weight was 1.5 kg (this is below the 3rd centile). Multiple anomalies were noted soon after birth, including microcephaly, club feet, high, narrow palate, low-set posteriorly rotated ears, 5th finger clinodactyly, and hypotonia. Both parents are phenotypically normal. The nursery resident asks if you would do interphase FISH studies because she has heard that rapid results can be obtained with this method. You suggest instead that a cytogenomic microarray analysis be done, to be followed if necessary by a full karyotype.

Questions

1 Why would interphase FISH not be the ideal test to perform in this case?

2 What is the difference between cytogenomic array analysis and karyotyping? What kinds of changes does each detect?

Five days later you get a call from the cytogenetics laboratory with the results which indicate the presence of extra material from the short arm of chromosome 17; karyotype shows that this material is attached to the end of chromosome 14.

3 How would you interpret this finding? Is the chromosome change balanced or unbalanced?

You explain the results to Betsy's parents and suggest that both of them have chromosomal studies. Her father is found to have the following karyotype: 46,XY,t(14;17)(p11.2;p11.2).

4 Why is karyotyping the preferred study for Betsy's parents rather than microarray analysis?

5 Betsy's father's karyotype is abnormal, but he is phenotypically normal. How would you explain this?

6 How does this finding explain the genetic change in Betsy?

7 Betsy's mother has had two miscarriages prior to Betsy's birth. Do these findings have relevance to those miscarriages as well?

Two years have passed. Betsy has had a difficult time, with major feeding problems and developmental delay. Her parents are interested in having additional children.

8 How would you counsel them regarding their recurrence risk of similar problems? What options are available to them to manage this risk?

Case 2: A metabolic problem

You get a call from the newborn screening laboratory about one of your patients, a girl named Sophia. You learn that her newborn blood screen test was abnormal, revealing a high level of phenylalanine. You have not met Sophia or her parents yet – one of your partners was on call when she was discharged from the hospital. Now you call her parents to arrange for them to come to the office for a repeat blood sampling, and also set them up to meet with a metabolic disease specialist the next day.

Questions

1 Why is it urgent to follow up on the abnormal metabolic screening test?

Sophia is seen in the Metabolism Clinic, and her parents meet with several members of the team. They are told that Sophia's phenyl-alanine level was 26 mg/dL (normal is <2 mg/dL). She is started on special formula food without phenylalanine, and blood and urine are obtained for tetrahydrobiopterin (BH4) analysis.

2 What is the underlying basis for phenylketonuria?

3 What is the purpose of the tetrahydrobiopterin analysis?

The tetrahydrobiopterin analysis is negative, and Sophia's parents gradually become familiar with the low phenylalanine diet. At the second visit to Metabolism Clinic they ask to speak with a genetic counsellor. They have learned that PKU is a genetic disorder, but are puzzled that they could have an affected child in spite of the fact that neither parent has ever heard of a relative with the condition.

4 How would you explain the lack of family history, and how would you counsel Sophia's parents about their risk of having another affected child?

Sophia's parents ask whether it is possible to obtain prenatal testing if they have another child.

5 What would be involved in providing prenatal testing?

Sophia is now 4 years old. Her parents are told that there is a medication that may help to lower Sophia's blood phenylalanine levels and allow her dietary restriction to be relaxed somewhat. She is tried on the medication, sapropterin, and indeed her phenylalanine levels do go down. She continues on the medication on a daily basis.

6 How does sapropterin work and why do only some patients respond to the medication?

Sophia is now 14 years old; she has remained on her special diet all these years, but is becoming increasingly independent and rebellious. Her parents ask for a counsellor to speak with Sophia, to discuss the need to remain on the low phenylalanine diet.

7 Is there a stage in life when the low phenylalanine diet can be relaxed?

8 What are the special issues faced by a woman with PKU as she reaches childbearing age?

Case 3: A child with skin spots

James is a 3 year old referred for evaluation of skin spots. His mother had noticed them when he was about 2 months old, but the spots have become more numerous and distinct over the past 2 years. At first the paediatrician dismissed these as 'birthmarks', but James's mother insisted that an evaluation be done as she began to do research on her own as to what they might be. On examination, James is found to have 10 'café-au-lait' spots ranging in size from 5 mm to over 2 cm. His examination is otherwise unremarkable, with no skin-fold freckling or other skin lesions, though his head circumference is in the 95th centile (i.e. large, but within the normal range). You suspect a diagnosis of neurofibromatosis type 1 (NF1).

Questions

1 Based on the information provided, can a definitive diagnosis of NF1 be established?

A complete family history is taken, and it is learned that no one else in the family has ever had multiple café-au-lait spots or any other signs of NF1. You examine both of James's parents, and neither has café-au-lait spots.

Medical Genetics at a Glance, Third Edition. Dorian J. Pritchard and Bruce R. Korf.

2 Does the lack of family history reduce your suspicion that James might have NF1?

You arrange for genetic testing of the NF1 gene from a blood sample. A missense mutation (i.e. a base substitution) is found in the coding sequence. This mutation has never been seen before, either in affected or unaffected. Most NF1 mutations are truncating mutations that lead to premature termination of translation, so the pathogenicity of this mutation is uncertain.

3 What kind of evidence would you require to determine whether this mutation is pathogenic or a benign variant?

After further studies, it is concluded that the mutation could well be pathogenic. You follow James on an annual basis, and by 4 years of age he is manifesting skin-fold freckling, confirming the clinical diagnosis. He does not have any visible tumours, and ophthalmological follow-up has not revealed signs of optic glioma. There is some concern that James is experiencing learning disabilities. His parents are interested in having another child, and ask about their risks of a second child having NF1.

4 How would you counsel James's parents regarding their recurrence risk?

James is now 14 years old, and has been doing well since his diagnosis was established. He is getting special help in school for learning problems, but is making good progress. He is now beginning to manifest small tumours on his skin, which appear to be cutaneous neurofibromas. His parents are asked to consider having him participate in a clinical trial involving use of an inhibitor of Ras signalling in treating the cognitive problems in NF1. Both his parents and James agree to participate, and he completes the study.

5 What is believed to be the mechanism for development of neurofibromas? Why does one see multiple individual tumours instead of development of tumours along every nerve?

6 Why would an inhibitor of Ras signalling be considered as a possible therapeutic intervention in NF1?

Ten more years pass and now James and his wife are considering having children. They ask whether prenatal testing is possible. They also inquire about the current state of treatment of NF1.

7 How would you answer the questions about prenatal testing and treatment?

Case 4: Muscle weakness

Luke is 4 years old and his parents are concerned that he is getting more and more clumsy rather than less and less as he gets older. At first their paediatrician was not concerned, but then, as Luke began having difficulty climbing stairs, he referred him to you for neurological assessment. Examination reveals a healthy looking boy who has difficulty getting up off the floor without using his arms for support. He has mild weakness of the hip flexors and prominent calves. Blood is sent for determination of creatine phosphokinase and the result is a staggering 25 000 U/L, normal levels being up to 170.

Questions

1 What is the significance of the elevated CPK?

Suspecting Duchenne muscular dystrophy, you send a blood sample for dystrophin gene deletion analysis. A few days later the test result comes back and reveals that Luke has a deletion of exons 44 to 47, which has resulted in juxtaposition of out-of-frame exons. You explain to Luke's parents that, unfortunately, the test reveals he has Duchenne, rather than Becker dystrophy.

2 What is the difference between Duchenne and Becker dystrophy, and how does the deletion test help to make the distinction between the two disorders?

After considerable discussion with Luke's parents, it is decided to start him on treatment with prednisone, an anti-inflammatory corticosteroid. He is also introduced to a programme of physical therapy.

3 What is the approach to management of Duchenne muscular dystrophy and what is the prognosis?

A genetic counsellor explains the genetics of the disorder to Luke's parents the day the diagnosis was established. Luke has one sibling, an older sister. His parents are well and his mother has a brother and a sister, both of whom are well. Luke's mother has no maternal uncles. Luke's maternal aunt is particularly worried when she hears about Luke's condition, because she has just learned she is pregnant.

4 How would you counsel Luke's mother and maternal aunt?

Dystrophin gene deletion testing is carried out on Luke's mother's DNA and that of his aunt, and both are found to carry the deletion.

5 What can be offered to Luke's aunt in terms of prenatal testing?

Luke's aunt's unborn baby turns out to be a girl, who is found to have inherited the deletion.

6 Is a female dystrophin deletion carrier at risk of developing muscular dystrophy?

Case 5: Cancer in the family

Ted is a 40 year old who is seeking counselling regarding genetic testing for breast cancer. He is concerned not for himself, but for his two daughters, who are 10 and 12 years old. Ted's sister has been diagnosed with breast cancer at age 36 and recently had a bilateral mastectomy. His mother died of breast cancer when she was 40; he has two maternal aunts, one of whom is currently being treated for ovarian cancer at age 65, while the other is in good health.

Questions

1 Would Ted's family history suggest an increased risk for hereditary breast cancer?

Ted is told that testing would be possible, but that it would be preferable to test his sister first.

2 What is the reason for testing Ted's sister before Ted is tested?

Ted's sister is tested for mutation in the BRCA1 and BRCA2 genes. Several weeks later the results are returned, and she is found to carry a stop mutation in the BRCA1 gene.

3 Would you expect that this mutation would be pathogenic?

4 What advice would you give Ted's sister based on this result?

Ted's sister has given her permission to communicate these results to Ted. Upon hearing of this, he explains that he is not concerned for himself, but is interested in having his daughters tested.

5 Does Ted face any cancer-related risks if he is found to carry a BRCA1 mutation?

6 What would you advise regarding testing his daughters?

Case 6: Targeted treatment

Mary is a 63 year old referred for evaluation of fatigue and weight loss. She had been healthy until about 3 months ago, but now has little energy and has lost 15 pounds (~7 kg). On examination she is noted to have a palpable spleen and slightly enlarged liver. Blood testing is done and she is found to have 22 000 white blood cells per cubic millimetre, and a mild anaemia. The blood smear shows myeloid cells at various stages of maturation. This explains the enlarged liver and spleen, which are probably similarly engorged with myeloid cells. A bone marrow aspirate is done, and chromosomal analysis reveals the presence of the Philadelphia chromosome.

Questions

1 What is the Philadelphia chromosome and what is its significance in this patient?

Mary is diagnosed as having chronic myeloid leukaemia. After consideration of her options, it is decided to start her on treatment with imatinib.

2 What is imatinib and how does it work?

Mary has been on treatment for 2 months, and her white blood cell count has returned to normal. Cytogenetic studies of her white blood cells failed to detect the Philadelphia chromosome, though PCR analysis still indicates presence of the translocation.

3 What is the basis of PCR testing for the presence of the Philadelphia chromosome?

4 Why would PCR testing detect the translocation when cytogenetic analysis was negative?

Mary has been doing well for 18 months, but recently she has begun to feel fatigued again. She is found once again to have increased white blood cells on her blood smear, and Philadelphia chromosome positive cells are once again found.

5 Why does relapse occur in patients with CML after treatment with imatinib?

Case 7: Worries about senility

Larry is a 54 year old whom you have been treating for mild hypertension for the past 4 years. His health is otherwise good, though he also has hypercholesterolaemia, for which he was recently started on statin therapy to protect him from atherosclerosis by lowering his cholesterol. At a routine follow-up visit he asks about testing for Alzheimer disease. His mother had been diagnosed as having presenile dementia several years ago, and recently died of the disorder. There is no other family history of which Larry is aware.

Questions

1 Is Larry at high risk of developing Alzheimer disease based on this family history?

Larry is told that there is no genetic testing that would be recommended at this time. He has no symptoms of Alzheimer disease and his examination is entirely normal. Not entirely satisfied, Larry goes on the internet that night and does some research on his own for genetic testing for Alzheimer disease. It doesn't take him long to find a lab that offers ApoE testing.

2 What is the relationship of ApoE to Alzheimer disease?

Larry calls the office the next day to ask if he can be tested for ApoE. You explain that this testing is not recommended as a screen for Alzheimer disease.

3 How would you evaluate ApoE testing in terms of clinical accuracy, clinical validity, and clinical utility?

Returning to the internet, Larry finds a lab that will accept a cheek brushing sample (mouth swab) without a physician's referral. The internet ad notes that the laboratory is 'CLIA certified'. He contacts the laboratory, which provides a kit in the mail. His wife helps him do the cheek brushing, and the sample is sent off to the laboratory.

4 Are there specific concerns about cheek brushing as a source of material for testing that would be different from blood?

A month later, Larry gets a report in the mail saying that his ApoE genotype is ε2/ε4. Now he calls your office again to ask what this means. Is he going to get Alzheimer disease?

5 How would you counsel Larry?

*Clinical Laboratory Improvement Amendments: an American accreditation of quality standards for laboratories providing medical diagnoses.

Case 8: A sleepy infant

You are called to see Kirsten, a 1-day-old girl, in the newborn intensive care unit. Kirsten was born after a 37-week pregnancy with birth weight of 2200 grams (4 lb 13½ oz). Her doctors are concerned because she seems to be unusually sleepy, with minimal responses to stimulation and very lethargic feeding. She is being fed by nasogastric tube and her vital signs are stable. Evaluation for infection has been negative, and she has no evidence of any metabolic derangement. On examination, she is breathing on her own and has no dysmorphic features. She is very lethargic and hypotonic, though there are no fasciculations (visible muscle flickering) and deep tendon reflexes can be elicited, which both argue against spinal muscular atrophy. The extreme lethargy and poor feeding are more typical of a central nervous system, rather than a neuromuscular cause for the hypotonia, though congenital myopathy or congenital myotonic dystrophy remain a possibility.

You suspect Prader–Willi syndrome and ask for chromosome analysis, FISH testing, and methylation testing.

Questions

1 What role do these tests play in the genetic diagnosis of Prader–Willi syndrome.

The chromosomes are normal female and the FISH test result is normal also. The methylation analysis, however, reveals only a maternal pattern. You suspect uniparental disomy.

2 What kind of testing can you do to confirm your suspicion?

DNA testing reveals that, indeed, Kirsten has two maternal copies of chromosome 15 and no paternal copy.

3 What is the mechanism whereby uniparental disomy causes Prader–Willi syndrome?

You explain the results to Kirsten's parents, and the natural history of Prader–Willi syndrome. Kirsten's parents are both 39 years old. They ask whether they would be at risk of having another child with the disorder, and whether their healthy 6 year old will be at risk of having affected children when she grows up.

4 What is the recurrence risk of uniparental disomy in this family?

5 Is Kirsten's sister at risk of having an affected child?

Kirsten's parents ask whether there are treatments available for children with Prader–Willi syndrome.

6 What would you advise Kirsten's parents about availability of treatments?

Case 9: Advance warning

Bill and Rita are interested in starting a family. Bill is 29 and Rita 27 years old. They arrange an appointment with Rita's obstetrician-gynaecologist to discuss prepregnancy issues. Bill's ancestors came from Germany and Rita's from Scotland. They are not aware of a family history of any specific genetic disorder and both are in good health. They are told that carrier testing for cystic fibrosis is available if they are concerned about this disorder for their future offspring.

Questions

1 What is the risk that Bill and Rita would have a child with cystic fibrosis?

2 How is cystic fibrosis carrier testing performed?

Bill and Rita decide to go ahead with testing. A few weeks later they learn that Rita carries the Phe508del mutation, but Bill's DNA contains no detectable mutation. The testing is estimated to reveal 88% of all pathogenic alleles.

3 Are Bill and Rita at risk of having an affected child?

4 How does the Phe508del mutation affect the function of the gene? *As an outcome of the tests, Bill's risk of being a cystic fibrosis carrier is reduced from 1/25 to approximately 1/200, making their risk of having an affected child 1/20000. Bill and Rita ask if there is anything available to be sure that Bill does not carry a CF mutation.*

5 How would you answer this question?

Case 10: Enzyme replacement

Tom is a 41 year old who is seen in the Nephrology Clinic. He was diagnosed as having Fabry disease at age 26 (see Figure 62.1). At that time, he had suddenly developed left-sided weakness and diplopia (double vision), and was diagnosed as having had a mild stroke. He was also found to have mild proteinuria. Over the ensuing years he has noted that he does not sweat and has had some difficulty with overheating in hot weather. This has caused him to limit his activity on warm days. He has occasional chest palpitations but no chest pain. Every 6–8 weeks he has attacks of vomiting and diarrhoea, which resolve within a day. He also notices pain and some numbness and tingling in his fingertips and toes.

Questions:

1 How could the diagnosis of Fabry disease be confirmed?

Tom has a brother and a sister. His brother is also known to be affected and is undergoing enzyme replacement therapy. His sister is well and has two sons, ages 9 and 11, who are in good health. Tom's mother is 65 years of age and is well. His father died of myocardial infarction at age 58. Tom's mother has a brother who is well, and she has two sisters who are also unaffected with Fabry disease. Tom has two daughters, ages 6 and 8 years, both of whom are well.

2 What pattern of inheritance for Fabry disease is suggested by this family history?

Tom is wondering whether he might also be a candidate for enzyme replacement therapy. His physical examination is notable for angiokeratoma on the palms of the hands and both knees. He has mild ankle oedema. Liver and spleen are not enlarged. He has mild weakness in his legs and some decreased sensation to light touch in the fingertips and toes. Laboratory studies reveal 2.68 g of protein/24 hours (normal is <150 mg/24 hours) in the urine and a creatinine clearance of 81.5 mL/min (normal: 97–137 mL/min). Blood pressure is normal. Ophthalmological examination reveals bilateral corneal opacities and dilated conjunctival vessels, although his vision is normal. Some left ventricular hypertrophy is indicated by ECG and echocardiogram, but cardiac function is normal.

3 What could be the pathophysiological mechanism by which these problems develop?

It is determined that Tom is eligible for enzyme replacement therapy, and when his initial evaluation is completed he is introduced to the protocol. This entails intravenous infusion of α-galactosidase every second week. He is re-evaluated 5 weeks later. His energy level has increased and he reports marked decrease in the pain in his fingers and toes. He has had no further episodes of vomiting or diarrhoea. Over the ensuing year, he is also noted to have reduced proteinuria. Gastrointestinal episodes are much less frequent than they had been in the past.

4 How does infused enzyme reach the normal site of action of α-galactosidase within lysosomes?

5 What other lysosomal storage disorders are currently treated by enzyme replacement therapy?

Case 11: Autism spectrum disorder

Jake is 4 years old and his parents have been increasingly concerned about him. Although he has achieved more or less normal motor developmental milestones, his speech and social development have been very slow. He says only a few words and does not put together sentences. He spends most of his time playing on his own, with very little interaction with others, either his parents, his sibs, or other children. He also tends to make repetitive movements and sounds for no apparent reason. His parents ask his paediatrician, who refers them to a developmental specialist. Jake is diagnosed as having autism spectrum disorder.

Questions

1 What is autism spectrum disorder?

Jake is next referred to a geneticist for evaluation. A family history is taken; no one on either side of the family had ever been diagnosed with autism. Jake is examined, and no dysmorphic features are identified.

2 What is the aetiology of autism spectrum disorder?

The geneticist draws a blood sample from Jake and arranges for testing of a number of things – these include a cytogenomic microarray and fragile X analysis, as well as analysis of amino and organic acids from plasma and urine.

3 What is the rationale for genetic evaluation of children with autism spectrum disorders?

A few weeks later, Jake's parents return to the geneticist to discuss the results of testing. Fragile X results were normal, but Jake was found to have a deletion involving chromosome 16, at 16p11.2.

4 What is the significance of the chromosomal deletion? *Both of Jake's parents are offered genetic testing; neither is found to have the deletion identified in Jake.*

5 What would you tell Jake's parents about the recurrence risk of autism if they were to have additional children?

Case 12: Exome sequencing

Zoe is 12 years old and has a long history of intellectual disability and congenital anomalies. She had a congenital heart defect that was repaired when she was an infant, as well as a cleft lip that was also surgically repaired. She was of normal birth weight, but has grown slowly since infancy and is now less than 5 feet tall. Her facial features are distinctive, especially with large, prominent ears. Over the years she has been seen by many specialists, but in spite of many genetic tests, no diagnosis has been achieved. Recently her paediatrician referred her back to a geneticist, who is unable to make a specific clinical diagnosis, but suggests that whole exome sequencing be done.

Questions

1 What is exome sequencing and what does it offer for clinical diagnosis?

Zoe's parents have a lot of questions about exome sequencing – how much does it cost, will the costs be covered, how likely is it that an answer will be obtained, are there risks involved in testing? They have a long conversation with the medical geneticist and a genetic counsellor about these issues.

2 How would you answer their questions?

Zoe's parents consider what they have learned, and ultimately agree to go forward. A letter is sent to their insurance company, which agrees to cover the costs of testing. A blood sample is obtained from Zoe and from both her parents.

3 Why is a sample obtained from Zoe's parents?

About 6 weeks later Zoe's parents go to the geneticist for a follow-up visit. They are told that Zoe was found to have a mutation in the gene MLL2. This is associated with the disorder Kabuki syndrome, which in retrospect fits with Zoe's phenotype.

4 What is Kabuki syndrome and why was the diagnosis not made clinically?

Zoe's parents are relieved to have a diagnosis, though they understand that the condition cannot be treated. They are particularly glad to know that Zoe is affected by new mutation, since neither of them was found to carry the same mutation.

5 What are the implications of this test for other family members?

Case 13: Direct-to-consumer genomic testing

Tom clicks 'enter' on the on the page of a web site for a company carrying out genomic testing, having provided his credit card information and setting up a user name and password. He had heard at a party about the possibility of arranging genomic testing on himself and after reading the information on the website, decided to go ahead. A few days later, he receives a kit in the mail, provides saliva in a tube, and mails it back to the company.

Questions

1 What does the company do with Tom's saliva sample?

About a month later, Tom is directed to a secure web site to see his results. He finds that he is at slightly increased risk of a number of conditions and decreased risk for many others.

2 How do you interpret the odds ratios provided by the company?

One of the conditions for which Tom is found to be at highest risk is Type 2 diabetes. He is not aware of any family history of the disorder and has never been told by his doctor that he has any signs of diabetes.

3 What is the significance of Tom's increased risk of Type 2 diabetes? Is there anything he can do to manage this risk?

In further exploring the web site, Tom notes that he can learn the results of ApoE testing for risk of Alzheimer disease. After thinking hard about this, he decides not to click on the box giving consent to receive this result.

4 What is the relationship of *ApoE* status to risk of Alzheimer disease? What might motivate a person to wish to know or not know of this result?

Tom creates a printout of the results from his testing and brings it with him to his primary care doctor the next time he has a routine appointment. His physician is surprised that so much information can be obtained without involvement of a medical professional.

5 What are the risks and benefits of direct-to-consumer testing?

Case 14: Treatment of genetic disorders

Marci is an 8-year-old girl who is affected with cystic fibrosis. The diagnosis was made when she was an infant, after she presented with failure to thrive and a respiratory infection. Over the years she has been treated with antibiotics, chest physical therapy and pancreatic

enzyme replacement. She has done well for the most part, but has required hospitalized for pulmonary infections on several occasions.

Questions

1 What is cystic fibrosis and how is it treated.

Marci is cared for at a cystic fibrosis specialty clinic. During one of her routine visits her physician speaks with her parents about a recent clinical trial that resulted in development of a new medication that is now approved for treatment of cystic fibrosis.

2 What is a clinical trial?

The medication is called ivacaftor, and is used to treat individuals with the Gly551Asp mutation in the CFTR gene.

3 What is the basis for ivacaftor treatment; why is it used only for individuals with this specific mutation?

Marci is tested and indeed has one copy of the Gly551Asp mutation (her other mutation is Phe508del, i.e. she is a compound heterozygote).

4 What is the mechanism of dysfunction resulting from these two mutations?

Marci is started on ivacaftor at a dose of 150 mg twice a day. She is monitored for side effects, and after 6 months of treatment has tolerated the medication well. She also has experienced an improvement in pulmonary function, though she still requires treatment with antibiotics and chest physical therapy.

5 What are the risks and benefits of ivacaftor treatment?

Case 15: Pharmacogenetics

Steven is a 45 year old in previously good health who is examined in the hospital emergency room with a painful and swollen leg. It began shortly after a long trans-Atlantic airplane flight. On examination his left calf is swollen, red and tender. A clinical diagnosis of deep vein thrombosis is made, confirmed by an ultrasound examination performed in the emergency room and then by a venogram in the radiology department. Steven is started on a course of IV heparin treatment.

Questions

1 What is deep vein thrombosis and how is it treated.

Steven is admitted to the hospital for treatment. After a few days he is told that he will be switched to an oral medication, warfarin. In preparation for this treatment, a blood sample is obtained for genetic testing.

2 How does warfarin work and what kind of genetic test would be done to prepare for treatment?

The genetic test shows that Steven is especially sensitive to warfarin, and his dosage is adjusted downwards accordingly. However, he is switched from heparin to warfarin without incident.

3 What would be the consequences of excess or deficient warfarin activity if too much or too little were administered?

Steven also has genetic testing to determine the cause of his deep vein thrombosis. He is found to be a carrier of the Factor V Leiden mutation.

4 What is Factor V Leiden and how does it predispose to thrombosis?

Given this result, Steven asks if other members of his family should be tested. The risks and benefits of genetic testing are discussed with him.

5 What is the clinical utility of Factor V Leiden testing in asymptomatic individuals?

Self-assessment case studies: answers

Case 1

1 Interphase FISH provides the ability to determine aneuploidy for any of the chromosomes for which chromosome-specific probes are applied. In practice, this usually means chromosomes 13,18, 21, X, and Y, since these are the chromosomes most likely to be responsible for aneuploidy in a liveborn child. Aneuploidy for other chromosomes and structural rearrangements would not be detected with the probes normally used. Therefore, interphase FISH is used to exclude major aneuploidy, but would not be useful in evaluation of a child where aneuploidy for those chromosomes is not clinically suspected.

2 Cytogenomic array testing involves competitive hybridization of isolated DNA from a patient and reference sample to oligonucleotides on a microarray, or quantitative hybridization of patient DNA to oligonucleotides on a microarray. Microarray testing provides very sensitive detection of copy number changes, i.e. deletions and duplications, but does not detect balanced rearrangements; the latter are better detected by karyotypic analysis of chromosomes visualized through the microscope.

3 The finding is indicative of partial trisomy for material from the short arm of Chromosome 17 (Case figure 1). The abnormality represents an unbalanced translocation.

4 Given the unbalanced translocation in Betsy, it is most likely that one of her parents carries a balanced translocation. Balanced rearrangements are not detected by microarray analysis, but are easily seen by karyotyping.

5 Although abnormal, the father's karyotype is balanced, with a reciprocal translocation between Chromosomes 14 and 17. This exchange resulted in transfer of the short arm of Chromosome 17 to the base of the short arm of Chromosome 14, and a small amount of material from Chromosome 14 to the base of the short arm of 17. No material was apparently lost or gained in this process, explaining why the father is phenotypically normal.

6 Betsy received the derivative 14 chromosome from her father (i.e. the copy of 14 with extra material derived from 17), as well as the normal Chromosome 17 from her father. This made her trisomic for most of the short arm of Chromosome 17 and monosomic for the short arm of Chromosome 14. Most of the short arm of Chromosome 14 encodes ribosomal RNA. Loss of this material is unlikely to be consequential, since other acrocentric chromosomes also carry ribosomal DNA. Trisomy of most of 17p, however, is likely to be clinically significant, given the large size of the region.

7 Although miscarriage is relatively common and may have been coincidental, the fact that Betsy's father is a balanced translocation carrier means that it is possible that an unbalanced chromosome complement was transmitted in either or both of these miscarried pregnancies. This would not be unusual for a couple where one partner is a balanced translocation carrier, since the father in this case faces a risk of creating sperm cells with unbalanced karyotypes. In some cases, the chromosomal imbalance is so severe as to lead to miscarriage.

8 The couple faces an increased risk of having another child with genetic imbalance regarding Chromosomes 14 and 17. The exact magnitude of the risk is difficult to know, since this is a very rare chromosome rearrangement, and risk of unbalanced gametes varies with different rearrangements. The couple can be offered prenatal testing by chorionic villus sampling or amniocentesis to see if a future fetus

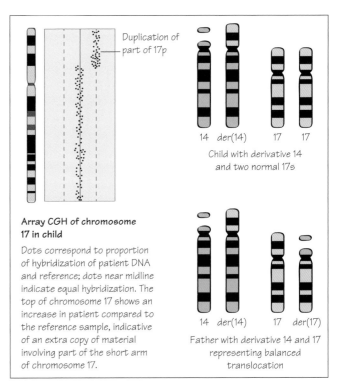

Case figure 1 Detection of duplication of 17p by array comparative genomic hybridization (left); idiogram of chromosomes 4 and 17 of child (showing derivative 14) and father (showing balanced translocation of chromosomes 14 and 17).

has inherited an unbalanced karyotype, or *in vitro* fertilization with preimplantation diagnosis.

Case 2

1 PKU is a disorder of amino acid metabolism in which there is a build-up of phenylalanine due to deficiency of activity of phenylalanine hydroxylase. Phenylalanine is cleared through the placenta *in utero*, and therefore does not begin to build up until after the first feed. Neurological damage begins to occur thereafter, provoking the urgency to restrict phenylalanine intake if the diagnosis is confirmed.

2 PKU is an inborn error of metabolism, most often due to mutation in the gene that encodes the enzyme phenylalanine hydroxylase required to convert phenylalanine to tyrosine (Case figure 2). In the absence of enzyme activity, phenylalanine builds up to toxic levels, and also is converted to phenylpyruvic acid, which is also toxic. In addition, there is a deficiency of tyrosine, and its metabolites, including the neurotransmitter DOPA and the pigment melanin. The former may contribute to neurological problems and the latter results in hypopigmentation.

3 Although most affected individuals have a mutation in the gene that encodes phenylalanine hydroxylase, a small minority have a deficiency of tetrahydrobiopterin, due to mutation in one of several enzymes required to synthesize this coenzyme. Tetrahydrobiopterin is a cofactor required for the conversion of phenylalanine to tyrosine (see Chapters 58 and 62).

Medical Genetics at a Glance, Third Edition. Dorian J. Pritchard and Bruce R. Korf.
© 2013 John Wiley & Sons, Ltd. Published 2013 by John Wiley & Sons, Ltd.

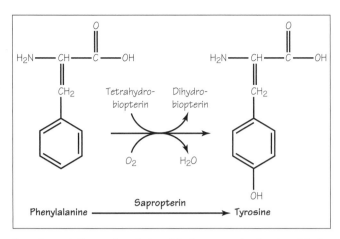

Case figure 2 Conversion of phenylalanine to tyrosine by phenylalanine hydroxylase requires the cofactor tetrahydrobiopterin; this reaction is stimulated by sapropterin.

4 PKU is inherited as an autosomal recessive trait. Both parents must be heterozygous carriers, and probably other members of their families are carriers as well. The carrier frequency in the Caucasian population is about 1/50, so the likelihood is low that other family members have also had a carrier partner. Sophia's parents, though, face a 25% recurrence risk with each pregnancy.

5 Prenatal testing is best done by molecular genetic analysis. This requires identification of the mutant alleles in the two parents, which now is possible to arrange on a routine clinical basis (see www.genetests.org for a list of laboratories). Once the mutations are identified, fetal tissue can be obtained by chorionic villus biopsy or amniocentesis and tested to determine if one or both mutations has been transmitted.

6 Sapropterin is a form of tetrahydrobiopterin that can be taken orally. In some patients with phenylalanine hydroxylase mutations, the BH4 can stimulate residual enzyme activity and reduce the need for dietary phenylalanine restriction. It is important to note, however, that some degree of phenylalanine restriction remains necessary and close monitoring of blood phenylalanine levels is critical.

7 It used to be thought that phenylalanine restriction could be relaxed in late childhood, as the nervous system matures. It is now recognized that phenylalanine restriction needs to be continued for a lifetime, as there are continued neurological consequences of high phenylalanine levels.

8 Women with untreated PKU have high blood phenylalanine levels that will cross the placenta if they are pregnant. This exposes the fetus to toxic levels of the amino acid, and results in low birth weight, congenital anomalies and abnormal neurological development. It is therefore critical that a woman maintains careful control of phenylalanine, beginning prior to conception and continuing throughout pregnancy.

Case 3

1 A clinical diagnosis of NF1 requires that any two of the following features be present:

    (a) six or more café-au-lait spots larger than 5 mm in a prepubertal child;

    (b) skin-fold freckling (e.g. axillary or inguinal);

    (c) two or more neurofibromas or one plexiform neurofibroma;

    (d) iris hamartomas (Lisch nodules);

    (e) characteristic skeletal dysplasia (orbital or tibial dysplasia);

    (f) optic glioma (tumour);

    (g) affected first-degree relative.

Based on the information provided, James fulfills one criterion (multiple café-au-lait spots), but not two, and therefore a definitive diagnosis cannot be established clinically. Many of the features, however, are age-dependent, so the diagnosis cannot be excluded at this point.

2 Approximately 50% of cases occur sporadically, without apparent family history of NF1. The lack of signs in the parents therefore does not exclude the diagnosis in James.

3 A missense mutation could be pathogenic, or might represent a benign variant. Given the fact that both parents are clinically unaffected and that the penetrance of known NF1 mutations is essentially 100%, the most powerful approach to determining the significance of the mutation would be to test both parents. If the mutation is not present in either of them, you can conclude that James has a new mutation, and this mutation would very likely be pathogenic. If the mutation is present in a parent, it would most likely be a benign variant, assuming no signs of the disorder in the parent. Other approaches would be to investigate more thoroughly if the mutation has ever been seen before in affected individuals, whether it segregates with the disease in families, whether it is seen in control individuals who are unaffected, and whether it affects the function of the gene product. The latter is difficult to do in a direct manner, but can be inferred from determination of whether the amino acid in question is conserved and by looking at the nature of the mutation in relation to the properties of the protein.

4 The penetrance of NF1 is essentially 100%, so if both parents are free of signs it is unlikely that they carry an *NF1* gene mutation. There is a possibility, though, of mosaicism, including germ line mosaicism. Therefore, one cannot counsel that recurrence is impossible, only that the risk is low. Since the mutation in the affected child is known, prenatal testing could be offered for a subsequent pregnancy.

5 The development of neurofibromas confirms the diagnosis of NF1. The *NF1* gene behaves as a tumour suppressor. Therefore, the tumor cells (Schwann cells in the case of a neurofibroma) have both the germline mutation and an acquired mutation of the homologous *NF1* allele (*c.f.* the 'Two-hit Hypothesis', Chapter 56). These mutations of the normal allele occur after conception, and account for the fact that neurofibromas are multifocal growths, and are not all derived from a single progenitor cell.

6 The protein product of the *NF1* gene, referred to as neurofibromin, functions as a regulator of the cell signalling molecule Ras (Case figure 3). Ras is activated when a growth factor binds to a membrane receptor; the activation involves binding of GTP to the Ras protein, which in turn then activates other proteins that eventually lead to transcription of specific genes in the nucleus. Neurofibromin stimulates the conversion of Ras-GTP back to Ras-GDP, effectively terminating the growth signal. If both copies of the *NF1* gene are mutated then no functional neurofibromin is present, and Ras signalling cannot be regulated. An inhibitor of Ras function might be useful in treatment if the primary biochemical mechanism of the disorder is hyperactive Ras signalling due to neurofibromin deficiency.

7 Assuming the pathogenic mutation is known, prenatal testing can be offered to detect the mutation, usually by chorionic villus sampling or amniocentesis. In some cases, single cell analysis is possible, enabling preimplantation diagnosis. Such testing would determine if the *NF1* mutation was transmitted, but does not predict the severity of the disorder. Regarding treatment, there are several clinical trials currently under way, including some that test drugs which target specific aspects of the Ras signalling pathway known to be involved

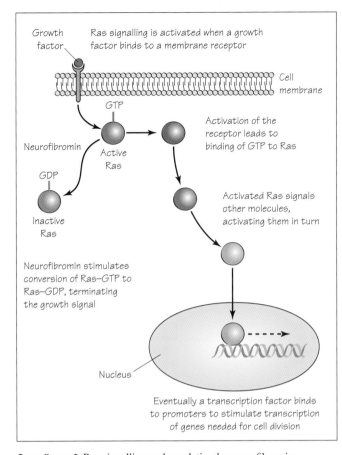

Case figure 3 Ras signalling and regulation by neurofibromin.

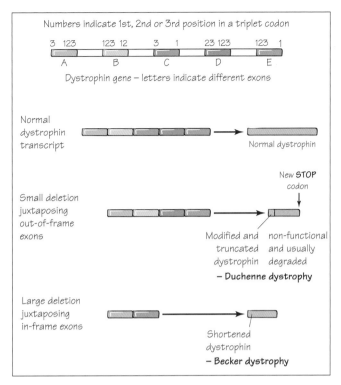

Case figure 4 Reading frame hypothesis involving dystrophin. Deletions leading to Duchenne dystrophy alter the reading frame of the protein (indicated by positions 1, 2 or 3 of the codon); those that lead to Becker dystrophy tend to preserve reading frame.

in the pathogenesis of NF1. The major current targets are neurofibromas and learning disabilities. It is expected that additional medication trials, targeted at a variety of clinical problems in NF1, will be launched in the coming years.

Case 4

1 CPK is an intramuscular enzyme that leaks out of damaged cells and the grossly elevated level suggests ongoing muscle damage. The examination reveals proximal muscle weakness, prominent calves and the difficulty getting up from a supine position referred to as the Gower sign. These features are all suggestive of Duchenne muscular dystrophy (see Chapter 11).

2 Duchenne and Becker dystrophy are both disorders in which there is gradual degeneration of muscle, but Duchenne tends to have earlier onset and more rapid progression. Both are due to mutation in the gene on the X chromosome that encodes the protein dystrophin (Case figure 4). Duchenne tends to occur when there is complete absence of functional dystrophin, whereas Becker results from mutations that result in abnormal quantity or quality of dystrophin. The most common type of mutation is deletion that affects one or more exons. If the deletion results in juxtaposition of exons with different reading frames (i.e. introduces a 'frame shift'; see Chapter 25), a modified protein results, resembling dystrophin up to the site of deletion, but with a completely different amino acid sequence after the deletion. If a stop signal (UAA, UAG or UGA) arises, a truncated as well as modified protein is produced. In either case, this results in Duchenne dystrophy. If a deletion juxtaposes exons 'in frame', dystrophin will be produced, albeit missing some protein domains due to the missing exons, resulting in the milder Becker muscular dystrophy.

3 There is no definitive treatment for Duchenne muscular dystrophy. The mainstay of management is physiotherapy, aimed at maintaining strength and mobility as long as possible. There is evidence that treatment with steroids slows progression of the disorder, and therefore its use is recommended, with careful monitoring for side effects.

4 Duchenne muscular dystrophy is an X-linked recessive disorder, and therefore usually affects males. Although there is no apparent family history of the disorder, there is a paucity of males in the mother's family who would have been at risk. Approximately two-thirds of the mothers of apparently sporadically affected boys are carriers; half of these mothers carry new mutations, half inherited them from their mothers. Both Luke's mother and his maternal aunt are therefore at risk of being carriers.

5 Given that Luke's aunt is a carrier, prenatal testing can be offered. This can include sex determination (since it is almost always males who are affected) as well as dystrophin gene deletion analysis. Fetal cells obtained by amniocentesis or chorionic villus sampling can also be tested.

6 Duchenne muscular dystrophy typically affects males, but on rare occasions a female can be affected. This may be due to non-random X chromosome inactivation, or the occurrence of a single X chromosome as in Turner syndrome. Some female carriers display mild signs such as muscle cramping and a proportion will develop a dilated cardiomyopathy.

Case 5

1 This family history suggests increased risk of breast and ovarian cancer (Case figure 5). Aside from having two first-degree relatives affected with breast cancer at a young age, he also has a relative with ovarian cancer. The most common cause of hereditary breast and ovarian cancer is mutation in the *BRCA1* or *BRCA2* genes (see Chapter 56). Approximately 7–10% of cases of breast cancer have a genetic basis, and of this approximately 52% is accounted for by *BRCA1* mutation and 32% by *BRCA2* mutation. The hallmark of a genetic predisposition to cancer includes the occurrence of cancer at a young age compared to the general population risk. There are several computer programs that are used to estimate risk of hereditary breast and ovarian cancer. One, called BRCAPRO, estimates Ted's risk at around 30%. Testing is usually offered to individuals whose risk is 10% or higher.

2 Current approaches to mutation testing do not detect all possible mutations in the *BRCA1* or *BRCA2* genes. Therefore, a negative test does not rule out the possibility of having a mutation. If Ted is tested and is negative, it may be that he did not inherit a mutation or it may be that the family mutation cannot be detected. On the other hand, it is very likely that his sister did inherit a mutation if there is one in the family, so a negative test in her would suggest that either there is no *BRCA1* or *BRCA2* mutation explaining this family history, or the mutation is not detectable with current approaches to testing. If she is found to have a mutation, Ted can be offered definitive testing to determine whether he inherited the same mutation.

3 Given that the mutation is a STOP, causing premature termination of translation of the protein, it is very likely to be pathogenic. The *BRCA* genes function as tumour suppressors, and the majority of pathogenic mutations lead to lack of expression of the gene product (see Chapters 17, 54–56).

4 Having had a bilateral mastectomy, Ted's sister does not face further risk of breast cancer. She does face, however, a risk of ovarian cancer (a lifetime risk of 28–44%). Her options to manage this risk include oophorectomy or surveillance with transvaginal ultrasound and cancer antigen 125 (CA-125) blood testing. CA-125 is a protein used as a biomarker for ovarian, endometrial, peritoneal and fallopian tube cancers. The normal upper concentration is around 35 U/mL.

5 Ted's risk of breast cancer is only minimally increased, though *BRCA2* mutation is associated with an increased risk of breast cancer in males. There may be a slightly increased risk of prostate cancer in males with both *BRCA1* and *BRCA2* mutations.

6 If Ted is a *BRCA1* mutation carrier, his daughters would each be at 50% risk of inheriting the mutation, in which case they would be at risk of breast and ovarian cancer. This risk, however, does not become significant until the middle of the third decade. Therefore, genetic testing for hereditary breast and ovarian cancer is not recommended for children. Rather, they should be offered counselling and the possibility of testing when they have reached an age when they can make an informed choice.

Case 6

1 The Philadelphia chromosome is created by translocation between Chromosomes 9 and 22 and is found in most cases of chronic myeloid leukaemia (CML). Not all cases of CML are Philadelphia chromosome-positive and it is also found in some other forms of leukaemia. The translocation juxtaposes the *abl* proto-oncogene on Chromosome 9 with the *bcr* gene on Chromosome 22. This results in production of a fusion protein with abnormal kinase activity, which helps to drive the abnormal growth of the tumour cells (see Chapters 39, 56).

2 Imatinib is a drug that was designed as a tyrosine kinase inhibitor (see Chapter 74). The drug binds to a site in the fusion protein with a high binding affinity for ATP (Case figure 6). It is a potent inhibitor of the abnormal enzyme and has been found to be highly effective in treatment of CML.

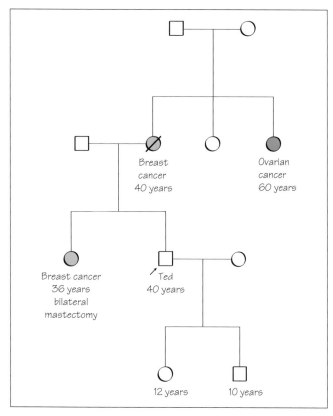

Case figure 5 Pedigree showing family history of breast and ovarian cancer.

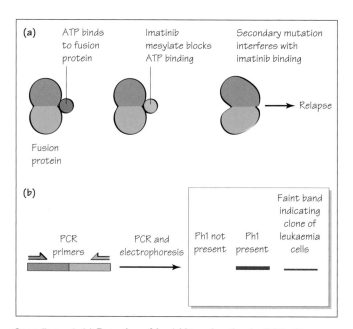

Case figure 6 (a) Detection of *bcr/abl* translocation by PCR; (b) inhibition of fusion protein by blocking of the ATP binding site with imatinib. Ph1, Philadelphia chromosome.

3 PCR testing for the *bcr–abl* fusion is done using PCR primers corresponding to the two genes that span the breakpoint. Normally, these primers would not cooperate in amplification, since the genes are on different chromosomes. In the typical translocation, however, the primer binding sites are sufficiently close for PCR amplification to occur and produce multiple copies of the sequence.

4 Imatinib can substantially reduce the number of leukemic cells, but typically does not completely eliminate them. PCR is significantly more sensitive than cytogenetic analysis, and therefore able to detect abnormal cells even in minute quantities.

5 Relapse can occur by proliferation of a small reservoir of leukaemic cells that undergo further mutation, resulting in a change in the conformation of the fusion protein, so that imatinib is no longer able to attach to the ATP-binding site. The period of remission can be prolonged if imatinib is used in combination with other chemotherapeutic agents.

Case 7

1 Alzheimer disease is a neurodegenerative disorder (Case figure 7) that presents with memory loss and behavioural changes. In about 2% of cases it is inherited as an autosomal dominant trait, but most cases are multifactorial. In families where autosomal dominant transmission does not occur, there is an empirical lifetime risk of Alzheimer disease of 20%. In first-degree relatives of patients that risk is doubled (i.e. 40%).

2 The *ApoE* locus is known to be associated with risk of Alzheimer disease. This is a polymorphic locus, with three alleles known as *ε2*, *ε3*, and *ε4*. The *ε4* allele is associated with increased risk of Alzheimer disease.

3 Testing *ApoE* genotype is highly accurate, but has limited clinical utility and clinical validity. Relative risk of Alzheimer disease is greatest in homozygotes for the *ε4* allele, but is increased also in those with just one *ε4* allele. Testing *ApoE* genotype is of limited clinical utility, since the presence of an *ε4* allele does not necessarily mean a person will develop Alzheimer disease. There is, moreover, nothing that can be offered to carriers to modify their risk, making the test of limited clinical utility as well. This is why *ApoE* testing is not recommended on a routine basis.

4 Cheek brushing is a way to obtain epithelial cells from the lining of the mucous membrane of the cheek, and is a convenient source of cells for DNA analysis. A relatively small quantity of cells is obtained, but sufficient to do targeted mutation testing. The major limitations are insufficient DNA for a large number of tests and lack of the RNA needed for some types of genetic tests. Cheek brushings however, provide adequate material for *ApoE* allele testing.

5 Larry has one *ε4* allele, which does increase his risk of Alzheimer disease. *ApoE* is a predispositional test, though, and not diagnostic, so there is still only a low risk he will develop the disorder. There is no recognized treatment so far available that will prevent Alzheimer disease, nor any special care plan based on the outcome of such tests.

Case 8

1 Around 70% of individuals with Prader–Willi syndrome have a deletion involving 15q11-q13, invariably of the paternal chromosome (see Chapter 27). Approximately 25% have uniparental disomy, with two copies of the maternal 15 and no representation of the paternal Chromosome 15. The balance are thought to have mutations within the Chromosome 15 imprinting centre, an unknown cause or are misdiagnosed. Methylation testing can distinguish the maternal and paternal copies of 15, which is abnormal in almost all cases of Prader–Willi syndrome.

2 Confirmation of suspected uniparental disomy is best done by obtaining blood from both parents and the child and using DNA polymorphisms to determine if the child has inherited Chromosome 15 markers from both parents. Finding genotypes inherited only from the mother would be indicative of maternal uniparental disomy.

3 Prader–Willi syndrome is thought to arise from lack of expression of a gene or genes on Chromosome 15 that normally are only expressed from the paternal chromosome (Case figure 8). If both copies of 15 are of maternal origin, these genes will not be expressed even if they are present.

4 The recurrence risk of uniparental disomy is very low. It is thought to arise from two consecutive non-disjunction events. First, non-disjunction in maternal meiosis gives rise to a trisomy 15 zygote upon fertilization. A second postzygotic non-disjunction restores the normal number of chromosomes, but if the paternal 15 is lost, maternal uniparental disomy results. This probably relates to maternal age, since the frequency of maternal non-disjunction increases with age.

5 Kirsten's sister is not at increased risk of having an affected child, since uniparental disomy is sporadic. Prader–Willi syndrome due to imprinting centre mutations can, however, be transmitted as a dominant trait (see Chapter 27).

6 Children with Prader–Willi syndrome are born with hypotonia, low birth weight and failure to thrive, but muscle tone and level of alertness tend to improve over time, as does feeding. In later childhood, however, a severe eating disorder usually ensues, along with behavioural problems and developmental delay. Without management, morbid obesity may result. There is now evidence that treatment with human growth hormone can result in control of the eating disorder, with significant improvement in somatic growth regulation and behaviour.

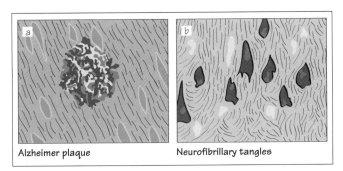

Case figure 7 Plaque (a) and neurofibrillary tangles (b) from the brain of an individual with Alzheimer disease.

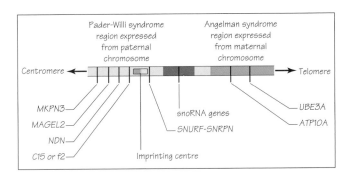

Case figure 8 Region of Chromosome 15 involved in Prader–Willi syndrome and Angelman syndrome. Regions expressed from the paternal chromosome are shown in blue, those expressed from the maternal chromosome in red.

Case 9

1 The frequency of cystic fibrosis among newborns of northern European ancestry is about 1/2500. The carrier frequency can be calculated from the Hardy–Weinberg equation (see Chapter 30). If $q2 = 1/2500$, $q = 1/50$, and the carrier frequency, $2pq$ is close to 1/25.

2 There is no biochemical test for cystic fibrosis carrier status. The testing is done by mutation analysis on a panethnic group of patients, using a panel of multiple (23) mutations that includes the top 99.9% of pathogenic mutations known to be associated with the disorder (Case table 9). Test sensitivity differs in different populations, depending on the frequency of those specific mutations in the population.

Case table 9 Panel of 23 mutations recommended by the American College of Medical Genetics for panethnic cystic fibrosis carrier screening.

3120+1G>A	Ala455Glu	G85E	Arg334W	1717-1G>A
3659delC	Phe508del	Arg347Pro	1898+1G>A	3849+10kbC>T
Ile507del	Asn1303Lys	Arg553*	2184delA	621+1G>T
Gly542*	Arg1162*	Arg560Thr	2789+5G>A	711+1G>T
Gly551Asp	Arg117His	Trp1282*		

3 Rita is found to be a carrier, but the testing is negative in Bill. There is still, however, a chance that Bill carries a mutation that was not included in the panel (approximately 12% of cystic fibrosis mutations are not detected in individuals of northern European ancestry on the standard 23 mutation test panel). There is indeed residual risk to this pregnancy.

4 The Phe508del mutation leads to abnormal processing of the CFTR protein, causing it to fail to be transported to the cell membrane. The physiological result is lack of protein at the cell membrane and in homozygotes, lack of chloride channel function.

5 If Bill carries a mutation, it was not one detectable on the standard mutation panel. In some cases now it is feasible to perform sequencing of the *CFTR* gene to search for mutations, though this would be costly and is not guaranteed to detect all possible mutations.

Case 10

1 The diagnosis of Fabry disease is confirmed by detection of deficient α-galactosidase enzyme activity in leucocytes or cultured fibroblasts. Although molecular genetic testing is possible, there is a wide variety of possible mutations, making molecular analysis more difficult than enzyme assay as a diagnostic test.

2 Fabry disease is inherited as an X-linked recessive trait, though some females manifest some signs of the disorder. Since Tom's brother is also affected, their mother must be a carrier. Their mother has only one brother, who happens not to be affected. We do not have information about the generation prior to Tom's mother. Tom's father's death from myocardial infarction is ascribable to unrelated causes.

3 The pathophysiology of Fabry disease is based on deposition of the GL-3 glycolipid, globotriaosylceramide, in endothelial cells due to lack of adequate α-galactosidase enzyme activity. This leads to chronic ischaemia (deficient blood supply) in tissues and obstruction of small vessels, leading to peripheral neuropathy (causing weakness, decreased sensation, and pain), renal insufficiency (causing ankle oedema, proteinuria and decreased creatinine clearance, indicative of decreased glomerular blood flow) and cardiac dysfunction. Deposition of storage material also occurs in corneal cells and the skin, leading to angiokeratomas.

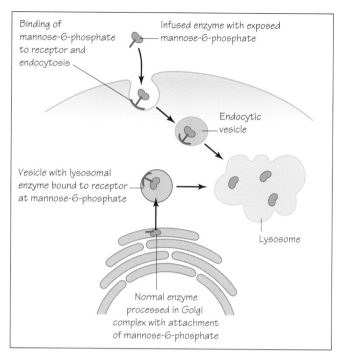

Case figure 10 Lysosomal enzyme is normally processed in the Golgi complex, where mannose-6-phosphate is attached. This binds to a specific receptor within a vesicle, which then fuses with a lysosome and delivers the enzyme. Infused enzyme with mannose-6-phosphate attached binds to membrane receptors, is internalized by endocytosis and the endocytic vesicle fuses with the lysosome.

4 Enzyme replacement therapy uses a purified, recombinant DNA-based enzyme synthesized *in vitro*. The infused enzyme is taken into cells by endocytosis before delivery to the lysosomes (Case figure 10).

5 Other lysosomal storage disorders currently treated with enzyme replacement therapy include Gaucher disease (β-glucosidase deficiency), Hurler syndrome (α-L-iduronidase deficiency), Hunter syndrome (iduronate-2-sulphatase deficiency) and Pompe disease (α-1,4-glucosidase deficiency). (See Chapter 62).

Case 11

1 Autism spectrum disorder is a family of developmental conditions characterized by a constellation of problems. Although there may be several distinct developmental disorders included under the 'autism spectrum' umbrella, they have in common three core features. These are impaired social interactions and communication skills and the tendency to engage in repetitive behaviours.

2 The aetiology of autism spectrum disorder is heterogeneous. Autism can be a component of many genetic syndromes, most notably fragile X syndrome, but many others as well, including Rett syndrome (in girls), tuberous sclerosis complex and inborn errors of metabolism such as phenylketonuria (if untreated). Single-gene and chromosomal disorders have also been identified in some with autism spectrum disorders. In many, the aetiology remains unknown.

3 Genetic evaluation is performed for a number of reasons. In some cases, albeit rarely, a treatable inborn error of metabolism may be identified. The effectiveness of treatment depends on the age at diagnosis and the condition, but metabolic disorders should not go

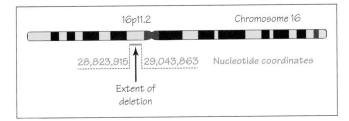

Case figure 11 Region of deletion on Chromosome 16p11.2, from nucleotides 28 823 915 to 29 043 863.

undiagnosed. Some conditions, such as tuberous sclerosis complex, can affect many body systems, and making a diagnosis provides a basis for anticipatory guidance and surveillance. Finally, recognizing a genetic aetiology provides a basis for genetic counselling of the family regarding risks of recurrence.

4 Chromosomal copy number changes are increasingly being recognized as cytogenomic microarray testing has become routine. It is now viewed as the first-line test in a child with developmental problems or multiple congenital anomalies, in preference to classical cytogenetic study. The microarray may detect copy number changes – deletions or duplications – that are well below the limits of resolution of the light microscope and may be pathologically significant. The frequency of detection of pathological copy number changes in children with autism spectrum disorder is now 15–20%.

5 The Chromosome 16p11.2 deletion (Case figure 11) in Jake has been described before in children with autism spectrum disorder and is likely to be responsible for Jake's problems. Both deletions and duplications of this region can occur in individuals with autism. The rearrangements occur at a site with repeated sequences that are prone to unequal recombination events. The deletion was not found in either of Jake's parents, indicating that this was a sporadic occurrence. Barring germline mosaicism, the risk of recurrence is likely to be very low.

Case 12

1 Exome sequencing involves use of second (or 'next') generation sequencing methods to sequence the entire protein-encoding component of the genome. This amounts to 1–2% of the genome, but includes the regions most commonly affected by mutation that lead to genetic disorders. It is accomplished by first isolating the exons from a DNA sample, sequencing all those exons, and then analysing the data to identify possible pathogenic mutations.

2 Exome sequencing is a new clinical diagnostic approach. The current (2012/2013) costs vary among testing laboratories; including both the sequencing and analysis, the costs in the US are currently $5000–$10 000. Such expenses are sometimes covered by insurance companies, mainly in circumstances where other diagnostic approaches have been unproductive. Although high, these costs may be less than those of multiple individual genetic tests, which may amount to $1000–$2000 each. Success rates depend on clinical circumstances – some reports suggest around 20–40%. The major risks of testing, besides not finding an answer, include discovery of variants of unknown significance, or findings in genes that predict medical problems, such as risk of cancer, that are unrelated to the original clinical question.

3 The success of exome sequencing depends on finding a mutation in a gene that might explain the clinical problem in the patient. Since Zoe is the only affected member of her family, this might be explained either by recessive inheritance, or by her having a new mutation with dominant inheritance. The former predicts that both her parents would

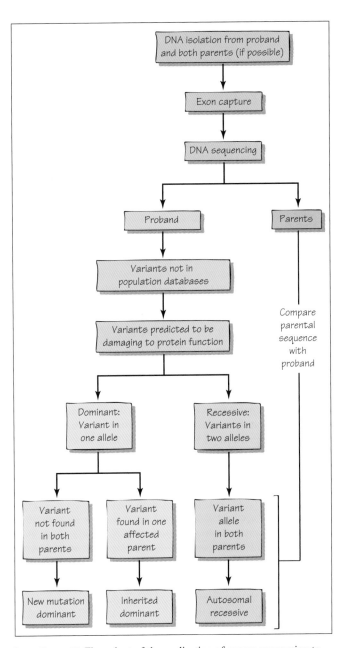

Case figure 12 Flow chart of the application of exome sequencing to identify the gene for an undiagnosed disorder, considering both dominant and recessive inheritance and comparing the proband's sequence to that of both parents.

be carriers; the latter that neither parent carries the mutation found in Zoe. In either case, it is helpful to have samples from both parents to compare with that of the patient (Case figure 12).

4 Kabuki syndrome is a rare multiple congenital anomaly syndrome characterized by intellectual disability, growth delay and characteristic physical features. The latter include elongated palpebral fissures with eversion of the lateral eyelids. Since it is rare it is not unusual for the clinical diagnosis to be delayed, or never established.

5 Kabuki syndrome is inherited as a dominant trait, but an appreciable number of cases are due to new mutation, as in this family. Excluding the possibility of germline mosaicism, in this family there would be only a low risk of recurrence. Any sibling would not be at risk, as they would already be showing signs of the disorder if they carried the mutation.

Case 13

1 DNA is isolated from the saliva sample and used to genotype approximately 1 million single nucleotide polymorphisms. The analytical validity (i.e. accuracy) of testing is very high.

Case table 13 Results of Tom's testing for five common disorders.

Condition	Odds of disease
Type 2 diabetes	1.24
Coronary artery disease	0.96
Parkinson disease	1.02
Asthma	0.85
Hypertension	1.13

2 The risk results are expressed as relative odds of getting disease, i.e. the odds of an individual with a specific genotype getting disease as compared to the odds of getting disease in those who do not carry that genotype (Case table 13). This can be used as an estimate of relative risk of disease in an individual with the specific genotype compared with risk in the general population. The risk estimates are based on outcomes of case–control studies. It is important to realize, however, that the quoted risks may not apply to all individuals, especially those with ancestry different from the populations in which the background studies were done. The risk estimates also do not take account of other non-genetic factors, such as body weight, smoking history, etc.

3 The results suggest a slight increase in odds of developing Type 2 diabetes. This does not mean that Tom definitely will develop the condition, as there are many other factors, both genetic and non-genetic, that contribute to risk. Aside from monitoring for signs, such as impaired glucose tolerance, and paying attention to diet and exercise, there is little that Tom can do to modify this risk.

4 Individuals who carry one or two *ApoE ε4* alleles have an increased risk of eventually developing Alzheimer disease. There is nothing that can be done to modify this risk, although some individuals found to be at risk have bought long-term care insurance. Some people choose to know their risk in spite of the lack of ability to reduce that risk, whereas others choose not to know.

5 Direct-to-consumer testing is a relatively new concept in genetics. Advocates believe that individuals have the right to explore their own genetic make-up and make decisions based on the information provided by the company. Sceptics fear that individuals may make medical decisions with inadequate understanding of the risks and benefits; for example, deciding not to pursue advice to maintain an ideal body weight if found to not be at high risk of diabetes. There is also concern that the test results can be misleading and are for the most part not useful in clinical management.

Case 14

1 Cystic fibrosis is an autosomal recessive disorder due to mutation in the *CFTR* gene that encodes a chloride channel protein. The major clinical signs are chronic lung disease due to obstruction of small airways as a consequence of thickened secretions, and malabsorption due to obstruction of the pancreatic ducts. Management typically includes treatment with antibiotics, chest physical therapy to improve pulmonary function and pancreatic enzyme replacement to manage malabsorption.

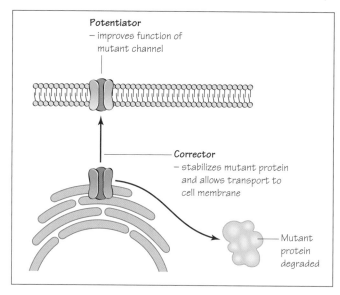

Case figure 14 Two strategies for therapy of cystic fibrosis, dependent on the nature of the causative mutation. Ivacaftor functions as a potentiator.

2 A clinical trial is a carefully controlled test of a new treatment or medical device on human participants. A Phase I trial is intended to identify toxicity and maximum tolerated dosage. A Phase II trial tests the safety and efficacy of the treatment in affected individuals. A Phase III trial compares the efficacy of the treatment with that of established treatments. A Phase IV trial consists of continuous monitoring for adverse effects, after a drug has been approved for routine use.

3 Ivacaftor was developed as an approach to improving the function of the chloride channel in the face of the specific Gly551Asp mutation (Case figure 14). This mutation substitutes aspartic acid for glycine at codon 551 in the CFTR protein, leading to dysfunction of the chloride channel. The drug improves the function of the mutant channel protein, and therefore functions as a potentiator.

4 The Gly551Asp mutation leads to production of a CFTR chloride channel that is transported to the cell membrane, but which does not function normally as a chloride channel. The Phe508del mutation leads to a protein missing the phenylalanine amino acid at codon 508. This mutant protein is transported to the proteasome (an intracellular organelle that degrades damaged and redundant proteins) and degraded within the cell, and therefore does not produce a functional chloride channel. Research is underway to identify drugs that will stabilize the mutant protein ('corrector' function) and allow its transport to the cell membrane.

5 Ivacaftor treatment has been demonstrated to improve pulmonary function and weight gain in individuals with cystic fibrosis who carry the Gly551Asp mutation. Serious adverse reactions include abnormal liver function, low blood sugar and abdominal pain. Other reported side effects include headache, mouth pain, respiratory infection and nausea. Happily, Marci has so far not suffered adverse side effects.

Case 15

1 Deep vein thrombosis is the presence of a blood clot that arises in a major vein, most commonly in the leg. It presents with a reddened, swollen and tender leg. The major concern is the possibility of part of the clot breaking off and causing embolism of the pulmonary artery, where it can obstruct blood flow from the heart to the lung (pulmonary embolus), which can be life-threatening. Deep vein thrombosis tends to occur in settings of prolonged inactivity, including long airplane trips. Some individuals are genetically predisposed (see below). It is treated with anticoagulation agents such as intravenous heparin in acute cases, but chronic coagulation requires an orally administered drug, usually warfarin.

2 Warfarin binds to and inhibits the enzyme VKORC1, which is involved in oxidizing NADH to NAD, in turn reducing vitamin K, a critical cofactor in activation of several of the proteins involved in blood clotting (Case figure 15). Inhibition of VKORC1 leads to lack of activation of these proteins, which inhibits blood clotting. Genetic testing can be done to determine the sensitivity of the patient's VKORC1 to warfarin, and also the activity of the major enzyme, CPY2C9, involved in warfarin excretion. Results of these tests can be used to predict optimal warfarin dosage, so avoiding trial-and-error dosing.

3 Excessive warfarin activity would lead to risk of haemorrhage; inadequate dosing would lead to risk of continued thrombosis. Optimization of dosage through genetic testing can reduce these adverse effects and more quickly lead to an appropriate dosage.

4 Factor V Leiden is a mutation of a single DNA base, substituting arginine for glutamine in the Factor V blood clotting protein. This leads to insensitivity to activated protein C normally involved in cleaving Factor V, which limits the extension of blood clots. Individuals who are heterozygous or homozygous for this mutation are at increased risk of deep vein thrombosis. The frequency of the Factor V Leiden mutation can be as high as 5% in some populations.

5 Factor V Leiden carriers are at significantly increased risk of deep vein thrombosis, but the clinical utility of knowing this is limited. The only known treatment is anticoagulation, but the risks of anticoagulation far outweigh the benefits in a healthy individual.

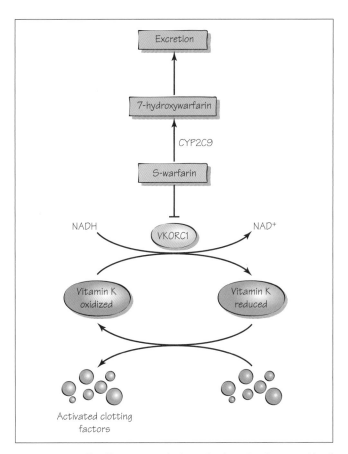

Case figure 15 Significant events in the activation of endogenous blood clotting factors and the site of action of warfarin.

Glossary

acceptor: a site at the 3' end of an intron concerned with its excision from hnRNA.

acrocentric: of a chromosome, with the centromere close to one telomere.

adenocarcinoma: malignant tumour of glandular tissue.

adenoma: non-malignant tumour of glandular tissue.

allele frequency: 'gene frequency'; the proportion of a given allele of all the alleles at a locus, in the individuals forming a specified population.

***Alu* repeat:** the most abundant repeat sequence in the human genome, found only in primates.

amelogenin: a protein component of the extracellular matrix of the dental enamel; its coding sequences on the X and Y chromosomes are used forensically in the molecular elucidation of sex.

anticipation: onset of genetic disease at younger ages in later generations, or with increasing severity in each generation.

anticodon: sequence of three bases within tRNA that is the base pair rule complement to a specific triplet codon and is utilized as such in the translation of mRNA into polypeptide.

antisense strand: template strand of DNA.

apoptosis: programmed cell death.

array: descriptive of techniques involving many samples dotted onto a small glass slide.

ascertainment: recognition of individuals with a specified phenotype.

assortative mating: mate selection on the basis of specific characters.

atherosclerosis: arterial hardening with deposition of lipid.

atopia: proneness to allergy.

autoimmune disease: disease caused by immune self-attack.

balanced polymorphism: genetic polymorphism maintained in a population by opposing selective forces.

Barr body: darkly staining DNA in the cell nuclei of female body cells derived from the X-chromosome.

Bayes' Theorem: a mathematical approach that refines probabilities by taking into account all relevant knowledge.

B cells: lymphocytes generated in the spleen or lymph nodes.

benign tumour: abnormal, compact mass of cells that does not endanger life.

bivalent: homologous chromosomes while pairing during meiosis.

Blaschko's lines: clonal boundaries revealed in the skin in some disease conditions.

branch site: a site within an intron concerned with its excision from hnRNA.

CAAT box: a common promoter of transcription; CAAT denotes its sequence of component nucleotides.

cachexia: serious debility and malnutrition.

cancer: breakdown in homeostatic control of cell growth leading to metastasis.

candidate gene: genetic locus plausibly involved in causing disease.

carcinoma: malignant tumour of the skin or epithelial mucus membrane.

Caucasian: of Indo-European ethnicity.

CCD camera: a camera that converts optical images into digital signals.

cellular oncogene: proto-oncogene.

centimorgan: genetic map distance between two loci that are segregated on average in 1% of meioses.

Central Dogma: concept that genetic information is transferred in the cell in the direction: DNA → RNA → protein.

centriole: cylindrical structure composed of nine sets of triplet microtubules concerned with synthesis of the mitotic spindle fibres and comprising half a centrosome.

centromere: the region of a chromosome that forms the spindle fibre attachment.

centrosome: an organelle that is an origin of, and peripheral anchor for, the mitotic spindle fibres.

chiasma: connection between the chromatids of homologous chromosomes where crossing over is occurring at meiosis.

chromatid: one of the two strands that result from duplication of a chromosome, found during prophase and metaphase of mitosis and meiosis. Each chromatid contains a single, very long molecule of DNA. They separate at anaphase and are then known as daughter chromosomes.

chromatin: the material components of chromosomes.

chromosome abnormality: phenotypically significant change in chromosome number or structure.

cirrhosis: degenerative liver disorder associated with fibrosis and loss of liver function.

***cis* conformation:** presence of alleles of different genes on the same strand of DNA, *c.f. trans*.

clone: two or more individuals (or cells) derived from one genome.

coarctation: narrowing of a vessel.

codominance: expression of both alleles in a heterozygote.

codon: a sequence of three bases within a gene, that corresponds to a specific amino acid in the corresponding polypeptide.

coefficient of kinship: the probability that an allele identified at random in one mating partner is identical by common descent to one at the same locus in the other partner.

coefficient of relationship: the proportion of genes shared by two individuals as a result of descent from a common ancestor.

complement: protein components of a complex that contributes to innate immunity to extracellular pathogens.

compound heterozygote: an individual with two deficient alleles at the same locus.

concordance: degree to which relatives, especially twins, share a particular trait.

consanguinity: genetic relationship.

consultand: individual who approached the clinician for genetic advice.

contiguous gene syndrome: a group of unrelated defects that are inherited together due to deletion of a set of genes in close proximity to one another.

continuous variation: variation in a character which forms a continuous series from one extreme to the other.

copy number variation: variation in the number of copies of a segment of chromosomal DNA.

coupling: *cis* conformation.

CpG: the sequence CG on one DNA strand, as distinct from C=G pairing between strands.

CpG island: a concentration of CpG sequences in chromosomal DNA.

Medical Genetics at a Glance, Third Edition. Dorian J. Pritchard and Bruce R. Korf.

CRASH syndrome: corpus callosum hypoplasia, retardation, adducted thumbs, spastic paraparesis and hydrocephalus due to mutation in the L1 CAM cell adhesion molecule.

cyclin: essential cofactor for activity of the cyclin-dependent phosphokinases (Cdks) responsible for operation and regulation of the cell cycle.

cyclopia: presence of a single central eye due to congenital malformation.

cyclosome: the 'anaphase promoting complex' which labels some redundant cell cycle proteins for destruction.

cytochrome P450: a superfamily of genes involved in eliminating chemicals from the body.

deletion: loss of some or all of a gene or chromosome.

diploid: having twice the haploid content of chromosomes, i.e. the normal full complement.

discontinuous variation: the existence of two or more non-overlapping classes with respect to a particular character.

DNA-binding protein: protein that affects gene activity by becoming bound to the DNA.

DNA chip: a small glass slide carrying an array of DNA samples.

DNA fingerprint: personally unique pattern of hypervariable minisatellite DNA repeats.

DNA hybridization: reassembly of complementary pairs of DNA single strands into a double strand by base pairing.

DNA probe: small fragment of single-strand DNA with the same sequence of nucleotides as the section of native human DNA of interest, labelled with a radioactive or fluorescent tag.

DNA profiling: derivation of a unique molecular description of an individual's DNA.

DNA renaturation: reformation of double helical DNA from complementary, single strands; DNA hybridization.

dominant: an allele is said to be dominant over an alternative allele at the same locus when it, rather than the alternative allele, is expressed in a heterozygote.

donor site: a site at the 5' end of an intron involved in its excision from hnRNA.

dot blot: DNA, usually amplified by PCR, applied directly to a membrane without electrophoresis.

dynamic mutation: transient or progressive change in the DNA that affects its coding properties or degree of expression.

dysgenic: relating to a deleterious genetic change.

dysplasia: abnormal tissue formation.

embryo: the developing individual at the stage 2–8 weeks, during which the rudiments of all the major organs are created.

empiric risk: observed frequency of disease in a given situation.

endocarditis: inflammation of the inner lining of the heart.

enhancer sequence: a chromosomal DNA sequence that binds a transcription-enhancing factor.

ethics: the science of morals and human duty.

eugenic: relating to a beneficial genetic change.

eugenics: the use of genetic measures to improve the genetic characteristics of a population.

exome: the protein-coding portion of the genome, excluding introns, control sequences, etc.

exon: an amino acid coding sequence of DNA within a gene.

expressivity: degree to which an allele is expressed in an individual.

fetus: the developing individual at the 8–38 weeks stage.

fibrillin: protein in connective tissue abnormal in Marfan syndrome.

fixation: elimination of alternative alleles in a population.

frameshift mutation: mutation involving loss or gain of nucleotides of a number not divisible by three, so that the translational reading frame is put out of register.

G0: a quiescent phase of the cell cycle into which proliferating cells can be diverted from G1.

G1: the first phase of the cell cycle, between M and S.

G2: the third phase of the cell cycle, between S and M.

G bands: pattern of AT-rich dark bands produced in chromosomes by special treatment followed by Giemsa staining.

GC box: a class of nucleotide sequence beside a structural gene that controls its transcription efficiency.

gene: the basic unit of inheritance.

gene expression: creation of a phenotypic character corresponding to a gene. It is frequently (but erroneously) considered as synonymous with transcription.

gene flow: geographical movement of alleles by migration.

gene frequency: see 'allele frequency'.

gene map: physical representation of the relative positions of the genes in the genome.

gene therapy: correction of an inherited defect at the level of the gene.

genetic association: occurrence of a specific allele with a specific phenotype at a frequency greater than expected by chance.

genetic code: set of correspondences between triplet codons of bases in mRNA and amino acids in polypeptides.

genetic drift: non-selective change in allele frequency.

genetic heterogeneity: similar genetic condition caused by different genes.

genome: genetic content of a haploid cell; the genetic makeup of a species.

genomics: the molecular study of all the nuclear DNA, together with its mRNA and protein derivatives.

genotype: genetic constitution of an individual.

germline mutation: mutation that can be transmitted to offspring.

Ghent criteria: accepted set of criteria used for diagnosis of Marfan syndrome.

haploid: possessing only one copy of the genetic material, as in a sperm or ovum.

haploinsufficiency: a condition in which the normal phenotype depends on activity of both alleles and reduction of 50% of gene function results in an abnormality.

haplotype: set of alleles of linked genes that tend to be inherited together.

Hayflick limit: a notional limit to the number of times cells of a particular species can undergo mitosis.

heritability: the fraction of phenotypic variation that can be ascribed to genotypic variation.

heterozygote: individual with dissimilar alleles of a particular gene.

heterozygote advantage: superior selective fitness typically shown by hetyerozygotes, as compared to homozygotes.

holoprosencephaly: failure of division of the forebrain into two hemispheres.

homeobox: characteristic DNA sequence found in genes for DNA-binding proteins involved notably in pattern formation.

homozygote: individual with similar alleles of a particular gene.

human genome: theoretical concept that includes the genomes of all normal human beings, as well as the idea of an 'average' or typical genome for a human.

Human Genome Project: a major international collaborative effort to map and sequence the entire human genome.

hypervariable DNA: fraction of non-coding DNA consisting of repetitive sequences that shows a great deal of variation in repeat number between individuals.

hypotelorism: abnormally closely spaced orbits.

imprinting: acquisition by a gene of a semipermanent modification that affects its expression. Imprinting can be changed in a subsequent generation.

inbreeding: breeding between individuals who share one or more common ancestors.

inbreeding depression: reduction in fitness caused by homozygosity of certain alleles due to inbreeding.

incest: sexual intercourse between close relatives, usually those sharing 25% or more of their genetic material.

inhibin: protein tested to screen prenatally for Down syndrome.

intron: a non-coding insert of DNA within a gene, *c.f.* exon.

isochromosome: chromosome with two arms of equal length and identical sequence.

isomerism: abnormal bilateral symmetry of body organs.

karyotype: a display of the somatic chromosome complement of an individual or a photomicrograph of his/her metaphase chromosomes arranged in standard order.

kinetochore: a class of organelles that become located at the sides of each chromosomal centromere and facilitates formation of the spindle fibres.

liability: inherited predisposition.

linkage disequilibrium: co-occurrence of closely linked alleles in a population more frequently than expected by chance.

linkage phase: situation of alternative pairs of alleles with respect to one another on homologous chromosomes.

linked: of genes, close together on the same chromosome.

lissencephaly: abnormally smooth surface to the brain.

location score: the equivalent in multilocus mapping of the lod score in two-point mapping.

lod score: a mathematical score of the relative likelihood of two loci being linked calculated at the most probable degree of linkage.

lordosis: exaggerated forward convex curve of the lumbar spine.

luciferase, luciferin: any of several enzymes and organic substrates found in luminescent organisms that undergo an oxidative reaction with generation of visible light.

macroorchidism: large testicles.

malignancy: ability of cells to sustain proliferation and invade other tissues.

malignant tumour: tumour with the capacity for unrestrained growth and shedding of invasive cells.

massively parallel sequencing: sequencing of DNA by techniques that handle millions of DNA fragments simultaneously.

meiotic drive: any meiotic mechanism that results in unequal fertilization by the two types of gametes produced by a heterozygote.

Mendel's laws: set of rules governing inheritance of single-gene features discovered by Gregor Mendel, sometimes presented as the 'Law of Segregation of Genetic Factors' and the 'Law of Independent Assortment of Genetic Factors'.

metacentric: of a chromosome, with the centromere near the middle.

metaphase plate: arrangement of chromosomes that forms across the main axis of the spindle apparatus at metaphase.

metastasis: transfer of cancer cells about the body.

microsatellite DNA: category of repetitive DNA with tandem repeats of a very short sequence, e.g. 1–4 base pairs.

minisatellite DNA: category of repetitive DNA with tandem repeats of a sequence of intermediate length, e.g. 10–15 base pairs.

mitosis-suppressor gene: tumour suppressor gene; the normal allele of such a gene suppresses cell division, usually at the transition from G1 to S, or G2 to M phase of the mitotic cycle.

Mondini defect: a defect of the cochlea in which the first two coils are merged.

monosomy: presence of only one copy of a chromosome.

mosaic: existence in the body of more than one population of genetically distinct cells derived from a common zygote.

M phase: the chromosome division phase of the cell cycle.

multifactorial trait: character that results from the joint action of several factors, including genes and environmental influences.

multipoint map: gene map based on several reference loci.

mutagen: environmental agent capable of causing damage to DNA.

mutation: process by which a gene undergoes a structural change to create a different allele; the new allele resulting from such a change.

mutator gene: faulty DNA repair gene.

myocardial infarction: death of heart muscle due to loss of blood supply.

neoplasia: ability of cancerous cells to proliferate in defiance of normal controls.

next generation technology: molecular genetic analysis of DNA sequence using new technologies, such as massively parallel sequencing.

nodal: a gene concerned with body patterning.

nuchal transparency: visual appearance of accumulated fluid at the back of the neck in a 12-week fetus.

nucleoside: compound of a purine or pyrimidine base linked to the sugars ribose or deoxyribose, e.g. adenosine, guanosine, cytidine, thymidine, uridine.

nucleotide: compound of a purine or pyrimidine base linked to ribose or deoxyribose, plus phosphoric acid, e.g. deoxyadenosine triphosphate, dATP.

obligate carrier: individual who, based on family history, must be a carrier.

ochronosis: bluish black discoloration of tissues.

odds ratio: the probability a disease will occur in a specific individual compared to that in a control individual.

oligogenic: resulting from the joint action of a small number of genes.

oligohydramnios: deficiency of amniotic fluid.

oligonucleotide: artificially synthesized DNA molecule.

oncogene: a modified proto-oncogene that contributes to a high rate of cell division, usually designated without a prefix, e.g. *myc*.

omphalocele: umbilical hernia.

otitis media: middle ear infection.

ototoxicity: chemical damage to the inner ear.

outbreeding: breeding with an unrelated partner.

penetrance: proportion of individuals of a specific genotype that shows the expected phenotype.

***PEX* genes:** genes involved in the assembly of the peroxisomes.

pharmacogenetics: the aspect of genetics that deals with variation in response to drugs.

pharmacogenomics: use of genomics to design new drugs or select drugs to treat disease.

phase: of linkage, the state of association of alternative alleles at one locus with those at a genetically linked locus.

phenotype: visible, tangible, or otherwise measurable properties of an organism resulting from the interaction of his or her genes with the environment.

pleiotropy: phenomenon of a single gene being responsible for a number of distinct and often seemingly unrelated phenotypic traits.

point mutation: substitution, insertion or deletion in DNA that involves only a small number of nucleotides.

polyadenylation: attachment of a 'poly-A tail' to an RNA transcript.

polygenic: resulting from the joint action of two or more genes.

polyhydramnios: excessive amniotic fluid.

polymorphism: presence in a population of two or more alleles at one locus at frequencies each greater than 1%; one allele of a polymorphic system, or its corresponding phenotype.

polypeptide: the first formed chain of amino acids created by transcription of mRNA, which when elaborated becomes a protein.

Potter sequence: a sequence of events that cause fetal abnormalities through oligohydramnios.

pre-embryo: the developing zygote from fertilization up to the end of week 2.

premutation: situation where there is expansion of triplet repeats beyond the normal range, but insufficient to cause disease.

preventive genetics: application of genetic insight for avoidance of disease.

proband: family member with specific phenotype who first came to the attention of the investigator or clinician.

progress zone: the region of the developing limb bud just behind the apical ectodermal ridge.

promutagen: a non-mutagenic substance that can be converted into a mutagen.

proposita: female proband.

propositus: male proband.

proto-oncogene: cellular oncogene; a normal allele that stimulates cell division, designated with the prefix 'c', e.g. *c-myc*.

pseudoautosomal region: homologous regions of the X and Y chromosomes where pairing and crossover occurs.

'rare': of genetic diseases, sometimes considered as occurring in less than 1/5000 births.

R bands: reverse bands, GC-rich parts of chromosomes that do not stain darkly with Giemsa stain, *c.f.* G bands.

recessive: an allele is said to be recessive to an alternative allele at the same locus when its expression is masked by that alternative in a heterozygote.

recurrence risk: risk a couple will have another child with the same disorder.

relapse: return of symptoms of disease after a period of apparent recovery.

remission: temporary abatement of symptoms of disease, literally 'sending back'.

repulsion: *trans* conformation.

restriction endonuclease: enzyme that specifically cuts double-stranded DNA at a defined base sequence.

restriction fragment: portion of double-stranded DNA released when DNA is cut with a restriction endonuclease.

reverse transcriptase: viral enzyme that creates DNA copies from an RNA template.

rickets: deficient ossification of bone epiphyses due to abnormality of calcium and phosphate metabolism related to vitamin D deficiency.

risk: the probability of occurrence of an event.

sarcoma: malignant tumour of mesodermal tissue.

second generation technology: see 'next generation technology'.

segmental aneuploidy: a chromosomal deletion of intermediate length.

sense strand: DNA strand complementary to the template strand and of sequence similar to that in the RNA transcribed.

sex chromosomes: X and Y chromosomes.

sex limitation: sex-related expression of an autosomal gene due to sex-related differences in anatomy or physiology.

sex linkage: inheritance and expression of an allele in relation to sex, by virtue of the gene being carried on a sex chromosome.

short tandem repeat: microsatellite sequence.

silencer: a sequence within the DNA that binds a transcription suppressor molecule.

silent mutation: mutation that causes no change in the corresponding polypeptide.

sister chromatids: two daughter strands of a duplicated chromosome joined by a common centromere.

somatic mutation: mutation that occurs in a body cell as distinct from the germ line.

SOX family: a family of gene transcription factors.

S phase: DNA synthetic phase of the cell cycle.

spindle: the tubulin fibre structure involved in separating newly formed chromosomes at mitosis.

SRY gene: a gene on the Y chromosome responsible for male differentiation.

START signal: triplet codon AUG that signifies where translation of mRNA should start.

statins: drugs that block cholesterol synthesis.

STOP signal: chain terminator, or 'nonsense codon'; triplet codon that indicates where on the mRNA translation should stop: UAA, UAG, UGA.

structural gene: a gene that encodes the amino acid sequence of a protein, as distinct from a regulatory gene.

submetacentric: of a chromosome, with the centromere between the middle and one telomere.

susceptibility gene: gene with an allele that confers predisposition to a disease.

synapsis: side-by-side association of homologous chromosomes at meiosis.

syndrome: set of phenotypic features that occur together as a characteristic of a disease.

talipes: club foot.

tandem repeats: two or more copies of the same sequence of nucleotides arranged in direct succession in DNA.

TCA cycle: tricarboxylic acid cycle.

T cell: a lymphocyte generated in the thymus.

telomere: specialized end of a chromosome.

template strand: antisense strand; the DNA strand along which RNA polymerase runs, producing an RNA molecule of complementary sequence.

test mating: mating with a recessive homozygote which reveals the genotype of that individual.

threshold trait: a character that shows discontinuous variation considered to be superimposed upon a continuously variable distribution of liabilities.

trans conformation: alleles of two linked genes are said to be in *trans* conformation when they are on opposite chromosomes at meiosis, *c.f. cis*.

transcript: initially formed RNA product of the action of RNA polymerase.

translocation: mutation that involves transfer of a piece of DNA to an abnormal site.

trimester: one of the 3-month divisions of a gestation.

triplet repeat: tandem repetition of a group of three bases in DNA.

tumour suppressor gene: mitosis suppressor gene; a gene responsible for arresting mitosis at the G1 or G2 block.

viral oncogene: oncogene derived from a viral insert, designated with the prefix 'v', e.g. *v-myc*.

wild type: naturally selected, theoretically with no significant overt abnormalities

Wright's inbreeding coefficient: the probability that two alleles in a homozygote are identical by descent.

xanthoma: yellow skin discoloration due to subcutaneous cholesterol deposition.

zinc finger protein: a protein of specialized structure stabilized by an atom of zinc, with the property of binding to specific DNA sequences.

Appendix 1: the human karyotype

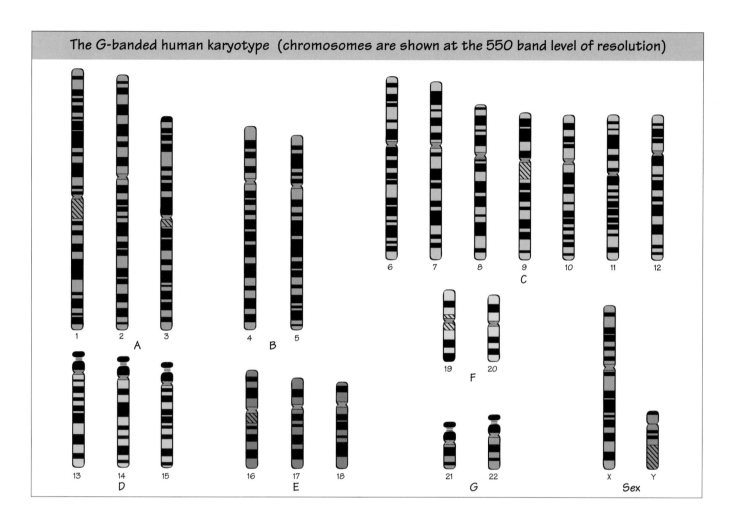

The G-banded human karyotype (chromosomes are shown at the 550 band level of resolution)

Medical Genetics at a Glance, Third Edition. Dorian J. Pritchard and Bruce R. Korf.
© 2013 John Wiley & Sons, Ltd. Published 2013 by John Wiley & Sons, Ltd.

Appendix 2: information sources and resources

Introductory general textbooks

Jorde, LB, Carey, JC and Bamshad, MJ. *Medical Genetics*, 4th edn. St Louis: Mosby, 2010.

Korf, BR and Irons, MB. *Human Genetics and Genomics*, 4th edn. Oxford: Wiley-Blackwell, 2013.

Nussbaum, RL, McInnes, RR and Willard, HF. *Thompson and Thompson's Genetics in Medicine*, 7th edn. Philadelphia: Saunders, 2007.

Sadler, TW. *Langman's Medical Embryology*, 12th edn. Baltimore, Philadelphia: Lippincott Williams and Wilkins, 2011.

Turnpenny, PD. *Emery's Elements of Medical Genetics*, 14th edn. Edinburgh: Churchill Livingstone, 2012.

Westman, JA. *Medical Genetics for the Modern Clinician*. Baltimore, Philadelphia: Lippincott Williams and Wilkins, 2005.

Advanced and specialized texts and reviews

Epstein, CJ, Erikson, RP and Wynshaw-Boris, A. *Inborn Errors of Development*, 2nd edn. Oxford: Oxford University Press, 2008.

Harper, P. *Practical Genetic Counselling*, 7th edn. London: Arnold, 2010.

Kinzler, KW and Vogelstein, B. Lessons from hereditary colorectal cancer. *Cell*, **87**, 159–170, 1996.

Lucasen, A, Parker, M. Confidentiality and serious harm in genetics – preserving the confidentiality of one patient and preventing harm to relatives. *European Journal of Human Genetics* **12**, 93–97, 2004.

Rantanen, E, Hietala, M, krisyofferson, U, Nippert, I, Schmidtke, J, Sequeiros, J and Kääriäinen, H. What is ideal genetic counselling? A survey of current international guidelines. *European Journal of Human Genetics* **16**, 445–452, 2008.

Rimoin, DL, Pyeritz, RE and Korf, BR. *Emery and Rimoin's Principles and Practice of Medical Genetics*, 6th edn. Oxford: Elsevier, 2013.

Speicher, M, Antonarakis, SE and Motulsky, AG. *Human Genetics. Problems and Approaches*, 4th edn. Berlin, Heidelberg, New York: Springer, 2010.

Strachan, T and Read, A. *Human Molecular Genetics*, 4th edn. New York, Abingdon: Garland Science, 2011.

Valle, D, Beaudet, AL, Vogelstein, B, Kinzler, KW Antonarakis, SE, and Ballabio, A. *Scriver's Online Metabolic and Molecular Bases of Inherited Disease*, vols 1–4, eds Scriver, CR and Sly, WS. New York: McGraw-Hill, 2012.

Young, ID. *Introduction to Risk Calculation in Genetic Counseling*, 3rd edn. Oxford: Oxford University Press, 2006.

Internet sites

American Society of Human Genetics (ASHG): www.ashg.org Website of major professional society dealing with research and education in genetics

American College of Medical Genetics and Genomics (ACMG): www.acmg.net Website of US professional society dealing with medical genetics and genomics.

British Society for Human Genetics (BSHG): www.bshg.org.uk A useful starting point with links to many other websites.

Clinical Genetics Computer Resources: www.kumc.edu/gec/prof/genecomp.html A valuable entry point to all the major genetics databases, for professional use.

Cold Spring Harbor DNA Learning Center: www.dnalc.org Educational materials related to DNA and genomics.

GeneCards: http://bioinfo.weizmann.ac.il/cards/ Database of human genes and their products.

GeneReviews: http://genereviews.org An online genetics textbook with reviews and educational materials, including guidelines for diagnosis and management of genetic conditions and database of diagnostic laboratories.

HumGen: www.humgen.org Site with information on ethical and legal issues in human genetics.

Human Genome Epidemiology Network Reviews: www.cdc.gov/genomics/gtesting/index.htm Identifies human genetic variations and reports their frequency in different populations; describes associated disease risks and evaluates relevant genetic tests.

Human Mutation Database: www.hgmd.org A compendium of databases of mutations responsible for human genetic disorders.

Infobiogen Database Catalogue (DBCAT): www.bio.net/bionet/mm/arab-gen/1997-February/005413.html A comprehensive public catalogue of biological databases.

National Center for Biotechnology Information: www.ncbi.nlm.nih.gov/ Provides links to many valuable genetic resources.

National Organization for Rare Diseases (NORD): www.rarediseases.org/ Maintains a list of rare diseases and affiliated groups.

Online Mendelian Inheritance in Man (OMIM): www.omim.org The standard and authoritative source of current knowledge of genes and single gene disorders. Presents links to relevant literature, map locations and clinical summaries.

POSSUM: www.possum.net.au/ Computer-aided diagnosis of genetic disorders and syndromes.

PubMed: www.ncbi.nlm.nih.gov/pubmed A service of the National Library of Medicine giving access to 11 million MEDLINE citations of standard publications on medical topics.

DNA-based techniques, gene mapping and gene therapy

European Bioinformatics Institute (EBI): www.ebi.ac.uk/ Access to nucleotide and protein databases.

ENSEMBL: useast.ensembl.org Eukaryotic genome database.

HapMap: hapmap.ncbi.nlm.nih.gov Website for international HapMap project.

HUGO Genome Nomenclature: www.genenames.org Website for Human Genome Organization Nomenclature Committee.

Human Variome Project: www.humanvariomeproject.org Website for Human Variome Project.

National Human Genome Research Institute: www.genome.gov Website for NIH National Human Genome Research Institute.

Pharmacogenetics Knowledgebase: www.pharmgkb.org Information about pharmacogenetic polymorphisms.

RefSeq: www.ncbi.nlm.nih.gov/RefSeq/ Standardized database of genomic sequence.

UCSC Genome Browser: http://genome.ucsc.edu Website for major human genome browser.

Medical Genetics at a Glance, Third Edition. Dorian J. Pritchard and Bruce R. Korf.

220 © 2013 John Wiley & Sons, Ltd. Published 2013 by John Wiley & Sons, Ltd.

University of Utah Genetic Science Learning Center: http://learn. genetics.utah.edu Educational materials related to genetics.

US Surgeon General's Family History Tool: www.hhs.gov/family-history/ Online tool for generating family pedigrees.

Embryology, development and birth defects

Common disorders of infants: www.marchofdimes.org

Images of normal and abnormal embryos: www.med.unc.edu/embryo_images/

International Clearinghouse of Birth Defects: www.icbdsr.org/page.asp?p=9895&l=1

Cancer

General: http://cancer.gov

Cancer Genome Atlas: http://cancergenome.nih.gov

Laboratory services

Clinical Molecular Genetics Society (UK): www.cmgs.org

European Directory of DNA Laboratories: www.eddnal.com

GeneClinics (USA): www.geneclinics.org

GeneTests: www.genetests.org

GeneReviews: www.genereviews.org

DECIPHER: http://decipher.sanger.ac.uk

Family support

Family Village: www.familyvillage.wisc.edu/ Information on medical disorders, targeted at the general public.

Genetic Alliance (USA): www.geneticalliance.org A good source of information on family support groups for genetic disorders.

Genetic Interest Group (UK): www.gig.org.uk A national alliance of patient organizations.

NORD: see above.

Index

Note: Page numbers in *italics* refer to figures.
Page numbers in **bold** refer to tables.

gonadal mosaicism 43
Gorlin syndrome 143
Gower sign *38*
gray (unit) 69
growth charts *124*, 126
growth factor receptors 139
growth factors 138, 139
    angiogenesis 141
    cancers 140
growth hormone, for Prader–Willi
        syndrome 209
GTPases 139
Günther disease 157, 158
Guthrie test 166

haem *156*, 157
haemochromatosis
    hereditary 153
    primary **26**, 174
haemoglobin 65
Haemoglobin Constant Spring 67
haemoglobinopathies 67
    α-thalassaemia **26**, 67, 77, 192
    see also β-thalassaemia
haemolytic disease of the newborn 77
haemophilia, gene therapy 195
haemophilia A 36, 38, 67
    allele frequency 80
    mutation *66*
haemophilia B 67
halothane sensitivity 21
haploidy 53
haploinsufficiency 99
haplotypes 82, 175
Hardy–Weinberg law 80
Hayflick limit 140–141
HB11 (snoRNA species) 71
head, shape abnormalities 126
heart
    congenital defects 116, 122–123,
        131–132
    embryology 109, 120–121
    Marfan syndrome *22*, 23
heat maps *144*
heavy chains, immunoglobulins 169
height (stature) *127*
helix-loop-helices 61
helix-turn-helices 61
helper T cells, antigen presentation *168*,
        169
hemidesmosomes 45
hepatic coproporphyria 158
hepatic phosphorylase deficiency 164
hepatic porphyrias **157**
hepcidin 153
HER2 *144*, 145
hereditary angioneurotic oedema 171, 196
hereditary coproporphyria **157**, 158
hereditary motor and sensory neuropathy
        20, 39, 45, 67
hereditary neuropathy with predisposition to
        pressure palsies 67

hereditary non-polyposis colon cancer *68*,
        69, 143
hereditary persistence of fetal haemoglobin
        67
heritability 128, 137
heterochromatin 47, 59
heterogeneity, genetic 130
heterogeneous nuclear RNA (hnRNA) 61,
        62
    splicing mutant 67
heteroplasmy 41
heterosis 35
heterotaxia 109
heterozygosity *16*
    allele frequency *79*, 80
    autosomal recessive inheritance and 25,
        27
    dominant inheritance and 19, 34, 35
    obligate 27
    X chromosome inactivation 97
heterozygote advantage 32, 77
hexosaminidases 32
HFE gene 153
high-resolution gene mapping 85
hip, congenital dislocation 118, **131**, **137**
Hippocratic Oath 197
Hirschsprung disease 116
histones 47, 57
history, medical 15
HLA-associated diseases, empiric risk 43
HLA system 173, 174–175
    diabetes mellitus 151
    tissue transplantation 78
    see also major histocompatibility
        complex
holandric inheritance 37
holoprosencephaly 109, 115–116
Holt–Oram syndrome 109
homocystinuria *146*, 147, 148
    vitamin B$_6$ for 196
homogeneously staining regions 139
homogentisic acid 147
homology, phenotypic 147
homoplasmy 41
homozygosity *16*, 19
    allele frequency *79*, 80
    autosomal recessive inheritance and 25,
        27
    compound, β-thalassaemia 67
housekeeping proteins 59
HOX genes *108*, 109
human chorionic gonadotrophin 192
Human Genome Project 83, 199
human immunodeficiency virus 172
    resistance to 77
human leucocyte antigen system *see* HLA
        system; major histocompatibility
        complex
humoral immune response 169
Hunter syndrome 162, **163**
Huntington disease **20**, 35, 73–74, *182*,
        198–199

Hurler syndrome 162, **163**
hybridization 177–178
    whole genome sequencing 87
hybrid vigour 35
hydrocephalus 116
hydrops, Turner syndrome 95
21-hydroxylase deficiency (OHD) 113, 174,
        175
hydroxymethylbilane 157
hydroxyurea 195
hyperargininaemia **159**
hypercalcaemia, infantile *98*, 99–100
hypercholesterolaemia, familial **20**, *22*,
        23–24, 154
hyper-IgE syndrome 172
hyper-IgM syndrome 172
hypersensitivity 171
hypertelorism 126
hypertension 134, **137**
hyperthermia
    malignant 21
    pregnancy 119
hypophosphataemic rickets 39
hypospadias **131**
hypotelorism 126
hypothyroidism, neonatal screening 192
hypoxanthine guanine phosphoribosyl
        transferase deficiency 159

I-cell disease 65, 147, 163
identification
    forensic 185
    genes 86–87
imatinib 145, 195, 208
immune complexes 171
immune system 168–169
    cancers, evasion 141
immunodeficiency 171, 172
    see also severe combined
        immunodeficiency disease
immunogenetics 13, 168–175
immunoglobulins *168*, 169
imperforate anus 116
imprinting, genomic 18, 70–72
imprinting centres 71, 72
inborn errors of metabolism 13, 147,
        166–167
inbreeding
    hybrid vigour 35
    see also consanguinity
inbreeding depression 28
incest 29
incidence, defined 81
incomplete dominance 35
incomplete penetrance 35, *42*, 43
incontinentia pigmenti *38*, 39
independent assortment, Mendelian
        17
index cases 15
individualized medicine 12
infantile autism **131**, 132
infantile hypercalcaemia *98*, 99–100

mitochondria *44*, 45
mitochondrial DNA 41, 45, 57
mitochondrial encephalopathy, lactic
    acidosis and stroke-like episodes 41
mitochondrial inheritance 18, 40–41
mitochondrion-specific RNA polymerase
    41
mitosis 48, 49
MN blood groups *79*, 80
mobile elements, frameshift mutations 67
modifier genes 35
molecular genetics 13
    cancers 145
Mondini defect 30
monogenic diseases 13, 191
monosomy 92
    Turner syndrome 95
monozygotic twins 136
Morquio syndrome 162, **163**
mortality 12
    twins 137
morula 107
mosaicism *96*
    gonadal 43
    prenatal diagnosis 190
M-phase 48, 49
M-phase checkpoint 51
mucopolysaccharidoses (MPSs) 161–163
Mullerian ducts 111
Mullerian inhibiting substance 111
multifactorial diseases 127–135
    defined 13
    twin studies 136–137
multi-hit hypothesis *142*, 143
multiple acetyl-CoA dehydrogenase
    deficiency 155
multiple births 136
multiple carboxylase deficiency, biotin
    196
multiple endocrine neoplasia Type 2 143
multiple exostoses **20**, 24
multiple sclerosis **137**
multiplex amplifiable probe hybridization
    (MAPH) 183
multiplex PCR 183
muscular dystrophy *see* Becker muscular
    dystrophy; Duchenne muscular
    dystrophy
muscular interventricular septum 121
mutagenesis 68–69, 192
mutations 13, 66–67
    DNA sequencing 180
    frequency estimation 21
    neurofibromatosis Type I 206
    nomenclature 67
    see also dynamic mutation
myoclonic epilepsy with ragged red fibre
    disease 41
myotonic dystrophy **20**, 73, 74–75, 118

N-acetyl transferase deficiency 21
natural selection 81, 197

neonates
    cystic fibrosis diagnosis 32
    diabetes **150**, 151
    immunity 169
    screening 192
neoplasms *see* cancers
neural crest cells 107, *108*, 109
neural tube 107
    defects *114*, 115, 131
        screening 191
    pattern of closure *106*
neurodegeneration, ataxia and retinitis
        pigmentosa 41
neurofibromatosis Type I **20**, 35, 143,
    206
neurofibromatosis Type II 143
neuronal apoptosis inhibitor protein, gene
        for 33
neutropenias 171
next generation DNA sequencing 87, 181
Niemann–Pick disease 161
nitrous acid 69
N-linked glycosylation 65
Nodal gene 109
noggin 109
nomenclature of mutations 67
non-allelic homologous recombination
        (NAHR) 99
non-coding RNA 62–63
non-histone chromosomal proteins (NHC
        proteins) 47
non-polyposis colon cancer 68, 69, 143
nonsense mutations *66*, 67
Noonan syndrome 115
normal distribution 128
normal range 128
NOR staining 90
Northern blotting 178
nose, embryology 125
nuchal transparency 192
nuclear factor kappa B 174
nuclear matrix 45
nuclei 45
nucleolar organizer regions 63, 90
nucleolus 45
nucleosomes 47
nucleotide-excision repair, DNA *68*, 69
nucleotides 55

obesity 135
obligate carriers 36
obligate heterozygosity 27
occupational screening 192
oculocutaneous albinism 25–27, 30, **147**,
    148, 166
oculocutaneous telangiectasia 172
odds ratios 133
oesophageal atresia 116
oestriol, unconjugated 192
Okazaki fragments 57
oligogenic diseases 130
oligohydramnios *114*, 115

oligonucleotides, synthetic, whole genome
        sequencing 87
O-linked glycosylation 65
omphalocoele 118
oncogenes 138, 139, 142, 143
    BRAF *144*, 145
oogenesis *52*, 53
opsonization 169
organelles 152
    lysosomes 45, 161
ornithine cycle disorders 159
ornithine transcarbamylase deficiency **159**
osteogenesis imperfecta **20**
ostium primum 121, *122*
ostium secundum *122*
otosclerosis **20**, 24
ototoxic deafness, maternally transmitted 41
ovaries
    cancers 208
    development 111
overdominance 18, 35
overlapping genes 59

p16 (protein) 51
p21 (protein) 139
p53 (protein) *50*, 51, 139
p63 gene, mutations 109
packing ratios, chromosomes 47
pair-wise concordance rate 136
palate
    cleft 129, *130*, **131**, **137**
    embryology 125, *130*
paramesonephric ducts 111
parasitic twins 137
parent–child matings *28*, 29
partial sex linkage 37
Patau syndrome 92–93
paternity, DNA profiling *184*, 185
pattern baldness 37
Pearson syndrome 41
pedigree diagrams 14–15
    autosomal recessive inheritance 25
    Li–Fraumeni syndrome *138*
Pendred syndrome 30
penetrance 18
    incomplete 35, *42*, 43
    twin studies 136–137
peptidyl transferase reaction *64*, 65
peroxisomal diseases 163
peroxisomes 45, 163
Pfeiffer syndrome *22*, 23
phagocytosis *170*
pharmacogenetics 12, 21
pharmacogenomics 194
pharyngeal arches 109
Phe508del mutation *see* cystic fibrosis
        transmembrane conductance regulator
phenotypes, defined 13
phenotypic homology 147
phenylalanine
    metabolism *146*
    restriction 206